Give us the chance

sport and physical recreation with
mentally handicapped people

Give us the chance

sport and physical recreation with mentally handicapped people

KAY LATTO DipPE MCSP

Illustrations by Elaine Batt

DISABLED LIVING FOUNDATION
London

First published 1981

ISBN 0 901908 38 X

Produced by
Davies Fleming & Associates Ltd.,
22 Kingsley Park Terrace,
Northampton

Contents

Preface

This book has been compiled as a result of the visits to hospitals, Adult Training Centres and clubs throughout the United Kingdom. The purpose of these visits was to see activities being practised and to discover the value, programme content, organisation and future development of physical activities and sports for mentally handicapped adults and children in their leisure time. Discussions took place with a variety of individuals, organisations, health, social service and local authority personnel. The content has been prepared with the following groups in mind:

> medical, nursing and other staff in hospitals who may have little technical knowledge about teaching sports and physical activities;

> physical education specialists and qualified teachers, instructors and coaches of individual sports and activities who may have little knowledge of the techniques of working with mentally handicapped people;

> the parent or volunteer who may lack background and training in both these areas.

The book is designed to assist these groups by including:

> the expert knowledge of a doctor and clinical psychologist — (see Chapters 1 and 2);

> the description of a number of programme activities, examples of projects and events, and general guidelines on organisation, presentation, facilities and resources.

The information is not exhaustive. It is designed to give readers sufficient confidence and impetus to try out new ideas and to extend their own knowledge in physical recreation and sport through experience, training courses and further study.

It is hoped that this publication will inspire all those working with mentally handicapped people, whether in hospital, training centre, club, at home or elsewhere to introduce a wider choice of activities in their programmes and to encourage a greater number of individuals to take part in them.

WE SHOULD GIVE MENTALLY HANDICAPPED PEOPLE THE SAME OPPORTUNITIES TO TAKE PART IN PHYSICAL ACTIVITIES, SPORTS AND OUTDOOR PURSUITS AS THE REST OF US.

Acknowledgements

In a project which entailed many visits in England, Northern Ireland, Scotland and Wales, and so much sifting of information, I am deeply indebted to my colleague Kay Evans, the Disabled Living Foundation's Project Officer for Physical Recreation. Her many years of experience enabled her to introduce me to many contacts and help with visits; above all she gave unsparingly of her time to discuss, read and check the type script. Kay's advice throughout these three years has made my task, as an inexperienced researcher and writer, possible.

So many people have welcomed this project and helped in our search to find out which sports and physical activities are practised in hospitals, adult training centres, Gateway Clubs and hostels, that we have found ourselves not only gathering information but disseminating it as well, such was the interest shown. Some people lent their dissertations and theses, other gave generously of their time to discuss work with, and projects for, mentally handicapped people, and many have contributed directly or indirectly to the text by committing their projects to paper or writing a chapter or article; others supplied photographs and videotapes.

We are indebted to the members of the DLF Steering Group for Sport and Physical Recreation for Mentally Handicapped People who have encouraged and advised us and to our staff colleagues who have helped to bring the publication into being.

We should also like to thank the Sports Councils for England, Northern Ireland, Scotland and Wales for their hospitality and help, and the British Sports Association for the Disabled who arranged the programme and transport in Yorkshire. This support was greatly appreciated.

Many organisations, both voluntary and statutory, have willingly shared their experience and expertise with us — health services, hospital administrators, consultant, medical and nursing staff, paramedical staff and sports and recreation officers; directors of social services and their staffs, managers and staff of adult training centres, Gateway Club leaders, play leaders and hostel wardens; voluntary organisations, associations and societies, the governing bodies of sport and members of the physical education profession.

We are grateful to the sports manufacturers who provided equipment, unihoc sticks and balls, balls of all sizes and textures, short handled bats and sponge balls which enabled us to introduce new games and variations on known games. Discussions on equipment of all kinds gave opportunity for experimentation with equipment simply adapted to enable mentally handicapped people to learn the games more easily in the early stages.

No acknowledgment would be complete without thanking all those, friends and relatives who gave us hospitality on our travels and never minded the late arrivals and early starts.

Our contacts have been too many to name each one individually, but Elaine Batt, for her delightful illustrations, Joan Duval and Hilde Wilsker who willingly typed and retyped the script, Diana de Deney, Editor of DLF Publications, who has in the past year guided and edited the script ready for publication, Dr Peter Sylvester and Mr. John Clements who spent time with us before and during the project and contributed to the text, must be named and thanked for their support throughout.

Author's Note

1. Before selecting activities or events from the practical chapters (6 to 14) of the book, please read chapters 1 to 5. These first chapters contain much background information to the rest of the text including a definition of mental handicap, problems which arise when teaching mentally handicapped people including those who are severely handicapped, general teaching methods, how to choose an activity and making the most of indoor and outdoor space available.

2. The illustrations are indicative of activities and skills and are **not** intended to show accurate technique. Female figures are shown with pigtails or appropriate head-dress.

3. Most of the activities and events described in the text are those actually seen by the author.

4. Activities suitable for severely mentally handicapped people are included in the index under *mental handicap, severe.*

5. Different terms are used to describe the same group of people in different areas of the country, i.e.:
    (i)   those who attend Adult Training Centres are trainees, clients or students;
    (ii)   those in hospital are patients or residents;
    (iii) those teaching in ATCs, hospitals or Gateway Clubs are teachers, instructors, leaders, recreation officers or coaches.

6. The term Sports Centre, Sports Leisure Centre or Recreation Centre denotes a large sports complex including facilities for indoor/outdoor sports and swimming on one campus or a centre for indoor and/or outdoor sports with swimming bath/pool in separate localities.

What is mental handicap?

(From Mental Handicap Fact Sheet 1 issued by the King's Fund Centre, 126 Albert Street, London NW1)

Mental handicap is a relatively new term. It is what the Scots call mental deficiency, the English and Welsh lawyers mental subnormality, and other countries mental retardation. It is usually defined by measuring the intelligence quotient (IQ). The average IQ is 100; anyone with an IQ of 50-70 is said to be mildly handicapped, and anyone with an IQ below 50 is called severely mentally handicapped, the group covered earlier by the unpleasant terms 'idiot' and 'imbecile'.

The World Health Organisation has produced these definitions:

Mild mental handicap (or subnormality, or retardation):
IQ 52-67. Slow development but children who can be educated within limits. Adults, with training, can work in ordinary employment and lead independent, normal lives.

Moderate: IQ 36-51. These people are backward, but can learn to care for themselves. Adults need to work in sheltered employment.

Severe: IQ 20-35. These people are backward in their physical skills, and their speech and language development, but aren't completely dependent on other people. They are often, but not always, physically handicapped.

Profound: IQ less than 20. They need constant care and supervision if they are to live, as they can't fend for themselves. Their physical co-ordination and sensory development are very much impaired, and again, they are often physically handicapped.

It is important to remember, however, that the IQ level is only a rough guide to a person's ability — few people would now claim that it tells us anything like as much as we need to know about potential skills and possibilities of development. Some people claim, too, that the IQ tests we use are biased against children of the lower social classes and immigrants; many of them seem to have a low IQ because they can't understand the cultural assumptions behind the test questions.

There is another point to remember when talking about mental handicap. People are only 'handicapped' in comparison with 'normal' abilities, and their handicaps only show up when they are asked to do things that society sets down as 'normal'. Before education was made compulsory, there was no such thing as an educationally subnormal child, because educational ability was not demanded of most people in England. So 'mental handicap' is a social and administrative definition, not a medical one.

Foreword

The able-bodied take physical activity for granted, whether as sport, games, outdoor pursuits, fitness training or dance. The Disabled Living Foundation tried to discover (from the Departments of Health, and of Education and Science, doctors, psychologists and physical education experts) what possibilities there are for mentally handicapped people to take part in these activities. It became clear that little is known about this subject and even less has been written about it.

The lack of opportunity to take part in sport and physical recreation deprives mentally handicapped people of enjoyment and prevents them from learning skills which may improve their concentration, their social awareness, their self control and their ability to make friends. The DLF, which has already produced a number of books and films about the problem of physical recreation for physically handicapped people, was therefore delighted when the Sidbury Trust agreed to fund the production of a work dealing with sport and physical recreation for mentally handicapped people. The Trust has also contributed to the cost of its publication thereby reducing the selling price. The Trustees of the DLF are deeply grateful to the Sidbury Trustees for finance and for their thoughtful encouragement in a difficult task.

The DLF was fortunate in persuading one of the few experts in the field, Mrs. Kay Latto, DipPE, MCSP, to make the study. She is a known expert in physical recreation, with many years experience in teaching physical recreation to mentally handicapped people and training students how to teach them. With the help of Miss Kay Evans, MBE, MCSP, DipPE, the project officer for our Physical Recreation Projects, Mrs. Latto made an intensive study which took her to all parts of the United Kingdom. The DLF is most grateful to Mrs. Latto, and also to Miss Evans for their help.

On page 00 the membership of the multi-disciplinary Steering Group to the project is listed. The advice of the group of volunteer advisers has made an important contribution to the author's success. This group of active working advisers have read and commented in detail on every paragraph. The author and Trustees unite to thank them for their most generously given and deeply appreciated help.

Particular mention must also be made of the help given by the Sports Council and their staffs for England, Northern Ireland, Scotland and Wales. This was not only with references, information and technical advice. The Sports Council for Northern Ireland and the four Area Health Boards funded travel and hospitality and arranged the programme of visits. The Sports Council for Wales arranged the itinerary of visits. The Scottish Sports Council for the Disabled, grant aided by the Scottish Sports Council, funded and arranged the visit to Scotland. All this support was greatly appreciated.

The doctor's contribution is by Dr. P. E. Sylvester, a distinguished psychiatrist, deeply interested in improving the quality of life for mentally handicapped people. The Trustees thank him warmly for the contribution and also for the important support on medical and hospital matters he gave the project workers throughout the Study. Mr. John Clements, who contributed the psychologist's chapter on the very severely mentally handicapped, is one of the few clinical psychologists who have worked in this difficult and demanding field. He also gave the project workers much support and the Trustees express their gratitude to him. The delightful illustrations are a voluntary contribution to the project by Mrs. Elaine Batt. The Trustees thank her warmly for her generosity and her interest, both of which have been a great encouragement to the project workers. Readers will agree that the illustrations contribute greatly to the readability of the book.

The book is intended for parents, for friends, for all those concerned professionally with the daily living of mentally handicapped people whether in hospital or in the community, for those concerned with the leisure time of mentally handicapped children, for the providers of physical recreation facilities whether in hospital or in the community, for the governing bodies of sport and physical recreation, for voluntary bodies in the field of mental handicap and for the interested public.

Give us the chance aims above all to be useful and practical. As it is a pioneer in its field, the author would welcome any comments, criticisms or contributions which would improve a second edition and so make it more helpful to those interested in sport and physical recreation for mentally handicapped people and especially to mentally handicapped people themselves and their families.

W. M. Hamilton.

CHAPTER ONE

A Doctor's View

Contributed by Dr. Peter Sylvester, Consultant Psychiatrist, St. Lawrence's Hospital, Caterham

A child whose mind fails to develop and mature adequately is said to be mentally handicapped. The child's intelligence is limited. He may grow normally but his mind remains slow in development and he is incapable of reaching and attaining the normal standards expected for a child of his age. Thus a child falls behind his peers in achievement. He may be unable to attend a normal school but should he do so he cannot keep up with the normal programme because of his difficulties in learning to read and write, and generally take care of himself.

There are different degrees of handicap. Some children are mildly handicapped and able to learn skills in reading and writing, while others are so severely or profoundly handicapped that they are unable to learn to speak and control their bodily functions.

Mentally handicapped people often have other problems. Physical handicap (cerebral palsy), blindness, deafness and epilepsy are common. Additional handicaps make it more difficult for a child to cope with living and he therefore needs special help from staff who are acquainted with his problems and specially trained to cope with them. Children may be so handicapped that they require assistance with feeding, washing, dressing and toileting. There are nearly half a million people in England and Wales, of all ages, with varying degrees of mental handicap.

It is important that mentally handicapped children be identified as early as possible so that they can be directed into suitable programmes of education and training. Sometimes the decision is easy; for instance, it is well known that children with Down's Syndrome (Mongolism) can be recognised at birth and a possible forecast of the child's future development predicted. Other children appear quite normal at birth and start to grow and develop in the normal way. It is only when they reach the age of 2, 3 or perhaps start school, that their handicap becomes obvious. There are different ways of detecting mentally handicapped children. One is by recording what are known as 'milestones of development', that is to say, the age at which a child is expected to achieve sitting up, crawling, standing, walking, talking and controlling his toilet habits. If these do not appear at specified times they may be the first important clues to a child's future mental disability. Fuller assessment requires complicated programmes of observation and testing and takes into account the social and educational aspects of a child's life.

Mental handicap sometimes goes by other names including mental deficiency, mental retardation and subnormality of mind. It is frequently confused with mental illness or psychosis but the two conditions are completely different. Mental illness affects the minds of an otherwise normal person — his thinking processes become disturbed or confused and he is amenable to treatment so that cure can be made; mental handicap, on the other hand, is often a symptom of some previous disease process and is a permanent condition which cannot be cured although it can be influenced and the person's mental and physical condition considerably improved. It must be said that the handicapped person can sometimes develop symptoms of mental illness in the same way as ordinary individuals. Legally, both mental handicap and mental illness are grouped together as mental disorder.

GENERAL HEALTH

Every mentally handicapped person is subject to the same type of physical illness and injuries as any other person. He is liable to get coughs, colds, influenza, pneumonia, skin infections, blood pressure, heart attacks and so on. A few conditions, not strictly speaking illnesses, occur more frequently in the handicapped person than in the intelligent — epilepsy, physical handicap, communication difficulties, blindness and deafness are common conditions. These complications are secondary to damage of the brain, which may also be responsible for the mental handicap. Clearly, if extra handicaps occur management problems are increased and can be very difficult.

Preventive measures against illness in childhood, including immunisation programmes against diptheria, tetanus, poliomyelitis and tuberculosis, have helped to give the mentally handicapped child a much better chance of enjoying good physical health. In times gone by, tuberculosis, chronic ear disease with offensive discharges, dental sepsis, chronic constipation, and skin conditions were common, but today these conditions can be largely controlled and do not constitute the menace they once did to physical well being.

If sport and recreation are to be enjoyed and result in further improvement in the physical and mental well being of the mentally handicapped person, it is important that he starts with the best possible health. Ambulant handicapped people can have poor posture and gait. It is not always clear why this is so, but in many it is connected with lack of participation in physical activities. Such people are likely to derive great benefit from sport and physical recreation and their posture improves.

A child handicapped either mentally or physically is less able to match his peers at all stages of development. At least two-thirds of children in a hospital for the mentally handicapped have multiple handicaps. Play for a child may be regarded as the nursery stages in preparing him for a sporting life. Normal children go through developmental programmes of play up to the age of 16 years and beyond. Play eventually merges with sport and physical recreation. Failure to meet schedules in development is likely to end with some degree of deprivation in emotional, social and possibly intellectual capacities. The handicapped child is unfortunately exposed to these risks. Nurses, teachers, play leaders, recreation officers and volunteers all have their part to play if the children are to take part in play, recreation and sports. Many handicapped children have to be taught how to play. Some years ago it was the fashion to have a rumpus room for children. One was created for a number of handicapped boys from 7 to 14 years and equipped with an array of expensive toys including tricycles, swings and climbing equipment. It was thought that that was all that was required and the day came when the children were allowed in to play. Unfortunately, they had no idea of how to use the equipment and within a few hours it was reduced to masses of twisted metal. Not only do the children need to be involved in play activities gradually and with suitable tuition, but more suitable equipment must be chosen to wean them from simpler toys until they understand the significance of tricycles and go-carts. As they grow older it may be necessary to teach them how to take part in sports and other types of physical recreation.

EPILEPSY

Epilepsy, like mental handicap, is not really a disease but a consequence of some illness, perhaps well defined perhaps not, which has left a persistent periodic manifestation. It can take many forms, the best known being grand mal and petit mal seizures. During a grand mal seizure the person falls unconscious to the ground and goes through a series of convulsions, recovery taking place after a few minutes. Someone suffering from petit mal has momentary lapses of consciousness which recur at frequent intervals. A child may have drop attacks during which he falls to the ground suddenly but recovers quickly, or salaam attacks during which he makes a bowing motion. Bizarre disturbances of behaviour may signify psychomotor epilepsy. Jacksonian epilepsy is revealed by local twitchings affecting an arm, leg or part of the face.

Epilepsy is common in handicapped people and afflicts 1 in 4 people living in long-stay hospitals. Fortunately there are drugs (anti-convulsants) which control the number of fits and their severity. In certain circumstances fits can be eliminated altogether.

Provided staff and organisers of recreational or sporting facilities are aware of a person's epilepsy and consultation with medical advisers is maintained, there is little reason to eliminate them from taking part in full programmes of sport.

It is well known that flickering light — possibly from the reflection of light from waves in a swimming pool — can provoke an epileptic seizure. However, only a few epileptic people are likely to have their fits triggered off by this sort of stimulation.

FITTING THE SPORT TO THE INDIVIDUAL

The mildly handicapped person who is physically fit can participate in any sport or recreational activity as he wishes. No limits need be put on his participation and he could compete with normal people. Many handicapped people are very competent and keen.

Looking at this problem from the opposite point of view one should choose and design sport for a particular candidate or group of people. The more severely mentally handicapped may find difficulty in accepting competitive games and those involving a great deal of training and skilled performance. However, they can participate in sports which are less intellectually demanding. Skittle matches have proved very exciting for less able participants who have enjoyed being members of a team and the spirit of competitiveness involved. Also, handicapped young women have formed very competent netball teams capable of playing not only other teams of handicapped people but inter-hospital teams and competing against schools and church groups outside the hospital. Once the fever of competition burns it is very difficult to extinguish.

Sport and recreation for mentally handicapped people who are also physically handicapped are more restricted but nevertheless many of these people can participate in swimming and events designed for their special needs. They can take part quite successfully in and enjoy to the full wheelchair scrambles, races and handball competitions.

Cricket, football and athletics can all be enjoyed by mentally handicapped people. Long-stay hospitals have long had a tradition of having a sporting calendar for these events. It is to be hoped that as long-stay hospitals run down and community ventures are developed they will not neglect to explore fully the sports and recreational requirements of the mentally handicapped person.

Once he has decided to take part in a sport, it is useful if the candidate can participate in some form of physical fitness training to help his general muscular strength and abilities and maintain flexibility of joints. The cardiovascular and respiratory systems improve their capacity to cope with increased physical demands. Also basic skill movements may need to be increased. Posture and the ability to walk, run, hop, kick, and catch may not be good or may even be absent in the severely mentally handicapped person. Simple exercises to improve these may therefore be the starting point before more advanced training can be attempted.

THE VALUE OF SPORT AND RECREATION

Parents, teachers, play and youth leaders all believe that physical recreation has health-giving qualities. Fashions in exercise such as jogging are claimed to reduce the risk of heart attacks. A fit sportsman is generally seen to exude health and vigour. Doctors, too, share in the general view that physical recreation has many special benefits to offer both to the handicapped and non-handicapped person.

How The Body Functions

To understand the bodily requirements for exercise it is necessary to know how the body functions:

1. The skeleton is a series of internal splints to which muscles are attached and through which they exert their forces when contracting.

Joints are necessary for movement to take place. Limb joints occur as ball and socket, and hinge joints. They act as fulcrums around which muscular action is effective. They are surrounded by ligaments. These surfaces are very smooth and bathed by fluid to reduce friction to a minimum.

2. Muscles have the ability to contract and relax. When contracted they exert a force of pull across a joint. They can act in groups to fix a joint for a particular action, e.g. bracing the bow arm when drawing the bow; others are prime movers, i.e. they flex or bend a joint, or extend or straighten a joint. Many muscular actions are complex and while some contract vigorously others have to relax in order to execute a desired movement, e.g. kicking a ball.

Muscles are controlled by nerves and have a rich blood supply.

3. To supply muscles in active exercise with nutrients and oxygen it is necessary that the blood supply be greatly increased. This happens through dilatation of the blood vessels to the muscles augmented by an increase in heart rate and blood pressure.

4. An important requisite to muscular action is a rich supply of oxygen from the atmosphere. To obtain this the rate of breathing increases in rate and depth so that more oxygen can enter the blood. This is further facilitated by an increase in the amount of blood circulating through the lungs.

5. When muscles are contracting they undergo increased chemical activity. More oxygen is used, more carbon dioxide produced and in severe exercise acid waste products get into the blood.

6. Smooth muscular actions producing competent athletic movements have complex nerve supplies. Some nerves control the state of the blood vessels, others record the state of muscular contraction while others are concerned with exciting muscular action. All this would be of little avail without the higher centres in the brain. Consider the position of a batsman in cricket: he takes an optimum stance for a strike at the ball, he has to watch the delivery, assess the flight and fall of the ball, judge his stroke, flex his muscles for the appropriate action and then, having struck the ball successfully, listen for his partner's call before taking off for runs. In the fraction of a second, numerous messages have been received and interpreted into appropriate actions through the brain mechanisms.

These systems can only function if they are supported by physical and psychological factors. Three important factors in sport and exercise are diet, attitudes and training.

Diet. A good balanced diet of proteins, carbohydrates, fats, minerals and vitamins is essential for all people. The total daily intake of food (calories) depends on the type of activity undertaken. Men need more calories than women and men doing heavy work need more than those doing light work. Sports people in training are likely to need a higher intake of calories than their jobs suggest. Proteins are used for tissue building and repair whilst carbohydrates and fats supply energy. Sugars, especially glucose, are one of the simplest forms of carbohydrates. It is easily absorbed into the body and a useful source of energy before an energetic event. Salt is an important mineral. It is lost in sweat during exercise. Unless a good reserve is built up prior to sporting events its loss results in muscular cramps.

Attitudes. Attitudes to sport and exercise are important. If a competitor wishes to succeed then he has to develop an element of aggression in order to win. The correct spirit will make him do his best. Conversely, if the attitude is one of helplessness and timidity then failure results. One thing all competitors have to overcome is anxiety and perhaps an element of fear while waiting to compete. Variation in personality types means that people overcome these problems individually. Those that do it best succeed. Support from team mates and coaches can be most supportive.

Training. All the points mentioned should be blended into a programme of training so that different bodily functions can be brought to harmonise with each other and result in the best possible performance of an individual. It would be reasonable when designing sporting programmes for handicapped people to match competitors with similar handicaps.

Social Benefits

There are also important social benefits. Playing in a team, competing in events and meeting other people both on and off the field can inspire loyalty and extend the scope of personal contacts and friendships. Sport provides a topic for conversation, therefore improving prospects of communication. The need to show and have clean underwear impresses cleanliness and a certain competitiveness in hygiene — one must be seen to have clean socks, pants and vest.

The post-match tea or supper is a common event after many team games. Handicapped people should indulge in this activity. They should be encouraged to bring their own followers, and to provide hospitality for the opposing team out of their own money; they should also be helped and encouraged to lay the tables, cut the sandwiches and undertake other chores. In this way they can be helped to develop an interest in looking after themselves at all times instead of relying on others to provide an ever-ready tea party. It should also be possibe for participants to have the customary 'after the match' drink in a pub.

It should be remembered that most handicapped people take longer than a normal person to do a given task, and that allowances for this must therefore be taken. For example, when a handicapped person is taken swimming he should be encouraged to undress, put on the swimsuit, dry off and redress by himself, but the person accompanying him must appreciate that these preparations can take a long time. This point should also be made to those providing the facilities.

Medication

Many handicapped people are prescribed anticonvulsants, tranquillisers, anti-physchotics and antidepressants, but this fact should not in general deter them from taking part in sport. The purpose of medication is basically to help people to lead a full and complete life. People on some medicines are told that their reactions may be slowed down and that alcoholic beverages should be avoided. This generalisation applies to handicapped people. However, the only person who can really advise in any particular case is the family practitioner and he should be consulted in all cases where there is any element of doubt.

Further Reading

ALLEN OF HURTWOOD, LADY. *Planning for play.* Thames & Hudson, London, 1975.

CRAFT, MICHAEL (ed.) *Tredgold's mental retardation*, (12th ed.). Bailliére Tindall, London, 1979.

HEATON-WARD, W. ALAN. *Left behind: a study of mental handicap.* Woburn Press, London, 1978.

CHAPTER TWO

A Psychologist's View

Contributed by Mr. John Clements, Lecturer in Clinical Psychology, Institute of Psychiatry, London.

The present text reflects the growing awareness that mentally handicapped people can lead a richer life given appropriate opportunites and help.

For a long time the handicapped person has suffered from the poor expectations held for him by others, and this in its turn has meant that he has been deprived of many of the opportunities open to other members of society. This book demonstrates that mentally handicapped people can participate in and enjoy every kind of sport and physical activity — the examples given are of work that has **actually** been done rather than what might be done in theory.

These examples highlight the many benefits which such involvement can bring. It provides the handicapped person with a wider and more normal experience of life. Although much has been done in recent years to show how even the most severely disabled can be taught greater social competence and independence there has been less emphasis on recreation and leisure. This has left an 'empty' part in the life pattern of many handicapped people, a part which these activities can help fill. Sport is a means whereby people from many walks of life can meet and grow to accept and understand each other. By increasing the involvement of the handicapped person in sport, it becomes easier for him to integrate with the rest of society. The more the contact between the non-handicapped and handicapped people the greater will be the understanding of and tolerance towards the disabled; many examples in this book, e.g. the Outward Bound courses, illustrate this process at work.

In Chapter One Dr. Sylvester discusses the many benefits which can be fostered by physical activities. These include improvements in general health and muscular co-ordination, encouragement of self care skills and social graces and the stimulation of imagination and communication and problem-solving abilities. These specific benefits can in their turn bring about more general improvements in self confidence and adjustment.

Few would argue about these benefits for most mentally handicapped people. And yet there are two groups which are often excluded from this kind of involvement — the multiple, profoundly handicapped, and those with severe disturbance in their behaviour. Whilst these groups present many practical problems, it can be argued that they will especially benefit from participation in organised physical activities.

For multiple handicapped people, the extent of their disabilities prevents them from influencing the environment for themselves — it encourages them to withdraw and become passive. It is therefore essential that they are kept involved in the world around them if they are not to become more dependent than necessary (see How to Choose an Activity, Chapter 4).

The solution to behaviour problems also requires active participation in positive programmes. This is not a question of using up people's energy — a model which attributes bad behaviour to an excess of energy is not appropriate in most cases. The benefit of a programme lies in the extent to which it helps people to behave well by giving them more skills, and by ensuring they receive plenty of attention and encouragement for so behaving. Those with disruptive behaviours often find themselves in situations where there is little to stimulate them and where they receive little attention from others, unless they act in a disruptive manner. A focus on teaching positive skills can break this cycle of events. In some specific cases, problem behaviour arises where an individual becomes very anxious. For these people some physical activities, e.g. yoga, music and movement may be particularly helpful in teaching them how to relax and prevent the 'explosions' in their behaviour.

The benefits are therefore very real and wide-ranging. Putting the ideas into practive, however, may not always be easy and it is useful to consider some of the general principles involved, and some of the common difficulties encountered in running such activities (see also Teaching Guidelines, Chapter 3).

BASIC STRATEGIES

1. Be open-minded. The whole content of this book highlights how handicapped people can be helped to engage in an enormous range of sports and activities. In selecting an activity it is important not to dismiss certain possibilities as being impractical for the mentally handicapped. If in doubt, try it out, and if it does not work one way, try in another way. This is not the same as being foolhardy. Throughout the book great emphasis is laid on having the right equipment and involving people skilled in the activity in question (even if they are not specialists in the field of mental handicap). But within these constraints, the horizons for handicapped people can be widened enormously by challenging traditional expectations.

2. Be specific. When planning a programme it is important to have a clear idea about what will be the result when the programme is successful. It is not enough to aim to 'develop potential' or 'enhance a sense of well being'. These are worthy aims, but before a programme can begin it is important to visualise what people will be doing after the programme is finished in what way will their behaviour be different.

3. Observe first, teach later. Once an activity has been selected it is tempting to start immediately to teach the skills involved. But it may be very useful to take the handicapped person through the activity and watch how he copes with various phases, given only minimal intervention (to prevent accidents, etc.). This kind of observation saves an enormous amount of time later — it may show that the person already has many of the necessary skills. It is important not to rely solely on what others estimate a person can do — give him the opportunity to demonstrate his capabilities. Conversely, he may show deficiencies in skills which people had assumed were present. For example, some people may have been brought up in an environment without steps and may therefore have no idea how to cope with stairs; therefore, if climbing activities are being planned it may be important to start at this very basic level.

4. Record the observations. Anyone closely involved in an activity can easily forget what people were like before teaching and training began. If slow, steady improvement goes unnoticed, this will lead to discouragement. Keeping a record — in the form of a diary — can serve as a reminder. The form it takes is not as important as the content, which should relate to observable behaviour rather than to processes that one guesses are going on inside the person.

5. Simplify complex tasks. Any activity can be broken down into a number of component steps. It has been shown many times that a handicapped person may fail to learn if a task is presented in too complex a fashion, but will progress when that task is broken down into small steps and he is taught one step at a time. Some of the examples in the sections on swimming and canoeing show how tasks can be split up. These are just examples — many more steps might be needed for one person, many fewer for another. There is no text-book recipe on how to analyse a task. The number of steps depends entirely upon the people involved. If they fail to make progress it may be necessary to split the item which they find difficult into several smaller steps. Progress to the next step should only take place after mastery of the previous one in the sequence.

6. Demonstrate the necessary response. It is important for the coach or instructor to continually demonstrate the response required from those with whom he is working. It is not enough just to describe it or to give a single quick demonstration; repeated modelling should rather be incorporated into the process of learning.

7. Maximise correct performance. Even with a good task analysis it may be necessary to help the person through the step being worked on. Such additional help may take the form of extra instructions and reminders (verbal or gestural), direct physical guidance, or use of a special aid, e.g. buoyancy aids in swimming. The section on swimming illustrates two ways in which extra help can be provided either by buoyancy aids or by the physical support of an instructor. It also illustrates an important principle that such aids should be seen as temporary devices, which are **gradually** removed until the individual becomes independent. If help is removed too quickly performance may deteriorate but, if it is never removed, the person will fail to achieve independence.

8. Ensure quick and comprehensible feedback. Many handicapped people have special difficulties with their language development so that they cannot learn just by instructions. They need to see the activities carried out and practise them in real life so that they can learn by their own experience. They need to try out a skill and judge its success by the feedback they receive, so that they can gradually learn the correct ways of responding and drop the incorrect ways. Providing meaningful consequences for behaviour is therefore an essential part of the development and practise of skills. Such feedback can be given in many ways and it is essential to find something which gets through to the individual or group with whom you are working.

For some, words of praise and social attention may be sufficient. Others may practise better if there are tangible prizes for achievement. Some may like to see a visible record of achievement, such as their improvements filled in on a chart or graph. The younger and more severely disabled may like certain kinds of physical contact (tickling, vibration) or sensory stimulation (lights, music) or direct material rewards (sweets, drinks, etc). For those lucky enough to possess videotape equipment, video feedback may prove a powerful motivator. The important point is to discover what an individual or group responds to, and to make that contingent upon their performance at the selected activity. It should be something which can be provided immediately and frequently, so that the person is encouraged to keep practising until mastery is achieved. Once an activity is mastered, it may provide its own satisfaction, but during the process of learning extra feedback and encouragement may be required.

SOME COMMON PROBLEMS

1. You can offer people the chance, but they just don't seem interested in the activity. It is important to recognise that personal enthusiasm for a particular sport will not automatically be infectious, and that initial response to a new situation should not be taken as a reliable guide to the value of an activity. A handicapped person may become very anxious about new situations because, in the past, these have been associated with confusion and failure. He may therefore seek to avoid such situations unless he is gradually and repeatedly exposed to them. This emphasises the need to structure his experience very carefully in the ways outlined in the section on basic strategies (see p. 8). Tasks need to be simplified, help given, and motivating feedback provided. Without this care in planning and presentation, avoidance and resistance may be increased, and the whole exercise will become unpleasant for all concerned. But as the description of the Pinewood Centre shows (see p. 148), interest can develop. A key element that this work also highlights is the need to involve the handicapped person in planning activities. He needs to participate; and participation is not just for those who can articulate their needs. It is valuable even for the most severely disabled people if the activities are structured around and involve their known strengths and preferences.

2. These activites are fine for the well behaved, but you cannot involve those who are disruptive. It has already been pointed out that sport and other physical activites may have special benefits for those with disruptive behaviour, but some thought must be given to strategies for managing the problems if they are to be involved. The first step is to recognise that many disruptive behaviours have been learned and persist because they achieve some kind of consequences or feedback for the handicapped person. This must be assessed by specifying the problem behaviour, studying the situations in which it occurs and the consequences which are achieved by it. It is important also not just to focus on the difficult behaviour but to ask the question 'What should the person be doing instead?' If he was not behaving badly, what would he be doing?

These two approaches lead to positive action to develop appropriate behaviour, and will suggest how the disruption might be 'unlearned' by making sure that it does not achieve the consequences maintaining it. Disruptive behaviour can lead to a lot of attention, or attempts to pacify, e.g. offering a cup of tea or sweets, and these may inadvertently be strengthening the problems. If so, it will be important to ignore the disruptive acts and focus all attention on appropriate behaviour. This may be very frustrating for the individual at first, and indeed his behaviour may get worse before he slowly learns that he can get what he wants by behaving constructively not disruptively.

These techniques may be neither appropriate nor feasible in some cases; it is then important to seek guidance on alternative ways of dealing with the problems. However, many problems can be solved by so planning a programme that participants have plenty to occupy and interest them, i.e. minimal waiting or 'empty' times, and by making sure that all attention is focused on to appropriate behaviour. This has sometimes been described as making sure you catch people being good.

3. All these ideas work well for the more able, but what can you do for multiply, severely handicapped people? This group of people, with physical and sensory handicaps in addition to their learning difficulties, present some of the greatest challenges to the ingenuity of parents, teachers, nurses and all others who work for them. There is little point in minimising the all too obvious difficulties of getting them to participate, but there is still much that can be done and progress is certainly possible. The first step is to ensure that adequate stimulation is received. This group of people often live in a state of sensory deprivation, both by reason of their own handicap and because of some of the environments offered to them. It is important to ensure that a good general level of stimulation is maintained to prevent withdrawal into a world of self-stimulation. The essence of such stimulation is that it be varied and adapted to the disabilities of the individual. Simply having loud music on, or hanging up coloured objects is not sufficient, because of the speed at which the nervous system adapts. Change and novelty are essential, and the exploration of alternative senses such as touch and smell, is needed. Maintaining stimulation is an important first step, but much more can be done.

The second step is to ensure correct positioning for the activity to be attempted. This positioning is critical in facilitating correct, voluntary movements and inhibiting abnormal, involuntary movements. This may necessitate finding a suitable position for the activity chosen, or choosing an activity which is suitable for the 'best' position of the individual concerned.

Selecting skills to teach and maintain them requires careful thought. The size of step into which a task must be broken may be infinitesimally small — one may be aiming for the eyes to follow a ball moving horizontally from left to right, or encouraging that half-inch movement of the hand that will move the chime bell. Teaching these basic skills requires great sensitivity in the level of help given. Progress may take the form of a very gradual reduction in the physical help required to grasp an object. The helper must be sensitive to the least movement from the handicapped person and reduce his prompting as he feels independent movement coming into play.

Providing comprehensible feedback may be difficult, and routine forms of social or material encouragement may be meaningless. In some situations vibratory stimulation has been found very useful in reinforcing good performance. In others some individuals show strong preference for particular kinds of music (both classical and modern).

Finally, there may be certain activities which more readily encourage responses from the multiply handicapped person. The sections on swimming, riding and music and movement may be particularly helpful (see also the sections on severely mentally handicapped people in Chapters 2 and 3). Some others which might not usually be called 'sport' are also worth considering, as is the potential of modern electronics to translate simple responses into complex forms of stimulation, e.g. modern fruit machines with light touch panels which lead to a range of changing visual and auditory effects.

These are only some examples and hints of avenues to explore. There is much still to be learned about involving this group, but enough is known for a start to be made.

4. You can teach handicapped people to do something one day, but you come back the next day, and they have forgotten all about it. Making generalisations about 'handicapped people' is always a dangerous exercise. The term mental handicap covers an enormous variety of learning problems in people who show large individual differences in personality. Some handicapped people may well be forgetful, as are some non-handicapped people, but this is not a general characteristic of those with a mental handicap. They certainly have difficulty in learning skills initially, and once they have been mastered they may need extra practice to consolidate the learning. But with careful teaching and plenty of practice, skills will be retained without an unusual degree of loss over a period.

There is another problem which may sometimes be interpreted as a memory problem. This arises where skills are taught in an artificial situation that cannot easily be related to the real situation. For example, later in the book (see p. 142) an example is given of teaching some handicapped people to use photographs as an aid in route-finding. The initial stages of this could have been taught in the classroom using a lot of verbal instructions and models of road junctions, houses, trees, etc. If so, it is possible that when placed in the real situation the handicapped person would be none the wiser. A far better strategy is that actually adopted, of going out into the real environment and teaching there. This is a good general guideline, to work in the real environment, using real equipment, rather than spending a lot of time on elaborate mock-ups of the natural situation, whose relevance may not be apparent to the learner.

5. These are all marvellous ideas, but you need enormous numbers of staff. In some situations high staffing is essential. But high staffing is not the only answer and, in some cases, too many staff can be as disruptive as too few.

It may be worth considering a few strategies which are useful in working with groups of people. If only one staff member is present for a group he will need to ensure that he uses activities in which all can participate to some degree, and he will need to rapidly move from person to person giving each one brief amounts of individual attention, rather than concentrating on only a few, or spending long periods with each person individually. If two staff members are available one can work with the groups whilst the other focuses on individual work. Roles can be swapped around and in this way each person gets periods of one-to-one work even in a situation where staffing ratios would seem to be low.

It may be useful to draw on other sources of help such as volunteers or handicapped members in the group who are competent at the skill. Sometimes this helping process can be facilitated by sub-dividing a large group into teams, and setting a goal for each team and a prize for achieving the goal. Of course, this situation must be handled carefully but it can be very powerful in releasing capacities for self-help.

6. You try and get this sort of thing going, but you get no support, and in the end you just give up. Many groups criticise each other for failing to support their new ideas. Parents, nurses, teachers and training centre staff all complain that they start a programme but this it does not get carried on by others, and many staff complain of lack of support from their colleagues, both senior and junior. There is no magical answer to this, but one key element is to decide, before beginning, who is needed to carry on the work, and who can sabotage it successfully. This list can be quite long and may include all sorts of people, not necessarily directly involved, e.g. supplies or transport officers. Everyone on this list must be consulted and involved **before** starting out. They need to feel that they have had a say and that the work is 'theirs' to some extent. Without this participative attitude in relation to the handicapped person, good ideas will fail to translate into good practice.

CONCLUSION

Involving mentally handicapped people in sports and physical activities is an exciting and under-developed area. This book highlights how expectations can be shattered and horizons widened by carefully planned determination and ingenuity. In the preceding sections of this chapter only a few general principles which may guide those setting out for the first time have been outlined. Putting these principles into practice requires great flexibility and responsiveness to individual needs, interests and abilities. There are no text book recipes for action but an enormous reservoir of untapped potential in both the mentally handicapped and those who can help them to a fuller participation in our society.

CHAPTER THREE

Teaching Guidelines

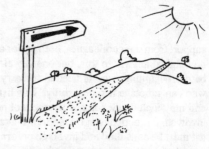

A coach in training should, if possible, work with very severely handicapped people for a few months so that he becomes used to their problems and adapts himself to helping them.

THE TEACHER'S SPECIFIC CONTRIBUTION

1. Keep verbal instructions short and simple. The group will learn through **doing** rather than listening.

2. A calm controlled voice creates a constructive working relationship. Avoid talking down to the group.

3. The teacher's efficient personal appearance and cheerful facial expression can do much to establish the confidence of those taking part.

4. Choose words carefully and test that instructions have been understood.

5. Rely predominantly on demonstration. Focus attention on what you want the class to look at, e.g. position of the feet — path of the ball. Be prepared to repeat the demonstration and test the class's understanding of the teaching point made. Demonstration may have to be taken very slowly to focus attention.

6. Reduce each skill to its simplest form so that each individual can achieve some success. Allow plenty of time to learn one skill before progressing to the next.

7. Constantly look for opportunities to praise class members, remembering that effort is as important to encourage as achievement. Create an atmosphere of success.

8. Teacher participation and demonstration are important motivating factors.

9. Discipline must be consistent, firm and clearly understood — 'say what you mean and mean what you say'.

10. Always position yourself where all can see and hear you and where you can see every individual in the group.

11. While thorough preparation of work to be attempted is essential the ability to adapt quickly in response to your **observations** of their capabilities and motivation is of equal importance.

ORGANISATION AND PRESENTATION

1. All equipment should be ready before the activity starts.

2. Active participation by all may be the ultimate goal, but some will take time to gain confidence and the opportunity to see others enjoying the activity is often a very necessary stage. Even spasmodic participation must be accepted in some circumstances.

3. Involve as many as possible in the preparation and organisation of activities — e.g. collecting and moving equipment, keeping the score.

4. Practice periods should be short with frequent change of activities to maintain motivation; on the other hand, when success is achieved repeat the activity so that those taking part can experience the joy of accomplishment.

5. Progression is not only measured by making an activity more difficult but also by improved performance, response and memory, e.g. folk dance sequence (see pp. 123-128).

6. Repetition plays a significant part in all stages when teaching mentally handicapped people, e.g. the importance or routine.

7. Encourage individuals and groups to work at their own variations and adaptations of activities and provide opportunities for them to talk things over with you, e.g. vary the size of bats and balls or working area — lower the net, etc.

8. Keep rules simple and adhere to them strictly, knowing that they are made for the safety and protection of all those taking part, e.g. athletics, swimming, games.

9. See that distracting influences are kept to a minimum during the session.

10. A short daily session of physical activity is of greater value than a longer one once a week.

(N.B. See Chapter 2 'A Psychologist's View' pp. 4-7, for a full discussion of some of the principles involved in teaching and organising physical recreation for mentally handicapped people).

SAFETY

'Nothing venture nothing win', but safety precautions must be taken at **all** times since some mentally handicapped people seem to have little sense of danger and equally some may suffer from irrational fears. Some safety measures have been included in the main sections of the book; nevertheless, the following points should always be borne in mind when preparing any programme of physical activity and sport.

1. Select the right equipment and ensure its care and maintenance.

2. Try to avoid injury caused by thoughtless organisation, e.g. running towards glass doors or walls, leaving equipment or other obstacles 'lying about', playing on uneven, splintery or slippery surfaces.

3. Make sure that suitable and adequate clothing and footwear are worn, e.g. for indoor work, socks and tights without footwear are always hazardous but working with bare feet on a clean, non-splintery surface has very specific advantages.

4. Maintain strict discipline and adequate supervision.

5. Choose activities suitable for the group and/or individuals.

6. Have a first aid box. The first aid box need not be a complex one. Most sporting adventures do not result in serious injury. Scratches, abrasions, bruises and occasional cuts are the most frequent types of injury. Anything more serious needs medical attention. The box should include:

   an assortment of bandages, e.g. 25mm (1″) cotton bandages for fingers, 50mm (2″) crepe bandages for sprains and bruises;

assortment of different sizes of adhesive plasters with sterilised dressings to cover cuts and abrasions;

a roll of cotton wool, useful for padding bruises and sprains and making firm pads to stem bleeding;

gauze squares 100mm (4") across, for toileting wounds;

safety pins;

scissors;

tweezers for removing splinters;

a box of tissues;

plastic incontinence pants;

sanitary towels — elastic and pins;

antiseptic cleaning lotion.

FURTHER CONSIDERATIONS

1. Programme. Offer a varied programme, e.g. some respond well to physical work with music while others may prefer work with balls. Provision for fitness training should be made, e.g. jogging, hiking, swimming.

Link sports and physical activities with current sporting events on television, e.g. World Cup, Olympic Games, 'It's a Knockout', 'Come Dancing'.

2. Transport. Mentally handicapped people may be denied the opportunity to take part in an activity or even to watch because there is no transport. If public transport is not available or is inappropriate, the provision of transport needs to be considered. In the case of England, Scotland and Wales legislation has given powers for this. *(See the Chronically Sick and Disabled Persons Act, 1970, section 2, and the Chronically Sick and Disabled Persons (Scotland) Act 1972, section 1).*

3. Integration. Where their social behaviour is acceptable and they have acquired the necessary skills, mentally handicapped individuals should be encouraged to join with other members of the community to enjoy all sporting activities, particularly those which are non-competitive. It is equally important that members of the general public should realise that some mentally handicapped people are capable of taking part with them in many sports, physical activities and outdoor pursuits (see Snowdon Report: *Integrating the disabled: report of the Snowdon Working Party.* National Fund for Crippling Diseases, Horsham, Sussex, 1976). Remember that mentally handicapped people can only successfully intermingle with the rest of the community if those in the community willingly accept them.

The timing of integration is vital to its success. An unsuccessful attempt at integration is counter-productive.

4. Resources. Make the best use of community resources, e.g. facilities and the people with expertise in sports and physical activities.

5. Volunteers. Volunteers can be drawn from many sources, e.g. parents, friends, voluntary organisations and students — the volunteers varying in background, experience and age. It is helpful if they can be given some form of advice as to the effective ways of working with mentally handicapped people.

6. Visual aids. Make full use of films — film strips, photographs, posters, charts, videotapes and other audio visual materials to reinforce the teacher's expertise. The resourceful teacher can find or improve other aids, e.g. models, diagrams, blackboard drawings.

7. Keep up to date. Continually examine teaching methods and make sure that you keep up to date in your knowledge of mentally handicapped peiple and the current developments in the world of sport and physical recreation.

CHAPTER FOUR

How to Choose an Activity

This book provides ideas on how to introduce physical activities and sport into the life of mentally handicapped people. Whether these ideas are effective or not depends to a great extent on whether the teacher is sensitive to the needs of individuals and to the community in which the work is being done. A good activity can be successfully introduced in one situation, yet fail in another.

Being aware of the varying needs of mentally handicapped people will help the teacher to make a wise choice of activity (see Chapter 1, pp. 1-3).

1. DEGREE OF PHYSICAL FITNESS

A group consisting of people with multiple handicaps may have to sit for most of the day. For these, non-weight bearing activities must be provided for body movement (see Severely handicapped people, below). Others may be ambulant and perhaps over-protected. These would need a more active programme, e.g. fitness training (see pp. 97-102), games (see Chapter 6) or swimming (see Chapter 8).

2. PLAY

Play is essential in the life of the child; through it he learns. In many instances play becomes recreation in adult life. Severely multiply handicapped adults may have missed many of the experiences play can provide and developmentally they may still need 'to play'. A teacher faced with this situation might consider using:

(i)   an adventure playground (see Chapter 13)

(ii) a soft play area (see p. 161)

(iii) a good floor for movement activities (see p. 11).

Having analysed the needs of the group and having found several suitable activities, the teacher must be practical and relate the choice to the facilities available.

3. MOVEMENT IS A LANGUAGE

Many mentally handicapped adults have severe problems of communication and have difficulty in relating to other people. Activities that involve some physical contact can help to build up relationships between themselves and the teacher and with each other. See, for example,

(i)   Veronica Sherborne's approach to movement (see p. 89)

(ii) folk dancing (see p. 114).

4. MOTOR SKILLS

Since these are less dependent on intelligence than many other activities, success which helps to build up confidence can be developed through the learning of specific skills:

(i)   ball skills (see pp. 18-25)

(ii) swimming (see Chapter 8)

(iii) gymnastics (see p. 99).

5. OPPORTUNITIES FOR INTEGRATION

To establish the confidence of those coming to help (e.g. parents, friends, students, coaches) is as important a consideration as the needs of the handicapped. Dancing is excellent for all ages (see Chapter 11). If the helpers are young it might be:

(i)   games (see Chapter 6)

(ii) gymnastics (see pp. 59 and 99)

(iii) swimming (see Chapter 8)

(iv) athletics (see Chapter 7)

(v)   outdoor pursuits (see Chapter 12)

The facilities available are crucial in choosing the activity (see p. 168).

6. IMPORTANCE OF GROUP MOTIVATION

When summer holidays are a topic of conversation and the weather is good, an interest in camping and other outdoor activities could be encouraging for the more able (see p. 137).

7. AGE OF THOSE TAKING PART

This is an important consideration especially if many are elderly. Activities in which music is used could provide the greatest encouragement for these (see pp. 91, 92).

8. SEVERELY HANDICAPPED PEOPLE

Staff dealing with severely handicapped people should not be 'put off' by the amount of material in this book which obviously relates to the more able.

While most severely mentally handicapped people will never aspire to many of the games, sports and leisure activities described, the text contains a fund of suitable ideas (see *Mental handicap, severe*, in Index) for such people. Any purposeful physical activity often seems to act as a stimulant to mental activity, and may itself be stimulated by the use of music or simple brightly coloured and interesting apparatus.

A first activity could be clapping in time to music — the rhythm being changed frequently in order to maintain interest and prevent a mechanical response. This may be expanded by alternate touching of some part of the body, such as 'Clap — touch head; clap — touch toes', etc. Such simple exercises can be undertaken with those who are also confined to bed or chair.

Adherence to a rhythm provides a kind of discipline which tends to promote more purposeful movements than might otherwise be achieved.

Equipment for very severely mentally handicapped people must be extremely simple; complicated apparatus only leads to confusion. Activities using bean bags, balls of various sizes, hoops and ropes encourage maximum effort.

Bouncing and catching movements are fairly easy to encourage, but throwing creates problems — 'letting go' the ball at the optimum point of the arm swing being the main one. A forceful arm swing is often produced, then — to the player's surprise — he finds he is still holding the ball. With practice this difficulty can be overcome, the aiming practice games described in Chapter Six (see pp. 38-42) could be helpful.

The bold entries in the index should provide ideas for a basic programme of activities from which it may be possible to lead on to more complicated exercises as improvement takes place. Appropriate material must be selected according to individual circumstances and potential. Other activities not specifically picked out in the index need not necessarily be precluded.

9. COMMUNITY LIFE

An establishment needs to develop its own community life. Carefully chosen physical activities play an important part e.g.:

(i)   dancing (see Chapter 11)

(ii)   'It's a Knockout' (see pp. 84-86)

(iii)   potted sports (see pp. 80-81).

10. CONTACT WITH NEIGHBOURING ESTABLISHMENTS

Such contact is not only stimulating for the handicapped but also for the staff. Carefully selected physical activities shared with others can be instrumental in 'building bridges' over a period of time, e.g.:

(i)   a shared gymnastic club;

(ii)   a folk dance club.

Annual events such as a dance evening or a sports day can also play their part in establishing contact with other organisations. This is also a way in which good facilities and teachers can be shared. To create and maintain lines of communication and close liaison with the health and social services and education departments of the local authority is vital.

11. FACILITIES

This book introduces teachers to many activites. It should enable them to select a sport or activity relevant to the facilities. Some need generous indoor or outdoor space, some are dependent on a good floor surface, while others can be practised on a fairly indifferent floor surface.

A resourceful teacher should be able to introduce some type of physical activity into the programme of residents and trainees even where facilities are comparatively poor, provided the establishment gives the necessary support. As progress is made so further consideration would need to be given to improving facilities (see p. 168).

12. SPECTATORS

The interest of the more severely handicapped people in sport and physical activities will mainly consist of watching others, although they should be continuously encouraged to 'move' and to share in some of the experiences, such as riding (if only in a pony trap), kite flying or swimming. The 'watching' can be made more worthwile by simple explanation and by ensuring an uninterrupted view.

For some spectators 'watching' may be the first stage in gaining confidence to **take part**, but there will probably be a wide variation in the length of time they take to become involved. The teacher's sensitive reaction to this unpredictable situation is all important if further progress is to be made. It can be useful if a note is made when someone joins in if only for a brief period of time.

Spectators at out-of-door events can become very cold, particularly if they are severely handicapped and the weather is cold and wet. Warm clothing should be worn including wheelchair mackintoshes and body and foot muffs when necessary. Spectators should be encouraged to sit or stand in as sheltered a place as possible.

If mentally handicapped people have the opportunity to watch sporting events on TV, some explanation of the activity being shown by parents or teachers will be invaluable.

CHAPTER FIVE

Landscape for Sport, Physical Recreation and Play

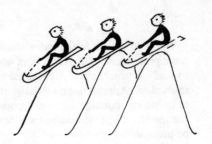

The grounds of schools, day and residential establishments for mentally handicapped people are very often examples of institutional landscapes which, unlike public open spaces, offer a rich opportunity to design specifically for a known group of people. The provision of open air facilities for sport, physical recreation and play should be an essential requirement of any design as it reflects the establishment's imaginative and caring role in the life of mentally handicapped people.

In addition, sites of suitable size may well offer opportunities to establish road safety training areas, gardening activities, pet keeping projects and such imaginative features as adventure play sites, camp sites, barbecue and picnic areas, quiet gardens and 'wilderness'. Although such items are space demanding, imaginative people have established them in surprisingly small grounds often with very little upheaval to an existing design; in fact, run-down Victorian gardens are often excellent starting points.

Few establishments will have ideal sites for every type of outdoor activity but some of the most successful facilities have been developed as a result of drive and initiative in what appeared to be very unpromising locations. If, however, no space is available near the hospital or ATC, a weekly trip to a nearby park or playing area might be arranged.

The various sites discussed below are intended to serve the major recreational activities which, in turn, stimulate different group and individual reactions and place different organisational and managerial demands upon the staff.

Anyone siting these activities should bear in mind their accessibility and distance from domestic facilities particularly toilets and stores although the noise generated by a group at play can be very disturbing both within and beyond the institution.

Convenient storage is a very important consideration as a 'long haul with the gear' is often the final deterrent or excuse for the faint-hearted. In addition, the safety of the participants must be considered particularly the risk of running on to vehicular roads in moments of excitement: nearby windows will also be at risk as there will inevitably be the occasional wild throw or kick. Finally, the ease with which such sites can be supervised and maintained must be considered and maximum use should be made of any existing landscape features.

Open air recreational sites are considered here under three headings: sports pitches, tracks and informal play areas.

SPORTS PITCHES

The construction and maintenance of high grade sports pitches, courts and tracks is a specialist subject: the skilled and qualified groundsmen concerned are well supplied with a technical literature relating to the needs and problems of supplying outdoor playing surfaces all the year round.

Further useful information is produced by the grass seed companies, the agricultural chemical industry, sports field construction companies, the Sports Council and the Sports Turf Research Institute.

In spite of such an array of technical data, many establishments are faced with adapting old grounds themselves, and the following general advice may be useful.

Most sports demand a pitch of a certain shape and/or size; it must usually be level or near level and have a reasonably true and smooth surface. These common requirements do **not** demand that the pitch be set in a rigid angular site. The somewhat harsh geometric features of sports pitches can be far more successfully integrated into surrounding leisure grounds if they are marked out from **within** a larger informal shape. This policy also has the great merit that it ensures that space for spectators is provided.

Pitch marking is a chore; one imaginative aid is to permanently mark out all corner points, etc., by sinking large nails or short metal bars safely below the surface and locating them when required by means of a metal detector. In practice this technique proves to be very straightforward and saves a great deal of time at the beginning of each 'season'.

Sports surfaces are all prone to wear. A grass turf which is cheap to establish and delightful to look at when in good condition must be respected as a living sheet of vegetation; over use, particularly under harsh weather conditions, inevitably results in fundamental, long term problems. The degree of damage varies with the season and is greatly influenced by the weather. Much of the current work on grass type selection, land drainage, the use of fertilisers, irrigation, moving, and aeration has helped schools and public authorities to increase the use of their pitches. The current literature contains some very useful hints on these topics. Tough hard wearing alternatives to grass have been developed: broadly speaking they are of three types, the bound mineral type, polymer bonded materials and 'plastic grass'. These materials can produce surfaces of excellent quality but they are very expensive to install and are by no means maintenance free. The general public often refer to them as 'all weather' pitches but this claim is rarely made by responsible manufacturers. Small courts with synthetic surfaces have been built at a few caring institutions but ashalt remains by far the most common hard alternative to grass. When carefully laid it can produce a tolerably safe and very hard wearing surface. Concrete is a far more 'vicious' material and should not be used.

TRACKS

Nature trails, trim tracks, follow my leader play — the list of linear or path activities has increased considerably in recent years. Ideally such play features are best constructed within, or, more accurately, between existing mature features, since part of their appeal is the visual separation of the 'stations'. Track designers should try to convey the feeling of a journey with a clear start and finish as this encourages participants to keep going to the end. The details of each station will undoubtedly be different but the common basic requirement is for a clear linking path, not necessarily of the same surfacing material throughout. The stations must have ample space for their particular activity or, where appropriate, house a prominent marker post; they must all have a clear way marker indicating the continuation of the track. Tracks offer the opportunity to use the landscape to provide **attainable** challenges combining physical obstacles with tests of initiative and independence (see p. 102).

INFORMAL PLAY AREAS

These multi-purpose sites serve as everything from kick-about areas to the open air venue for organised games and dance.

The landscape demanded by these activities is far less precise in both size and form than that required by 'formal' sports. Indeed, in contrast to the sports field, there are considerable advantages in developing an informal play site within mature grounds, as slopes, banks, robust trees and shrub masses can add greatly to the range of activities.

The first requirement is for a reasonably level, **well drained** area of tough turf or hard surface which is free from obstacles. The strongest argument in support of any necessary redesign — the removal of intruding paths, flower beds, shrubs and small trees etc. — is to remind objectors that the grounds are an integral part of the caring institution.

The features and the planting that surround the play area must be robust; inevitably people and play equipment stray, and tough shrubs like *Symphoricarpus* 'Hancock' and ground cover such as *Hypericum calycinum* will survive the occasional wanderer while a regiment of tulips will not.

When the site is used for ball games a lot of time can be saved if a retieval net, possibly in combination with grass banks, is used. Many types of cheap twine and plastic garden net are now obtainable, and are preferable to the cage-like appearance of wire netting or chain link fencing. Temporary nets can be removed when not in use but if they are to be successful they must be easy to assemble and quick to dismantle. Uprights should be designed to slip into permanent sockets and any horizontal cross pieces can be linked by the simple devices sold in garden shops for the construction of fruit cages.

If possible informal play areas should be within reach of mains electricity and water; for special occasions a **long** length of heavy duty garden hose fitted with a shut off nozzle and a similar length of high quality extension lead with outdoor fittings will suffice, although of course these items require an outdoor tap and a weatherproof socket — facilities which are often absent. It is also important to know how temporary services are going to reach the play area: preferably they should be 'round the back' so that they are out of harms way and cannot trip anybody up. Such services provide the opportunity for a large number of special events, for example music, lights, paddling pools and play fountains.

Permanent water features, no matter how shallow, are not acceptable to some caring authorities while others take great pride in showing off their pools and fish ponds. There is much to be said for **temporary** water which can be made a special play feature in very hot weather. Sand pits and deliberately constructed hollows in the grass can be turned into shallow pools by simply spreading out and flooding a sheet of 500-1000 gauge plastic or, better still, butyl rubber; a spray jey on a hose pipe is all that is necessary to complete some very wet entertainment for suitably clad youngsters.

The basic movements of running, swinging, climbing, sliding and see-sawing can be set into verdant backgrounds, a point often made by the adventure play movement. Both traditional and adventure play use fixed equipment, but the visual impact, interest and safety of such equipment varies enormously. There is little doubt that on all three counts some of the best designs currently available come from Scandinavia, Holland and Germany. The range is frequently and well reviewed in the journals of landscape architecture which also carry many trade advertisements.

Unfortunately, fixed play equipment often looks as if it has been 'dumped' in the middle of a ten acre field, but it is best to avoid exposed open sites, and shrub screens and shade trees are valuable as they help to tie the apparatus into the landscape. On the other hand small strips and patches of turf easily become mud; they should be dispensed with as they are expensive and awkward to maintain. All fixed equipment should be securely and safely anchored with no exposed footings or protruding bolts; their surrounds should be well drained, mud free and soft enough to cushion accidental falls.

In most European countries fixed equipment is set within loose sand or, if this is anappropriate, flexible tiles. Slides are often built into the side of a play mound while sand pits can be integrated into the landscape by simply contructing them rather like golf bunkers within turf. Alternatively, they are sometimes bounded by a low palisade of vertical logs.

FURTHER READING

BENGTSSON, A. *Environmental planning for children's play.* Crosby Lockwood, St. Albans, 1972.

Playing fields and hard surface areas. Department of Education and Science. Building Bulletin 28, 1966.

THODAY, P. R. *Hospital grounds utilisation.* University of Bath, 1974.

CHAPTER SIX

Games and Sports

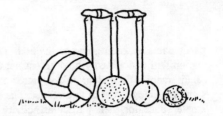

Planning a games session – Adaptations – Scoring – The teaching of skills – Activities using hoops, ropes, balls, beanbags and quoits – Activities using improvised equipment – Forms of tag – Team races – Team races using various formations and equipment – Group games without equipment – Easy games in circle formation – Fun games without equipment – More difficult games – Skills leading up to minor and major games – Examples of minor games – Games with a difference – Trampolining – Gymnastics

Practically all the major games and sports can be played with success by some mentally handicapped people, provided the required skills are sufficiently mastered and the appropriate adaptations are made. It is important for the teacher to know the up-to-date rules of any game and sport that is to be taught, since the ultimate aim is to play the game to the official rules. However, mentally handicapped players should never be thrust into an activity or game before they are ready for it — ready mentally as well as physically, socially and emotionally.

The following is a list of games and sports which the author has seen played to a greater or lesser degree in adult training centres and/or hospitals and clubs (the list is increasing yearly):

archery	golf	skating
association football	gymnastics	skiing
athletics	handball	snooker
badminton	hockey	squash rackets
bagatelle	indoor bowls	swimming
batington	judo	table tennis
basket ball	karate	table skittles
billiards	karting	ten pin bowling
bowls	lawn tennis	trampolining
cricket	netball	tug-of-war
croquet	petanque	unicurl
darts	quoits	volley ball
frisbee	rounders	weight lifting
fencing	rowing	

Some games and sports require only one or two participants, e.g. badminton, bowls, table tennis, archery, skating. Since these can become leisure pursuits throughout life, opportunities to play some of these should be encouraged.

Games and sports can be played:

as a session devoted to games;

as recreation in a lunch hour;

at camps and holidays;

at sports leisure centres;

at parties and social evenings;

at sports meetings and tournaments (see Chapter 9);

as an item in displays of physical activity.

National games and sports have not been included. The national governing body of each sport will provide the current rules, coaching manuals, films and charts (see Appendix 3).

The following games and variations are included in some detail because they are less well known but are enjoyed enormously and can be played by people with a wide variety of abilities: batington, petanque, unihoc, play with boomerangs and frisbees, skittles.

Games and sports are valuable because they:

1. train dexterity and co-ordination particularly of eye and hand

2. develop the necessary skills which serve as training for all games and sports such as football, netball, unihoc, athletics, badminton, bowls

3. channel excess energy into purposeful skills and provide an outlet for repressed emotions

4. stimulate the less active to move

5. help to develop alertness, perseverance, self-control, optimism, courage and confidence

6. increase the will and the ability to play to the rules, to be a good loser and to co-operate with others

7. create opportunities for competition of varying types

8. give the players responsibilities e.g. helping with the organisation and care of equipment, leading a team, training them to take care of their own personal sportswear. (See also Chapter 1, p. 3.)

Before planning a games session consider:

1. the physical and mental abilities, likes and dislikes and the difficulties of the group of players;

2. the facilities — indoor and outdoor — the size of the surface and the nature of the playing space;

3. what equipment is available, is it safe and in good repair?

4. any hazards e.g. low ceiling lights, glass windows; unstacked chairs and out of doors obstructions such as trees, posts and broken glass;

5. the play area and the markings within it; the dimensions will naturally influence the number of players taking part and the type of equipment being used;

6. the playing area must be contained and be clear of obstacles if ball games are to be played. If the ball is lost under obstacles, the game stops and the aim of continuous activity is defeated.

PLANNING A GAMES SESSION

A games session will only prove successful if it is carefully prepared and presented. The number of practices and games will depend on the length of the period and on the number and ability of the players. The presentation will, of course, need to be adapted to the ability and mood of the class.

Select activities, practices and games which provide activity for:

1. everyone rather than those in which the majority of players are quickly 'put out';

2. the less able players.

Organisation (See Teaching guidelines p. 8).

1. Make sure that equipment is available;

2. make any floor markings before the session starts (players may well be able to help);

3. mark the boundaries of the playing space clearly. If it is **smaller** than the whole space — by chalk lines, 'masking' tape or rope, benches, chairs (even skittles can be used, providing they are sturdy and do not create a hazard).

A Suggestion for the Plan of the Session

A session of half an hour to one hour working time should include:

1. a warming up activity with or without apparatus (individually with a partner or in small groups) (see pp. 16 and 89);

2. one of more skill practices (see pp. 16-27);

3. a team race, a group, a minor or a major game.

Presentation (See Teaching guidelines p. 8).

Game-like activities and games are an important part of the whole programme of recreation. The following are further suggestions to remember when preparing a games session:

1. know how to play the game yourself in order to demonstrate and coach effectively;

2. it is better to start with a small group of 'would be' enthusiasts who, through their enjoyment, naturally encourage others to join in;

3. decide the least number of skills the players need to know before they can take part in the game or a modified form of it;

4. practice these skills individually, in pairs or group activities, then 'have a go' at the game;

5. teach the players to understand the meaning of and obey the whistle or the word 'stop';

6. be firm in enforcing the rules and encourage the players to accept the referee's decision with good grace;

7. collect a variety of game-like activities and simple games which can be used in unpredicted circumstances;

8. remember the less skilled who are unable or incapable of playing the more complicated team games; modified, or your own invented, games can be successful for these players;

9. introduce one game or one skill at a time.

ADAPTATIONS

Adaptation is often necessary. Here are some examples:

1. substitute walking for running;

2. substitute equipment of different size and weight;

3. adapt equipment e.g. shorten handle of badminton racquet;

4. reduce or increase the size of the playing area;

5. restrict players to definite zones;

6. hit the ball on the second bounce;

7. allow players to hold the ball for a longer period;

8. use a bounce, roll or underarm throw to replace an overarm throw;

9. simplify scoring.

SCORING

1. 'Beat your own standard' method — useful when practising simple activities e.g. increase the distance or height of a throw.

2. Count the number of goals e.g. football; points e.g. table tennis; games e.g. tennis; runs e.g. cricket.

3. Count 1 point for achieving a part of a complete rounder e.g. in rounders or Danish rounders: 1 point for reaching 2nd base, 2 points for reaching 3rd base, 3 points for reaching 4th base, 4 points for a rounder — without being out.

Only adapt the scoring when necessary, e.g. badminton, volley ball and lawn tennis scoring can be difficult to understand; a simplified method such as the points system in table tennis might be used at first. It is essential that the players understand the method of scoring at every stage.

WARMING UP

It is vitally important that the body is warmed up and prepared for more vigorous activities — games and sports.

Different ways of achieving this are:

1. easy jogging;

2. general body exercises (see pp. 89-90);

3. carefully selected games of tag (see p. 27);

4. activities using various equipment — practised individually or in pairs.

The warming-up period should be short and at the beginning of any games session; it should start easily building up to more vigorous movement e.g. before going outside to play football or netball — a short warm up session might be taken in the hall/gym.

THE TEACHING OF SKILLS

First and foremost, players must be taught to play with e.g. balls bats and hoops of different sizes, weights and types, so that they feel at ease with them. By degrees the skills of throwing, catching, kicking, fielding, intercepting, dodging, aiming and hitting — which are common to all games — can be introduced. These skills are based on certain fundamentals learnt largely through experience, practising and playing, and once reasonably well mastered, players will be able to grasp new games more quickly. Sometimes, at an earlier stage, it is advisable to play the games with the least possible number of rules.

When practisingh, players can work individually, in twos or small groups. As the fundamentals of the various techniques and skills are understood and mastered, competition can be introduced on an individual, partner or team basis. The teacher, by experimenting with such apparatus as beach-balls, balloons, old shuttle-cocks, bean bags, quoits and improvised apparatus, and later balls and bats, can discover many enjoyable and interesting ways of using them, thereby inventing an endless variety of activities. Often the players themselves will offer ideas.

ACTIVITIES USING HOOPS, ROPES, BALLS, BEANBAGS AND QUOITS

1. Sit in the hoop with one part of the body touching the floor outside it, e.g. foot – elbow; change to another part, e.g. hand, knee.

2. Sit outside the hoop with one or more parts of the body touching the floor inside it.

3. Hold the hoop up like a mirror 'look through'. Repeat holding the hoop high – move it high, low and side to side.

4. Sit with hoop on the floor in front, touch the hoop in different places, one hand, then the other, then alternately – make the touch light, touch near, touch the far side.

    Variations: (i) clap after each tap – touch and clap, touch and clap – clap high; (ii) move hoop further away and to one side, then the other. Stretch as much as possible in all directions.

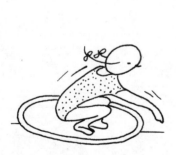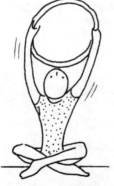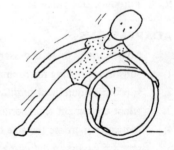

Activities using hoops

5. Stand with the hoop on the floor. Step in and out of the hoop in different directions. Right in, left in – left out, right out – forwards sideways and backwards.

    Variation: jump with and without a rebound – hop in and out of hoop.

6.   Stand with feet apart, hoop in front, one edge resting on the floor, hold the hoop loosely with both hands on top – 6-9 in. apart. Roll the hoop from side to side keeping hold of it, gradually increase the movement – rolling it from one hand to the other and swaying from foot to foot.

7.   Bowl the hoop, keeping close to it.

8.   Bowl the hoop forwards – move to catch it before it drops.

   Variation: roll the hoop to a partner who catches it and rolls it back.

9.   Stand, spin the hoop, let it nearly 'die', then pick it up.

   Variation: spin the hoop, run to a line or run round the hoop, catch it before it drops.

With Partners

10.   Stand with feet apart, one hoop between two partners facing each other, holding the hoop loosely with both hands at waist level (hoop parallel to the floor). Swing the hoop from side to side letting the body weight sway from foot to foot (easy knees) – gradually increase the width and height of the swing.

   Variation: look through the hoop as it swings high – develop it into a 'pancake turn'.

11.   One partner holds the hoop at right angles to the floor; the other partner gets through the hoop without touching it, change over.

   Variation: one partner holds the hoop parallel to the floor between knee and hip height, other partner gets through by stepping over the hoop – curling up and coming out from underneath, repeat from underneath coming out over the top, change over.

12.   Spread hoops out on the floor – use the hoops as stepping stones – step from hoop to hoop, leap from hoop to hoop. Many other ways of using hoops will be discovered. Hoops, beanbags or balls can be used together bouncing and throwing through a hoop from varying distances, in pairs or threes – one holding the hoop when necessary.

Long Ropes, 6-8m (20-26') long

   Two ropes stretched across room, held at knee height (hold the ropes lightly).

1.   Two or three at a time step forward over the rope, moving on to next rope; repeat, turn and run back to place.

2.   Step sideways over the rope and back again and over again, along the rope – move on to the next rope. Repeat.

3.   Rope on the floor, spring over it; gradually raise the height.

4.   Swing rope from side to side, jump over low swinging rope. Jump as the rope swings towards you.

5.   Hold ropes at hip height, move forwards under the first rope and sideways under the second. Move under the rope with a turn or backwards. Try not to touch the rope. Gradually increase the speed.

6.   As (5) in pairs, one guiding the other with a twist – one moving forwards the other moving backwards. Vary the speed.

7.   Turn the ropes in unison slowly and quickly.

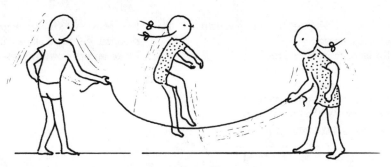

Activities using ropes

8.   One rope turned across the centre of the room, with the rope turning towards them, the players run under the turning rope – one at a time at first, later two at the same time. Progress to 'keeping the pot boiling'.
   Progress to skipping.
   Remember to change the 'rope turners'.

9.   **Skipping individually**

   Mentally handicapped people can learn to skip individually. Skipping ropes should be long enough to touch the ankles when the arms are fully stretched sideways. If handles are available they should have ball bearings to allow the rope to turn freely without twisting – if ropes are provided without handles, then the ends should be bound. Practise –

   (i)   skipping on the spot with a rebound;

   (ii)   skipping on the spot without a rebound;

   (iii)   combine (i) and (ii) 4 skips with a rebound followed by 8 skips without a rebound;

   (iv)   skip moving forwards and backwards;

(v) stand, turn the rope overhead to one side followed by the other.
Rope turn 4 turns on left, 4 on right. Rope turn 2 turns on left, 2 turns on right. Alternate turns left, right, left, right.

Dance steps, for example, polka, step and hop, pas de basques can all be performed in a skipping rope. The rope can be turned either forwards or backwards (practise both). To change from backwards to forwards skipping, practise 7 skips with a rebound, 'check' the rope by dropping the handles downwards. This checks the rope in front as the 8th skip is performed. The next 7 skips are then performed with the rope turning forwards, check the rope on 8 and skip backwards again.

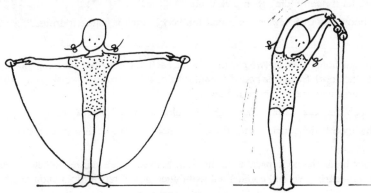

Activities using ropes

10. **Skipping with short ropes** or long ones, 2 turning – 1 skipping; use skipping rhymes. Here are some examples:

(i) I am (Edward) dressed in (blue),
These are the things he can do,
Clap his hands, touch his toes,
Skip one more and out he goes.
Increase the number of skips 2 – 3 – 4 etc.

(ii) Sally's in the garden,
Doing some skipping,
Along comes Peter,
And out goes Sally.
(Use individual skipper's names when possible.)

(iii) Two little sausages frying in a pan,
one went pop (clap) and one went bang.
(Jump with feet astride the rope.)

(iv) House to let
Apply within
When you go out
I come in.

(v) Keep the kettle boiling *(running under a turning rope)*
Miss the beat – you're out
next in.

(vi) All in together
This fine weather
When it's your birthday please jump out,
January, February, March, April, May . . . etc.
(Skipper runs out when the birthday month is called.)

(vii) Using 'name of person skipping' twice to give two skips between each action.
Rosemary, Rosemary touch the ground
Rosemary, Rosemary turn right round,
Rosemary, Rosemary climb upstairs,
Rosemary, Rosemary say your prayers.
Rosemary, Rosemary switch out the light,
Rosemary, Rosemary say good night.
run out.
(Many other actions could be substituted.)

(viii) Salt, Mustard, Vinegar, Pepper – 4 slow skips with rebound – 8 quick skips without a rebound.
Make up your own rhymes.

THE BALL

Playing with a ball fascinates all ages; the ball is 'alive'. Even before any specific skills have been mastered a ball can be used to stimulate movement. At the same time the properties of the ball are being explored and demands on concentration are being made. At this stage it is preferable to use larger size balls. The teacher initiates activities and works with the group. Variety of task is more important than the developing of specific motor skills.

An example of an activity session

Each with own ball including the teacher.

1. Hold it with both hands, roll it from right to left hand etc. Feel its shape and texture. Hold it as high up as possible – look at it.

2. Put it very carefully on the floor. Creep round it very quietly, jump round it etc.

3. Sit with the ball; use hands to roll ball across or round you, under knees etc. – make patterns.

4. Stand with ball in hands. In contrast to previous activity use the ball to make a noise, i.e. big bounces which encourage vigorous body movement; do not be too concerned with catching the ball.

5. Throw and catch – encourage carefulness and quietness in contrast to 4.

6.   Place the ball on the floor, dribble it using the inside of the feet, then try using other parts of the body, hand, and from sitting, elbow, seat, head, etc. Notice the range of body movement, the effort involved.

7.   Stand, make up a game keeping the ball **off** the floor as much as possible; regard effort to do so as success.

8.   Roll the ball and run after it to retrieve it.

9.   Use flat of hand to pat-bounce downwards or upwards.

Climax: Free choice alone or with partner.

Observe the capacity to play without specific direction. This will help the teacher to plan the next session. This approach can be adapted to the use of other small apparatus, e.g. hoops, ropes, quoits, bean bags.

Activities can be adapted to suit indoor or outdoor activities e.g. if working on asphalt the players cannot be asked to sit or crawl on the ground.

Getting the feel of it

In the early stages, let each member of the group choose a ball from a box of balls of different sizes, weights and colours. Help them to feel the weight and shape of the ball, also its texture. Talk about its shape and texture. Let them discover what can be done with a ball.

Ball practices for specific skills can be devised with:

1 ball for each person; 1 ball between two; in small groups.

Players can develop skill with a ball if they are given the opportunity to learn the technique of: rolling – throwing – bouncing – controlling and stopping – passing – catching – dribbling – kicking – batting (hitting) – heading – trapping – with all kinds of balls, large, small, heavy, light, hard, soft.

As players become familiar with the ball and can perform most of the skills, more difficult activities can be taught involving more than one skill, e.g. bouncing and throwing, hitting, catching and throwing.

Rolling the ball

1.   Roll a ball between partners.

2.   Roll a ball to the side of a partner to pick up and return.

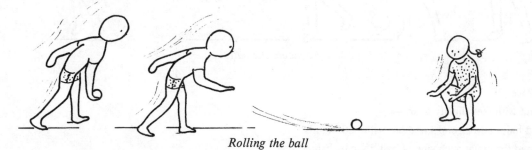

Rolling the ball

3.   Roll different size balls between skittles.

4.   Roll balls through the legs of a chair placed between two players. Count the number of balls which go through – which couple can get 2 – 4 – 6 balls through in the shortest time – which pair can roll two or more balls through consecutively.

5.   Sit with knees bent – hold the ball in both hands, resting on knees – let it roll down to the ankles – kick it up with feet and catch it.

Variation: kick the ball up to a partner.

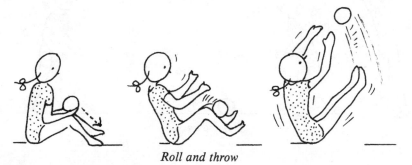

Roll and throw

Bouncing the ball (different sizes of ball)

●   Hold the ball in both hands with fingers spread at the sides (hands take the shape of the ball);

●   press with the hands to make it bounce;

●   watch where the ball bounces and move to catch it.

1.   Bounce the ball
       (i) with both hands – catch after each bounce;
      (ii) at waist level continuously;
     (iii) as high as possible;
      (iv) as low as possible;
       (v) right hand only;
      (vi) left hand only
     (vii) alternate hands;
    (viii) as (vii) travelling;
      (ix) 3 times with right hand, 3 with left;
       (x) as (ix) travelling;
      (xi) to a partner (vary the distance apart);
     (xii) into a chalk circle to partner (vary the distance apart).
      When bouncing a ball and travelling, bounce the ball forward (ahead).
2.   Bounce the ball with either hand walking round a circle (5 m (16.5′) diameter) repeat running.
3.   Bounce the ball on the floor and catch it as it rebounds off a wall.
4.   Bounce the ball with a two-handed bounce to partner. Start the bounce high overhead. Start as 4, aiming to bounce ball in a circle (1 m diameter).

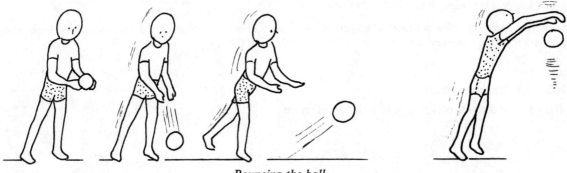

Bouncing the ball

Bounce Pass

   Stand with feet slightly apart —

- hold ball between waist and hip with both hands;
- spread fingers at each side of ball, thumbs behind ball;
- extend elbows and wrists and push ball to the floor to bounce about 1 m (3.25′) in front of team-mate or partner;
- follow through with hands, thumbs pushing the ball and elbows close to sides.

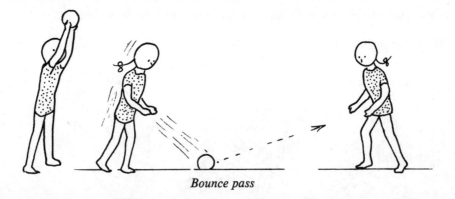

Bounce pass

Dribbling (as in Basket Ball)

   Stand with one foot slightly in front of the other; hold ball in hands (as in bounce pass), push forward and downward, bouncing the ball; keep ball close to the hand in a continuous bounce movement on the spot. The fingers controlling the direction of the bounce and the wrist supplying the force; move along a straight line dribbling the ball, keeping the body erect; move along in a crouched position guarding the ball with your body.

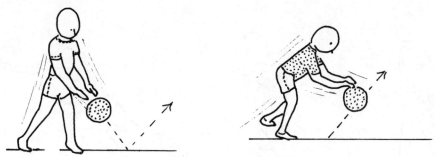

Dribbling the ball

Throwing

A good throw depends on a number of points such as the size and weight of the ball, the accuracy of the direction in which it is thrown, the distance and speed. The whole body weight must go into the throw. The right stance is important to enable the weight of the whole body to supplement the arm movement in a forceful throw. The underarm throw is valuable when only a short distance is to be covered.

Single underarm throw (right-handed) (small ball)

Step onto the left foot towards the target; swing the right arm backward transferring the weight onto the right foot; swing the right arm downward and forward towards the target transferring the weight to the left foot; follow through, stepping onto the right foot in line with the ball, and extending the wrist and elbow in the direction of the throw. Let each player find out which hand is easiest to use but practise with both.

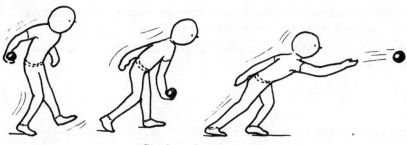

Single underarm throw

Overarm throw (right handed)

Hold the ball in the fingers; step onto the left foot with the left shoulder pointing towards the target; extend the right elbow backward behind the shoulder (away from the body) transferring the weight to the right foot; with the elbow leading, release the ball in front of the shoulder (transferring the weight from right to left foot during the throw; follow through with the whole body extending the arm, wrist and fingers and stepping onto the right foot in line with the ball.

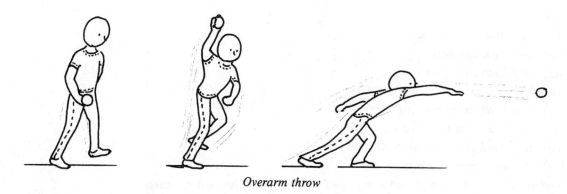

Overarm throw

Quoit throw (right handed)

Hold the quoit flat, thumb on top of the quoit; bend the wrist and elbow towards the body; step forward onto the right foot at the same time as the elbow and wrist are extended in the direction of the throw; the quoit should travel through the air 'flat'. Rubber quoits are smooth and easier to handle than rope quoits.

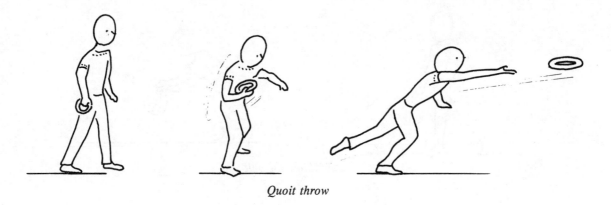

Quoit throw

Practices

Practise —

(i)   throwing and catching in twos, catching with both hands at first;

(ii) throwing quoits over an object – cricket stump, skittle – or stick held in the air.

Catching

Watch the ball carefully, note its rise and fall and move towards it; extend the arms and hands to meet the ball, spread the fingers in the direction of the ball; close the fingers round the ball and pull it towards the body as it is caught; the whole body, particularly the arms, must 'give' so that the ball is caught softly in the hands.

Catch with both hands at first, then with alternate hands. Beanbags are easier to catch particularly for older people. If they are made of bright colours they are often more easily seen than a ball.

The basic principles of throwing and catching are the same as for small balls. One advantage of a beanbag is that it drops rather than rolls away if it is not caught.

Practices

1.   Throw the beanbag up and catch it – increase the height;

2.   throw the beanbag up and clap once and catch it; repeat increasing the number of claps;

3.   throw the beanbag ahead, run and catch it.

A beanbag can be substituted for a ball in all activities except bouncing, batting and kicking.

Throwing, passing and catching practices

Examples – beanbags, beach balls, balloons or quoits can be used when appropriate. Use both underarm and overarm throws according to the players' ability.

Individual

1.   Standing: throw the ball up with:

   (i)   two hands and catch it;

   (ii)   right hand catch in two hands;

   (iii)   left hand, catch in two hands;

   (iv)   right hand, catch with right hand;

   (v)   left hand, catch with left hand;

   (vi)   right hand, catch with left hand;

   (vii)   left, hand, catch with right hand.

   Variation: (i) – (vii) against a wall with a bounce between the throw and the catch.

2.   Throw ball against a wall and catch before bouncing, with right, left, or both hands. As they improve, introduce a bounce back.

3.   Throw ball upward and forward and catch it on the run with right, left or both hands.

4.   Throw and catch over measured distances; A holds the ball, B stands at a stump or mark 3m (10′) away; 3 or 4 other stumps are placed in a line behind B at intervals of 1½-2m (5-7′). A throws overarm to B, B returns it to A, moves back to next stump and so on. The aim being to increase the length of throw and to return the ball accurately.

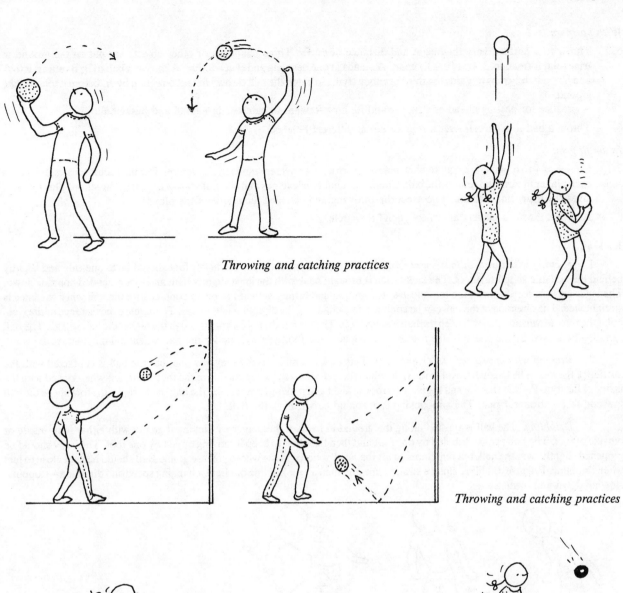

Throwing and catching practices

Throwing and catching practices

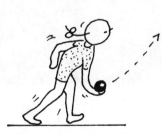

Throwing and catching practice moving

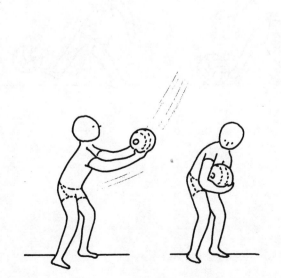

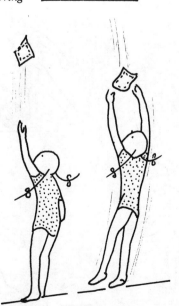

Catching

With partners

5.   Throw to a partner, vary the height and distance of throw. Three beanbags or other objects are put on the ground in triangular formation, 3-4m (10-13') apart. A stands at one beanbag and B at another. A throws a ball to B; B returns it to A and immediately runs towards the third beanbag trying to catch the ball thrown in that direction by A, before it touches the ground.
      A practice for passing ahead of a player and running forward to catch as in netball and basketball.

6.   Throw a ball to a partner over a rope or net at different heights.

In small groups

7.   Circles of 4 to 6 players, 1 ball to each player. Instructor or helper stands in the centre. The instructor throws the ball to each player in turn who returns the ball. Count the number of catches and accurate throws. Change direction. This practice gives the instructor a chance to correct the throwing and catching technique of the players.

8.   As 7 but throw to players anywhere round the circle.

Kicking

1.   *Kicking with inside of foot (right foot).* Place ball in front of the feet. The left foot should be to one side and slightly behind the ball as a supporting foot. The kicking leg is brought back with the knee slightly bent and toes extended pointing down. The leg is brought forward with the toes close to the ground and turned outward to make contact with the ball when the knee is straightened. The direction of the ball can be controlled by changing the direction of the toes. To increase the distance of the kick, point the toes downward, this will keep the ball low and fast. The further the leg follows through the higher the ball will go. The ball can also be kicked by the inside of the foot by making sure the foot gets well under the ball when making contact.

2.   *Kicking with outside of foot (right foot).* This kick is similar to the previous one, but the ball is contacted with the outside of the foot. The ball will travel to the right when flicked or kicked by the outside of the foot: to the left when kicked with the inside of the foot. Pointing the toe and keeping the foot straight and making contact with the ball on the top of the foot keeps the ball low and fast – strongest kick. The non-kicking foot should be ahead of the ball.

3.   *Dribbling.* The ball is pushed along the ground in front of the player by kicking it gently with either foot, inside or outside of foot. The ball can be dribbled by one foot and then the other to keep it moving or just by one foot. The body should be crouched slightly over the ball, but remember to lift the head at times to see where you are going. Ball should be kept close to feet when dribbling. Practise dribbling along a straight line and then a crooked line or circle, changing speed and direction – stopping, slowing down and turning.

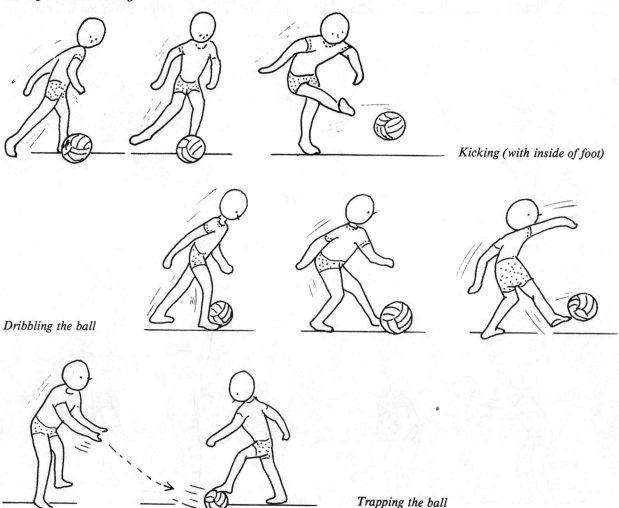

Kicking (with inside of foot)

Dribbling the ball

Trapping the ball

4. *Trapping with the sole of foot*
  (i)   throw the ball up slightly in the air to a partner;
  (ii) keep the eye on flight of ball;
  (iii) move forwards as the ball descends;
  (iv) lift the foot slightly to make contact with ball as it strikes the ground;
  (v)   the sole of foot traps the ball by placing it on top of the ball.

With outside of foot (right foot)
  (i)   throw the ball up into the air;
  (ii) keep the eye on the flight of ball at all times;
  (iii) move forwards and to the side as the ball descends;
  (iv) lift the right foot slightly off the ground;
  (v)   right foot is bent over at the ankle, knee moving outwards when making contact with the ball as it strikes the ground;
  (vi) body should be moving to the right in a slightly crouched position. Hands to be used for balance.

Other parts of the body

  (i) *Calf or thigh.* When the ball is descending or bouncing high the leg contacting the ball must remain limp and give with the ball so that it will drop immediately in front of the player. Pull the thigh back and inward, cushioning the momentum of the ball as it makes contact with the thigh.

  (ii) *Chest or stomach.* Balls coming at you quickly or slowly above waist height are usually trapped by the chest and sometimes the stomach. To cushion the ball, the body must move back with back arched, arms by sides or slightly in front bent position. This reduces the ball's momentum and, therefore, helps direct the ball to the ground near the feet of the player. Body should be wrapped well round the ball, arms and hands should not touch the ball.

5. *Heading*
    The ball should be contacted at all times with the front of the forehead at the hairline. The neck and spine are held rigid and feet should be off the ground although at the start this is not necessary. Eyes follow the flight of the ball until contact is made between the head and the ball. Greater distance can be obtained by using the neck muscles and driving the ball away. It is good practice to try and place the ball by heading it in different directions and also to get above it and head it down to a partner's feet.

Dribbling practices
1.   Dribble a ball with right foot and then left foot for a distance of 8m (26′ 3″) round an obstacle and back – walking.
2.   Dribble, on the trot, as above.
3.   Dribble, using both feet, continuous passing, round an obstacle at 8m (26′ 3″) distance and back.
4.   Dribble a ball out and in and around four skittles in a line each about 600mm (2′) apart without touching them with the ball. Inside and outside of foot to be used.

    It is difficult to dribble or control the ball while running. If possible, therefore, this should be done out-of-doors on a grass surface. The ball should never be passed so far ahead as to be out of control.

Kicking practices
1.   Kick a ball against a wall while standing and stopping it on the return.
2.   Kick a ball at an angle to a wall and run on to ball on return and stop it.
3.   Kick ball against a wall and move on to the return and kick it back against the wall. Use alternate feet.
4.   Kick ball to partner and receive it back.
5.   Kick ball between two skittles about 600mm (2′) apart.
6.   Kick ball inside circle or hoop on the wall.
7.   Kick the ball a distance of 10m (11yds).
8.   Kick the ball a distance of 15m (16.5yds) two times out of four.
9.   Distance is measured to the point where the ball stops rolling.
10.   Kick the ball continuously with either foot as it rebounds off a marked area on a wall. Try to do this ten times without stopping the ball.
11.   Practise kicking the ball from penalty spot on football pitch between the goalposts. Then introduce a partner to act as goalkeeper.

Heading practices
1.   Head ball back to partner using the forehead.
2.   Head ball with side of the head to partner.
3.   Head ball on forehead down to feet of partner.
4.   Head ball on forehead against a wall.

ACTIVITIES USING IMPROVISED EQUIPMENT

NOTE: The games described on pp. 26-34 are only a selection, many more can be devised by the teacher.

1. **Tyre stepping**

    Equipment: 10 car tyres 500mm (20″) apart.

    Rules: 1. Players step from tyre to tyre without stepping anywhere else other than within the tyres. 2. The course shall be from point A – B and back again to A as illustrated. 3. The player completing the course in the shortest time is the winner.

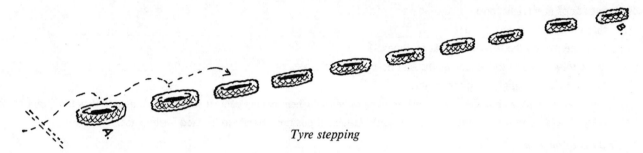

Tyre stepping

2. **Drums**

    Equipment: 5 car tyres 500mm (20″) apart.

    Game: Start line is 1.20m (4′) wide. Player rolls tyres and endeavours to knock down drum or drums. Each drum has a point score. If a drum is knocked it is immediately reset in position. Each competitor has five tyres and two attempts.

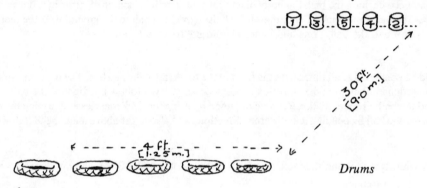

Drums

3. **Horse shoe throwing**

    Equipment: Five pieces of 25mm (1″) dowelling (broomstick handle), 300mm (12″) high and 500mm (20″) apart set into a base board 12mm (½″) thick. Five horse shoes 300mm (12″) high and 200mm (8″) wide made from hardboard.

    Game: The player tries to score as many points as possible by throwing shoes onto the peg or landing between lines (see diagram).

    Rules: 1. Each peg and square carry a score rating. 2. Each shoe must land within the designated playing area. Shoes outside are out of bounds (see diagram). 3. One foul throw, i.e. out of bounds, is allowed. 4. The player with the highest number of points is the winner. 5. If a shoe is more than halfway on the peg but not the full way, the full peg value is scored. 6. In the event of a draw a throw off will take place.

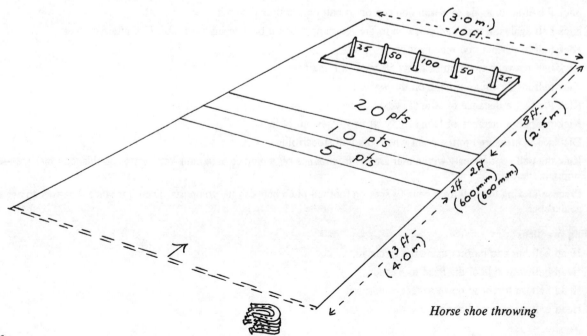

Horse shoe throwing

4. **Skittles variation**

Equipment: 10 painted coke tins (empty), circle marked on ground, medium sized plastic ball.

Game: Each tin has a given value of 1-10 points. The competitor endeavours to knock as many tins as possible from the circle.

Rules: 1. The tins are placed in a triangle shape – within the circle. 2. Only tins knocked completely outside the circle score. 3. The radius of the circle shall be 450mm (18″). 4. The throwing distance will be 350mm (12″). 5. Each competitor shall have three attempts at the full set of skittles each time, the total number of points being the final score. 6. The competitor with the greatest number of points is deemed the winner. 7. In the event of a tie. a throw off will take place until a winner is found.

FORMS OF TAG

1. **Tag**

Equipment and formation: A coloured band for each player, one, the catcher, wearing her band, the remainder holding theirs.

Game: The catcher tags a player who puts her band on and becomes a catcher. The game continues until everyone has been caught.

Variation: All players tuck their band loosely in the back of the skirt or shorts.

Game: Everyone tries to take the others' bands. The winner is the player who has taken the most bands.

2. **Release**

Equipment: None.

Formation: Free.

Game: One or more catchers. When caught a player bobs down. Continue until all are caught.

Variation: Other players can 'release' a 'caught' player by touching them. They then rejoin the game.

3. **Arches**

Formation: Players in pairs round the room. One couple hold hands forming an arch.

Directions: On a signal the players run under the arch and round the room. They try not to be caught under the arch when the whistle goes. Any couple caught under it stands by the first arch and makes another one. This continues until only one couple is left running under the arches. When the whistle goes any number of couples can be caught under the arches. The last couple to be caught are the winners.

4. **Chain Tag**

Formation: Players run freely in the play area. One catcher.

Game: The first player caught joins hands with the catcher and they chase the rest. When another player is tagged the catchers join hands to make a chain of three. When the next player is tagged the chain divides into two pairs and so on, until all the players are caught.

TEAM RACES

Presentation

1. The race should be simple.
2. Be sure there are the same number of players in each team; arrange for a player to run twice if the teams are uneven, rather than have one standing out. If some players are unable to take part, make use of them as scorers or markers.
3. Teams should never be longer than 6 players – long teams mean long waits and very little activity which defeats the purpose of the race; moreover, some players will lose interest and be a nuisance, spoiling the fun for the rest. Where helpers are available, the number of players in a team can be reduced (more teams).
4. The course should be clearly indicated and conditions must be fair for all.
5. Players must play to the rules e.g. (i) feet behind the line before being touched off (ii) finish as directed (iii) lines to be straight and the players in the right order.
6. In races in files make it clear on which side of their teams the players run – remember it is easier to run round an object such as a chair or skittle rather than round a ground marking.
7. Explain exactly how the race starts and finishes and the method of scoring. Check that the players *understand.*
8. Indicate teams either by names or colours, but in group games minor or major games, teams should be marked by coloured bibs or bands.
9. Demonstrate the pathway of the race and what specific skill is used, e.g. running to pick up an object. Let No. 1 in each team walk it through while you prompt, then No. 2 and so on until each player has had a practice turn. Repeat this if necessary, then let them 'have a go' increasing the speed as they improve. Announce the winner.

Scoring

1. The team as a unit scores at the end of the race.
2. The individual players may score on behalf of the team – e.g. score a point for the winner each time Nos. 1, 2, 3 or 4 has run. Each player needs to remember his number.

TEAM RACES USING VARIOUS FORMATIONS AND EQUIPMENT

Formations

For team races a variety of formations can be used, e.g. circles, files (one behind the other), files divided into two, triangular, ranks (side by side), one formation v. another (circle, line etc.), star, free formation.

Here are some simple team races using these formations.

Circles

'Shopping' Small circles.

Equipment: Four or less objects of any suitable kind for each team, e.g. a beanbag, a quoit, a ball, a coloured band.

Formation: Each team of 4-6 players sits in a circle formation. The objects are placed in the centre of the circle. Players are numbered.

Directions: The instructor calls out a number and an object, e.g. No. 2 – beanbag. No. 2 gets up, picks up the beanbag, runs round the outside of the circle, replaces the beanbag, returns to place and sits. The first player to be sitting receives a point and the team scoring the highest number of points is the winner.

Variations: 1. 4 different coloured beanbags replace the 4 objects. The call then is no. 3 and a colour. The player then picks the beanbag of that colour and runs. 2. 2 objects replace 4, each one represents a shop, e.g. grocer, greengrocer or butcher etc. The call is No. 1 plus some article purchased in either of the two shops. This can be built up to 3 shops. 3. 1 object representing a shop. The call is No. 4 plus a commodity which may or may not be purchased in that shop. If it is, the player picks the object up and runs as before. If not, the player sits still.

This game has many possibilities and can be used to help colour identification, shopping knowledge. Start with a small number of objects and build up.

Large Circles

Wandering Ball

Equipment: 1 beanbag or ball.

Formation: The players form a circle with one or more in the middle.

Directions: A beanbag is thrown from player to player while those in the centre try to intercept it. The beanbag should be thrown quickly and passes vary in height. When one of the middle players intercepts the beanbag he changes with the player who threw it. Other ball passing and bouncing games can be played in this formation, e.g. Circle Dodge Ball.

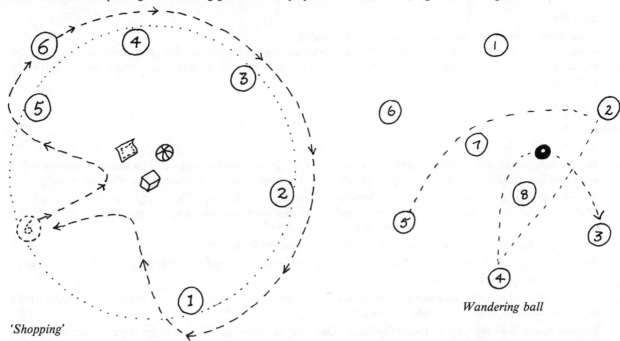

'Shopping'

Wandering ball

Files

Band Relay

Equipment: 1 coloured band for each player. 1 suitable chair for each team.

Formation: Each team of 4-6 players stands in a file behind a marked line. A chair is placed 8-10m (26-33') in front of each team.

Directions: 1. No. 1 runs to the chair and loops (ties) the band onto the chair (on most chairs there is a place where this can be done; it may have to be upside down). No. 1 runs back and touches off No. 2. Continue until all players have tied the band onto the chair and are back in place. The first team to be sitting in a straight line is the winner. 2. Repeat the running, but untying the band, the first team sitting with their bands on is the winner.

Variation: Complete 1. and 2. in one race.

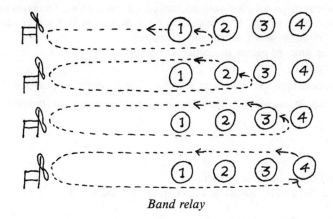

Band relay

Files divided into two

Roll and Run Relay

Equipment: One ball for each team.

Formation: Each team of 8-12 players is divided into two sections which face each other. No. 1 holds the ball.

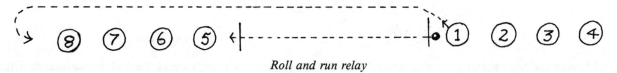

Roll and run relay

Team of 8

Directions: No. 1 rolls the ball to No. 2 and runs across to stand behind No. 8. No. 5 rolls the ball to No. 6 and runs across to stand behind No. 1. The game continues until all are back in their correct order but on the opposite side to which they started. The ball is thrown to No. 1 who holds it up.

N.B. If there is an odd player, Nos. 1-4 facing Nos. 5-7 at the finish, No. 1 will be in possession of the ball and no extra throw will be needed.

Variations: 1. throw the ball; 2. bounce the ball; 3. roll the ball through the legs of a chair placed between the two half files.

Free Formation

Pat and Bounce

Equipment: One tennis, or plastic or sponge ball for each player. A number of obstacles e.g. chairs, skittles.

Formation: Each team of any number of players stands in free formation and the obstacles are placed anywhere in the room.

Directions: Each player bounces the ball 5 times on the spot and then runs completely round 2 obstacles holding the ball in his hand. Repeat the bouncing and runs round two more obstacles, excluding the last obstacle used. Repeat the bouncing again and sit. The Instructor calls 'Stop!' at the end of a given time and each player who is sitting scores one point for the team. The team scoring the greatest number of points is the winner.

Variations: Vary the size of ball, the number of bounces and the number of obstacles to run round.

One Formation v. another

Circle Passing v. Team Running

Equipment: 1 large ball or beanbag, 1 chair or more chairs.

Formation: Two teams of 6-8 players. 1 team stands in a file behind a marked line, the other round a large marked circle.

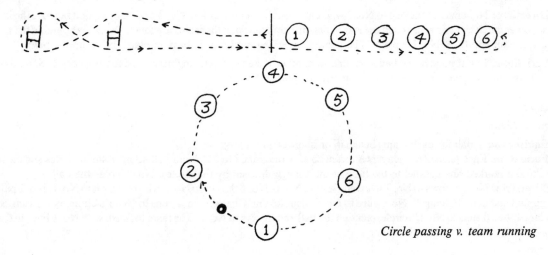

Circle passing v. team running

Directions: The team in the circle pass the ball anti-clockwise from one to another counting each pass, while the other team run a set course one after another, No. 1 running first. When No. 6 has completed the course he calls 'Stop!' The centre players stop and announce the number of passes made; if the ball is dropped:

1. the counting is continuous, dropped passes **not** being scored, or
2. counting must start at 1 again.

Teams change over and the game is repeated. The team with the highest number of passes is the winner.

Variations: 1. Vary the shape of the course. 2. Vary the direction of the running and throwing. 3. Bounce the ball instead of throwing.

Ranks

Quoit passing

Equipment: 1 quoit (beanbag or ball can be used).

Formation: Each team of 6-8 players stands in a rank (players stand side by side in a line).

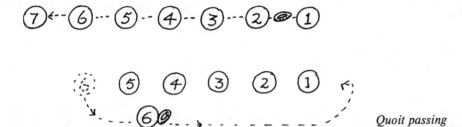

Quoit passing

Directions: No. 1 has the quoit. Pass the quoit from one to the other to the end of the rank. Each player must handle it, the end player runs up behind the rank to No. 1's place, all move down 1 place. Continue passing the object down the line until each player has had a turn, and they are all back in their original places. To finish, No. 1 runs up to the top and holds the object up. The first team to finish is the winner.

Variation: Pass the quoit behind the back.

Star or Wheel

Star Trek

Equipment: 1 ball for each team.

Formation: Each team of 4-8 players stands side by side in a rank forming 1 spoke of the star. No. 1 in each team is at the centre of the star.

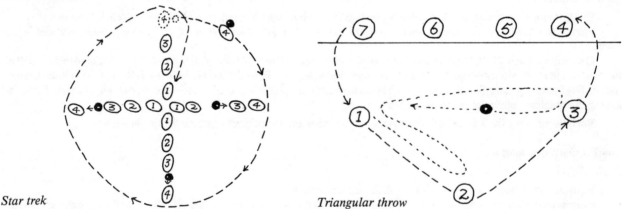

Star trek   *Triangular throw*

Directions: No. bounces the ball to No. 2 who catches it and bounces it to No. 3 and so on until it reaches the last player. The last player catches it and runs round the star in the direction in which the teams are facing, back to the end of the team, up in front of the team and takes No. 1's place. The game is repeated until No. 1, back in place, holds up the ball.

Variations: 1. Pat bounce the ball from one to another instead of catching between each bounce. 2. Spread out (more distance between players). Throw the ball from one to another.

Triangular

Triangular Throw

Equipment: 1 ball for each team (beanbag or quoit can be used).

Formation: Each team of 6-8 players is arranged as in diagram. Nos. 1, 2 and 3 standing in small circles and the rest of the team behind a marked line parallel to the base of the triangel formed by the circles. No. 1 holds the ball.

Directions: No. 1 throws to No. 2 who returns it to No. 1. No. 1 throws to No. 3 who returns it to No. 1. No. 1 puts the ball on the ground and calls "Change!" No. 1 runs to No. 2's circle. On 'Change' No. 2 runs to No. 3's circle. No. 3 runs behind the line by No. 4. No. 6 runs to No. 1's circle, picks up the ball and throws to No. 1. The team to finish with No. 1 back in the original position with the ball held up is the winner.

TEAM RACES WITH EQUIPMENT

Belisha Beacon

    No. in team: 4-6 players.

    Equipment: Cardboard tubes 300mm (1') long, some black, some white, 1 orange ball for each team.

    Formation: Teams stand behind the starting line, each player has a white or black tube alternately – the last player has the ball.

    Directions: The leader runs to a given mark and stands the tube on end. Each member of the team runs and builds the tube on the one before (alternate black and white). The last player puts the ball on top. The team with the Belisha Beacon built and standing is the winner.

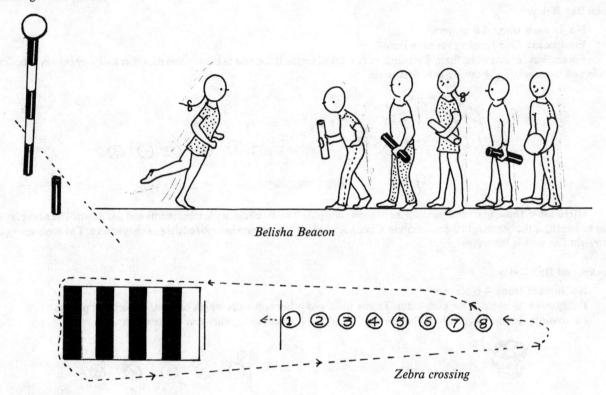

Belisha Beacon

Zebra crossing

Zebra Crossing

    Using black and white strips of hardboard a Zebra crossing can be built as in Belisha Beacon.

Building Bricks

    No. in team: 4-6 players.

    Equipment: Plastic building bricks which fit into each other 1 for each player.

    Formation: Teams line up behind the starting line. The leader runs and puts the brick on a given mark and returns to place. Each player runs in turn and builds on the previous bricks until the 'tower' is built. The team completing the tower first wins.

    Variations: 1. Build on a table. 2. Crawl under the table and then build, crawl back under table and run to touch off the next player. 3. Build on a chair placed on the table. Players may have to step on to another chair to reach the top. Make it a little more difficult each time.

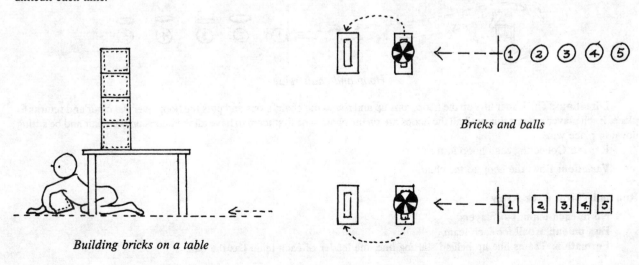

Bricks and balls

Building bricks on a table

Bricks and Balls

No in team: 4-6 players.

Equipment: 2 bricks and 1 ball for each team.

Formation: Put 2 bricks 10-15 m (33'-50') apart on the floor in front of each team. 1 ball 150 mm (6") diameter is placed on 1 brick.

Directions: Each member of the team runs in turn to move the ball from one brick to the other as directed.

Variations: 1. Move 2 balls between 3 bricks. 2. Increase the number of bricks. 3. Increase the number of balls. 4. Vary the way the balls are moved on the bricks.

Bean Bag Relay

No. in each team: 4-6 players.

Equipment: One beanbag for each team.

Formation: Teams sit on floor. Two circles are marked on the floor, one at the top and the other half way between the first circle and the team. The beanbag is in first circle.

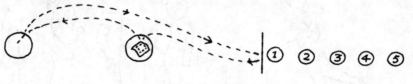

Bean bag relay

Directions: The leader runs, picks up the beanbag and puts it in the circle at the top, returns and sits down. The next player runs and changes the beanbag to the other circle. Continue until the whole team has moved the beanbag in turn. The team sitting in a straight line first is the winner.

Bucket and Ball Relay

No. in each team: 4-6 players.

Equipment: Buckets, 1 for each team. Tennis balls and other soft balls which bounce, **1 for each player.**

Formation: Teams stand behind the starting line with a bucket at the other end of the room.

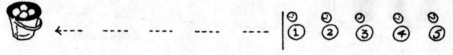

Bucket and ball relay

Directions: The leader bounces a tennis ball up to and into the bucket and returns to place. Each player repeats this in turn. The last player brings the bucket of tennis balls back to the front of the team. The first team to be in line with the bucket of balls in front is the winner.

Hoop and Chair Relay

No in each team: 4-6 players.

Equipment: 1 chair for each team. 1 hoop for each player.

Formation: Teams sit in a line. A chair is placed in front of each team some distance away. Each player has a hoop on the floor at the side.

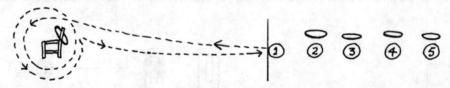

Hoop and chair relay

Directions: The leader lifts up the hoop, runs up and round the chair, stops and puts the hoop over the chair and returns to place. Each player repeats this until all the hoops are on the chair. The first team to have all the hoops on the chair and be sitting down in place wins.

Repeat: Collecting each hoop in turn.

Variation: Bowl the hoop to the chair.

Run and Throw Back Relay

No in each team: 4-6 players.

Equipment: 1 ball for each team.

Formation: Teams line up behind starting line, the leader of each team has the ball.

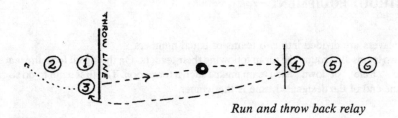

Run and throw back relay

Directions: The leader with the ball runs to a mark or line a short distance away, stops, turns and throws the ball to the next player who catches it and runs up to the line and throws to the next player – then stands behind the leader. Play continues until all the team are lined up behind the leader who has the ball. Each player must go to the **end** of the line **after** throwing. Repeat the relay until team is back in the original place.

Basket Ball Relay

No in each team: 4-6 players.
Equipment: Plastic footballs, 1 for each team, 1 set of uprights (4) for each team (skittles).
Formation: Teams stand in a line; uprights are set up in pairs – the course is 15-16m (approx. 50-55') long.

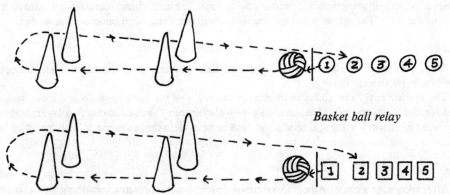

Basket ball relay

Directions: The leader bounces the ball (basket ball style) – passing between the uprights and runs back to give the ball to the next player. The team finishing first wins.

TEAM RACES WITHOUT EQUIPMENT

Circle Weave

No in team: 4-6 players.
Formation: Each team stands in a circle. Each team member is numbered.
Directions: The leader runs and weaves in and out through the team members to the right, the leader touches off No. 2 and stands in No. 2's place. No. 2 does the same and this is repeated by each player until the last player finishes in No. 1's place. The first team to finish and sit down in the circle wins.

Leap Frog Relay

No. in team: 4-6 players.
Formation: Teams stand in a file at least 'two arms' length apart. All players except the last in each team bend over in leap frog position (keep heads tucked in).
Directions: The last player leaps over the 'frogs' in the team to the front and takes up the leap frog position – the rest of the team repeat this from the back of the line. The first team to finish and sit down wins.

Numbers Relay

No. in team: 4-6 players.
Formation: Teams stand in a line – numbered.
Directions: The teacher calls a number. The player in each team with the number called runs up round a marker (chair) and back to his place. The first runner back in place scores 1 point for the team (see that all the numbers are called). The team scoring the greater number of points wins.

Variations: The action may take various forms, e.g. walking, skipping, hopping, crab walking, jumping with two feet together.

Trains

No. in team: 3-4 players.
Formation: Team stands in a line facing a marker (chair) 8-10m (26-33') from line.
Directions: The leader runs round the marker, back round the end oif the team and picks up the next player who holds hands (round waist), both run, pick up the next. The 'train to finish back in line without losing the 'trucks' wins.

GROUP GAMES WITHOUT EQUIPMENT

Quick Formation

Formation: The players are divided into two teams of equal numbers.

Directions: The two teams skip round the room following their leaders. On the signal from the teacher who may shout the words 'file', 'straight line', 'circle', 'sit down', each team makes such a formation. The first team to do so gains a point. The team gaining most points at the end of the designated time is the winner.

Simon Says

Formation: Free.

Directions: The teacher or a player chosen by the players to be leader stands in front of the rest. Commands are given such as 'jump', 'sit', 'turn round', 'clap hands', 'stamp feet'. If the command is preceded by 'Simon says', then the players must obey. If 'Simon says' is omitted the command must be ignored. If the player makes 3 mistakes he is either eliminated or takes the place of the leader. The winner is the last one out.

Grandmother's Steps

Formation: Free.

Directions: The teacher or 1 player chosen to be leader stands at one end of the play area – the rest at the other end, standing behind a line. The aim is to creep up to tag the leader without being seen. The leader turns round from time to time and anyone seen moving is sent back to the start. The player who tags the leader without being seen becomes the leader.

The Fish in the Sea

Formation: All players sit in a circle on the floor or chairs. Each player is given the name of a fish, kipper, haddock, cod, mackerel etc., several players to each fish.

Directions: The teacher says 'The cod is swimming in the sea' (all the cods jump up and move round the circle anti-clockwise). 'The sea is calm' – players walk. 'The sea is choppy' – players run. 'The sea is rough' – players leap and spring. At any stage the words can bring other fish into the sea, send some back or have all in the sea together. The condition of the sea can also change.

The Animal Farm

Formation: All players sit in a circle on the floor or chairs. Each player represents something found on a farm. The farmer, the farmer's wife, the children, the cockerel, hens, sheep, goats, cows, dogs, cats, horses, ponies, a plough, combined harvester, barn, etc.

Directions: The teacher tells a story about a farm bringing in all the words. The players, when their word is said, run round the outside of the circle and back to their place. Make the story as realistic as possible and have more than one sheep, goat, cow etc. . . . It may be necessary for some players to represent two words.

Variations: 1. Marketing — players represent different kinds of shops — grocer – baker – butcher – chemist etc. The teacher calls out a commodity and the 'shop' which sells it stands up and runs round. 2. Substitute the Zoo or Circus for the farm.

Noughts and Crosses

This is a very popular quiet game based on its namesake. With nine chairs in the centre of the hall thus:-

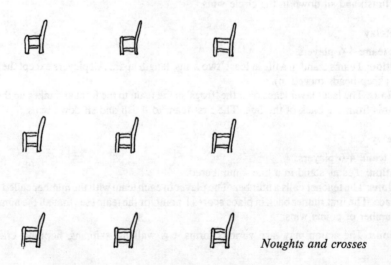

Noughts and crosses

Two teams stand on each side of the hall identified either by sex or a band. The teams in turn are asked a question suitable to the ability of the player on any subject, i.e. general knowledge, local knowledge, hygiene, sport, etc. If the correct answer is given the player sits on one of the nine chairs, if the answer is wrong the question is then given to the other team and so the game proceeds until one team or the other has completed a line of three as in the paper and pencil version.

EASY GAMES IN CIRCLE FORMATION

The following games can be used as practices in one circle or one circle and another. This depends on the number and skill of the players.

Circle Pass Ball

Equipment: Football or smaller ball.

Formation: Circle.

Directions: Pass ball round circle in various ways: 1. Clockwise – anti-clockwise. 2. Bounce round circle. 3. Throw and catch with one hand. 4. Throw high and low. 5. Throw to alternate players (miss one player).

Centre Pass Ball

Equipment: Football or smaller ball.

Formation: Circle. 1 player in centre.

Directions: The centre player passes the ball in various ways to each player who returns it in the same way: 1. Throw underarm – overarm. 2. Bounce. 3. High, low. 4. On the move.

Circle Gap

Equipment: Football or smaller ball.

Formation: Circle. 1 player in the centre.

Directions: The centre player passes the ball to No. 1 on the outside of the circle. No. 1 returns it and runs to a new position between Nos. 2 and 3 where he again receives the ball from the player in the centre. He returns it and moves to a position between Nos. 3 and 4 and so on until he reaches his own place.

Wide Legs

Equipment: Football.

Formation: Circle(s). 1 player in the centre.

Directions: Players on the outside of the circle. Stand with legs apart. The player in the centre tries to roll the ball through the legs. The ball can be stopped with hands or arms.

Variation: No player in the centre – try to roll the ball through other players' legs.

Call Ball

Equipment: Football or smaller ball.

Formation: Circle with teacher or player in the centre.

Directions: Teacher or player in the centre throws the ball up in the air and simultaneously calls out the name of a player on the outside of the circle who runs in and tries to catch the ball before it touches the ground.

FUN GAMES WITHOUT EQUIPMENT (competitive and non-competitive)

Stand Up

Start with pairs sitting on the ground, back to back, and arms linked. Stand up together (push against each other's back) next time add a friend and all three stand up together. See how many you can add . . .

Line Tug of War

Two teams line up facing each other on either side of a centre line; each member of the opposing team grasps the hand of the player opposite and tries to pull him over the line. The team which has the most players on its side of the line at the end is the winner.

Crusts and Crumbs

Two teams stand in files facing the teacher:

X	O
X	O
X	O
X	O
X	O
CRUSTS	CRUMBS

The teacher calls c-r-r-r-ust or c-r-r-r-umbs rolling the r's – when the crusts or crumbs are called, the players run to the wall. A player who fails to run or a player of the wrong team runs – they lose a point.

Knots

Form a circle with everyone facing inward, shoulder to shoulder. Everyone puts their hands out and grasps two other hands. Do not grasp the hands of a person next to you, or two hands of the same person. Now unravel yourselves, without letting go of any hands. (You may pivot on your handholds, but do not let go). Another version is to make one break before you start, especially if your group is younger.

Spirals

Form a circle, with everyone facing inward, holding hands. Ask one person to break his right hand hold, and start to walk around the person he just broke with, in a large circle, with everyone holding hands and following him. Thus, a spiral is formed, with people being wrapped around the person who stands still. When all persons are wrapped around, the innermost person, still holding hands with the others, ducks down and comes out through the group until the spiral is totally unravelled.

Slip and Through

Formation: 2 circles.

Directions: Each player faces a partner holding hands and forming two circles (inside and outside circles). All the couples slip step round the room. On a signal the players in the inside circle stand still, with their feet apart. Those on the outside run round the circle and through their partner's legs. They finish by sitting, cross-legged, behind their partners (who have now formed the outer circle).

MORE DIFFICULT GAMES

The Devil's in the Middle

Equipment: 5 beanbags.

Formation: Place the 5 beanbags equidistant across the playing area. Two teams – numbered. Try to ensure that the players with the same number are of equal ability. Teams stand – as in diagram.

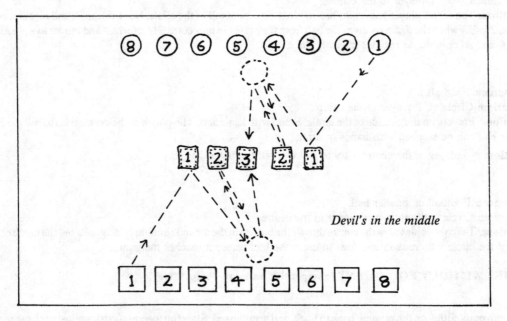

Devil's in the middle

Directions: On 'go' the first player in each team runs and picks up bag No. 1, runs back with it and puts it in a circle in front of his team. The same player repeats this with bag No. 2. He then runs for bag No. 3 but as this is the only remaining bag, the first player to pick this bag and put it in the circle wins a point for the team. To make the competition even keener, replace No. 3 bag with a wrapped sweet! Repeat until all players have had a turn.

Variation: Place circles in a different position.

Balloon Tennis

No. in team: Any number.

Equipment: A balloon or beach ball, a net or tape fixed at 'reach' height or slightly lower.

Formation: 2 teams, one on either side of the net.

Directions: Toss for 'Service'. The aim is to 'ground' the ball on the opponent's side of the net. The server bats the ball over the net with a flat hand. It is batted with one or two hands back and forward over the net until it is 'grounded' when one point is scored.

Serving: The server continues to serve from alternate sides at the back of the court until a point is lost; then the other side serves. Give everyone a chance to serve. Decide how many points make up a game, 7 – 11 – 15 – 21.

Practices: 1. Practise batting, throwing and catching a balloon or ball in pairs. 2. As 1. over a net at 'reach' height.

N.B. As the players improve the game can be played to Volley Ball rules.

Awkward Hockey

Equipment: 2 broom handles – 2 wood blocks approximately 100 x 50 x 25mm (4″ x 2″ x 1″).

Formation: Two teams are numbered. Wood blocks are placed in the centre of a drawn circle in front of each team. The broom handles are placed in the centre of the playing area.

Directions: The players whose numbers are called run to the centre, pick up the broom handle, run back to the wooden block and propel it across the floor to place it in the opposite circle. The first player to put the block in the circle wins a point.

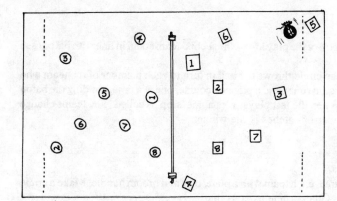

Balloon tennis

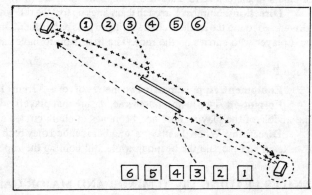

Awkward hockey

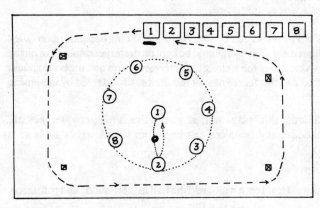

Count down

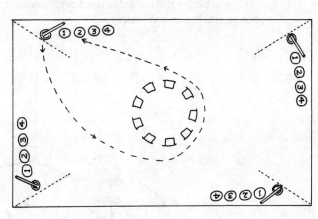

Grand prix

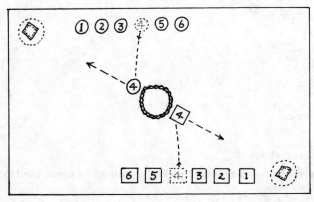

Rope pull

Count Down

Equipment: Frido Ball – baton.

Formation: Two teams. One team forms a circle in the centre of the play area – the second team stand in line with baton (see diagram).

Directions: On the word 'go' the player in the centre of the circle throws the ball in turn to each member of the team who returns it. Each catch is called and counted. The team with the baton run round a planned course, one at a time, handing the baton to the next in line (relay fashion) until the whole team has run. When the last player gets home 'stop' is called. The teams change places and proceed as before. The team with the highest number of catches is the winner.

Grand Prix

Equipment: 4 tin plates or old trays – 4 broom handles.

Formation: 4 equal teams based in 4 corners of the play area, each team with a plate/tray and broom handle. Make a circle of chairs in the centre to mark the track, seats turned inward. Chalk a line as start line.

Directions: Number 1 in each team lines up for 'the off' with tray/plate on floor with broom handles in 'dished' side. On 'go' 'drivers' go round the circle of chairs trying to pass each other. On reaching team pit, the driver hands over the broom handle to the next player who carries on the race. The first team to have raced all team members, wins.

Rope Pull

Equipment: Approximately two metres of rope, 37 mm (1½") diameter, ends tied together to form circle. Two beanbags.

Formation: Two teams, numbered, ensure that players with the same number are of equal strength. Put rope in a circle in the middle of the playing area and beanbags in chalk circles diagonally opposite to each other.

Directions: When the players' number is called they both run, take hold of the rope and try to pull each other back to their own team and pick up the beanbag while still holding the rope. The team with the most successes wins.

SKILLS LEADING UP TO MINOR AND MAJOR GAMES

Aiming Practices

Aiming at targets of various kinds and with different types of apparatus can be fun. Accurate aiming depends upon quick observation, controlled action, good footwork and co-ordinated movement. The eye should be kept on the target rather than on the object being kicked, thrown, rolled, hit or pitched, while the follow-through of the kicking leg or throwing arm and the body should also be directed towards the target. Progress can be easily measured and the degree of skill required easily adapted by increasing the distance and decreasing the size of the target.

Many indoor games involve aiming, e.g. darts, quoits, billiards, skittles, as well as games like bowls, croquet, netball, basketball, football, cricket and ten pin bowling. With imagination many practices can be set up which are valuable as a preparation for these games and sports.

The following are some examples.

1. Roll, throw or pitch a ball towards a small circle drawn at ground level on a wall, field the ball as it rebounds and roll, throw or pitch again. Increase distance.

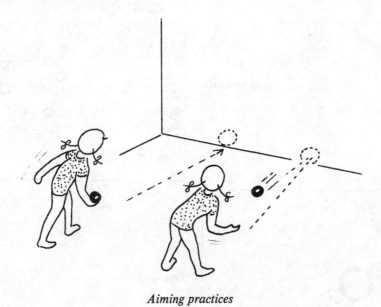

Aiming practices

2. Pitch a ball at a skittle a metre in front of the wall, field as it rebounds.

3. Throw a ball at a target of several concentric circles painted on a wall — the highest to lowest score from the centre point to the outer circle.

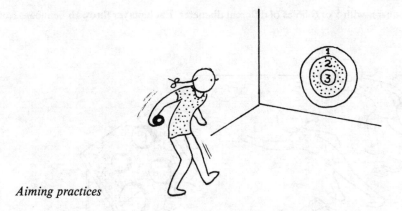

Aiming practices

4.   Draw circles on the floor and throw or slide beanbags or quoits or shuttlecocks onto them. Score as for 3.

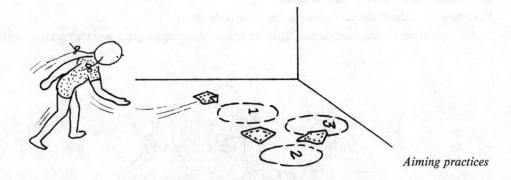

Aiming practices

5.   Hang a piece of wood with hooks on it on the wall and throw quoits onto them. Each hook has a different score

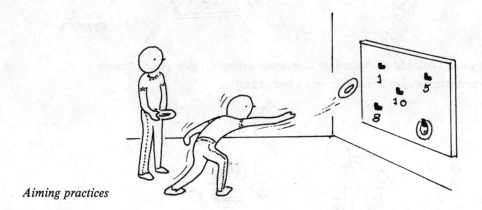

Aiming practices

6.   As 3 on the floor at an angle.

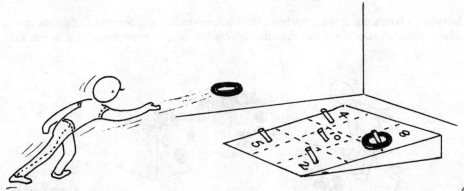

Aiming practices

7. Strong pice of wood 1 metre square, with 5 or 6 holes of different diameter. Each player throws 6 beanbags from a given distance.

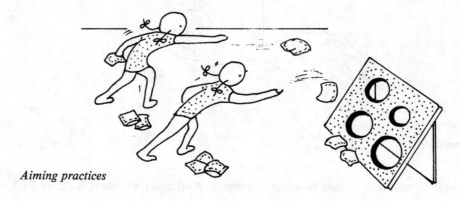

Aiming practices

Score according to difficulty (size of hole).

Variation: use balls of different sizes e.g. tennis or table tennis.

8. Throw a quoit over a stump from various distances; start by dropping the quoit over the top and gradually moving back step by step.

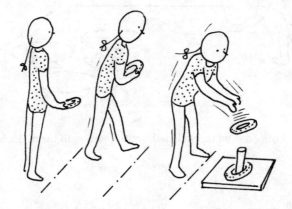

Aiming practices

Targets of different colours could be introduced (a) to increase difficulty; (b) in place of number.

9. Throw balls of the same size or of different sizes into a box or basket.

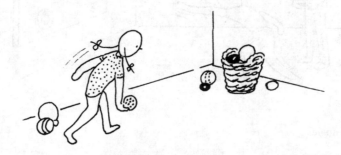

Aiming practices

10. As 9 but paint faces on the boxes, e.g. clowns, cowboys, Red Indians, ducks, cats, dogs etc. Cut out the mouth and/or eyes (make the holes large enough for the size of ball to go through easily). Aim to throw through the mouth and/or eye holes.

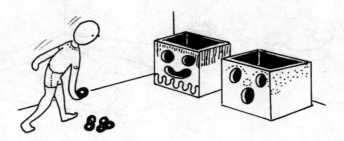

Aiming practices

11. Throw a ball through a hoop fixed at various heights with a partner.

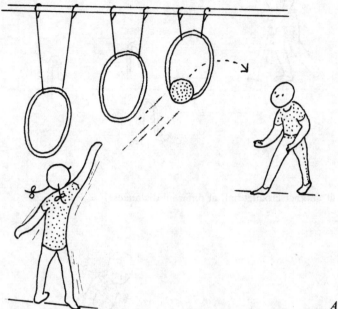

Aiming practices

12. Throw a ball into a basketball or netball net (shooting action), from different distances within the shooting area. It is an advantage if the net can be lowered on the post in the early stages of practice.

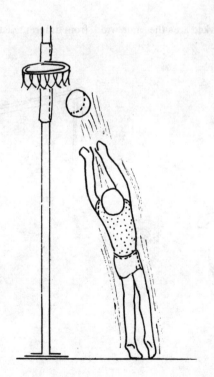

Aiming practices

13. Throw or roll a large ball to hit a skittle from 2m (6'): gradually increase the distance and decrease the size of the ball.

14. Throw or roll a ball between two skittles at different distances — gradually increase the throwing distance and decrease the distance betweeen the two skittles.

15. Hit a croquet ball with a mallet through a hoop at different distances.

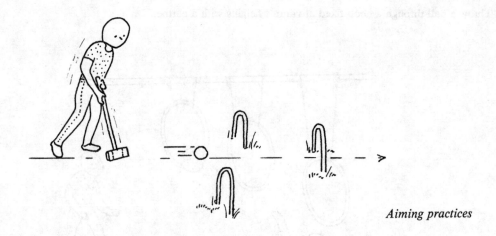

Aiming practices

16. Hit a croquet ball to hit another croquet ball at different distances.

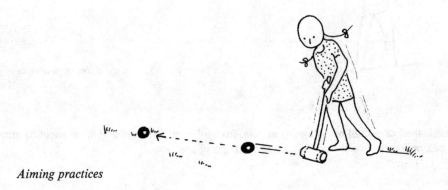

Aiming practices

17. Kick a ball through goal posts or marked area the same width from different distances and angles within the football goal area.

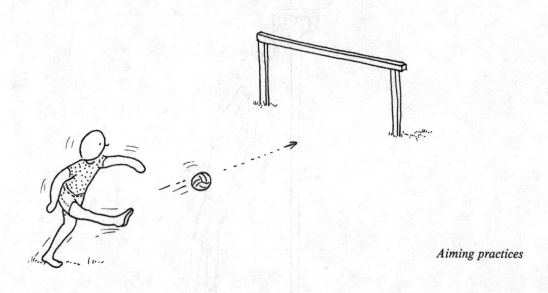

Aiming practices

In pairs

18. A and B face each other with a small chalk circle drawn between them. A pitches ball to B aiming to make it bounce in the circle. B repeats. When 2 or 4 consecutive balls have bounced in the circle, both players move 1 pace backwards. The couple which has successfully pitched at the greatest distance from one another at the finish of the practice is the winner or score 1 point each time the ball bounces in the circle.

19. A and B face each other some distance apart, each behind a line, with a skittle between them. A rolls or pitches the ball at the skittle; B fields it and repeats. The couple gaining the greatest number of hits is the winner.

In small groups

20. 4-6 players stand outside a large marked circle. A skittle is placed in the middle of the circle. A ball is thrown across the circle from player to player; on the signal, the player with the ball aims at the skittle. The game continues without a break. The team scoring the highest number of hits is the winner. Alternatively, the throw at the skittle may be made after each 2 or 3 consecutive passes.

21. One basketball or netball ring and 1 football for 4 players. From a given mark or on the run each player shoots in turn, while the other 3 stand round the post ready to jump for the ball if the shot is unsuccessful. Players score 2 points for each goal they shoot and 1 each time they succeed in holding the ball after having jumped for it.

22. Each team of 4-8 players stand in a circle round a box or basket. 3 chalk circles of incrasing diameter are marked round the basket at an appropriate distance from it. Each player has 3 beanbags or other small objects. Working at the same time, each player aims to throw the beanbags into the box, one from each circle. If the beanbag misses, it must be collected and thrown again from outside the circle until successful. The team first having all the objects in their basket is the winner.

Footwork Practices

Practically every game involves some movement of the feet — hence the importance of footwork. When waiting to move whether to catch, field, bat or run a course the player should be alert, ready to move in any direction, e.g. the sprinter, tennis player or footballer. The feet should be mobile and strong.

For mobilising and strengthening the feet and ankles, with bare feet.

1. Small lilting movements both feet together and toes on the ground, gradually increasing to high springs with a rebound. The strong extension in the ankle joint should alternate with relaxation, heels being lowered as far as possible between each rebound. (For other footwork exercises see Chapter 10).

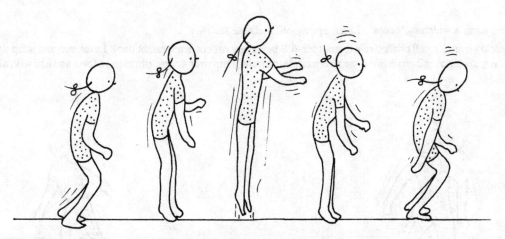

Footwork practices – training spring

For training quick response

1. Spring forward with long strides aiming to cover the ground with as few strides as possible.

2. Run forward on signal, turn and run in the opposite direction or sideways as directed.

3. Run forward on signal, jump and land on both feet or one foot followed by the other.

For training spring

1. On the run, spring over marked spaces each wider than the last.

2. On the run, jump to touch 3 hanging articles each suspended at a greater height than the last.

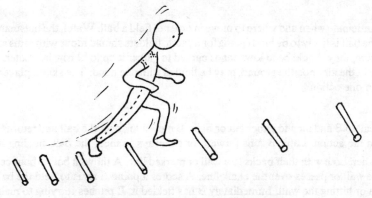

Footwork practices – training spring

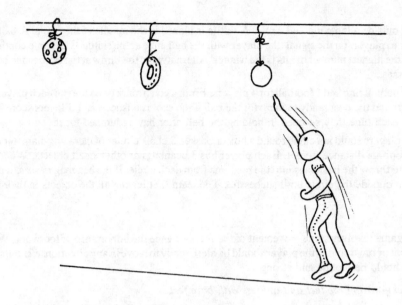

Footwork practices – training spring

3. Run and jump a widening 'brook'. Later, spring off alternate feet.
4. Step quickly from 1 small chalk circle to another, 6-8 being drawn (not in a straight line). Later, run and jump a set obstacle course, e.g. spring over 2 chalk lines, step from circle to circle, jump over a rope, run along a form and end with a high spring.

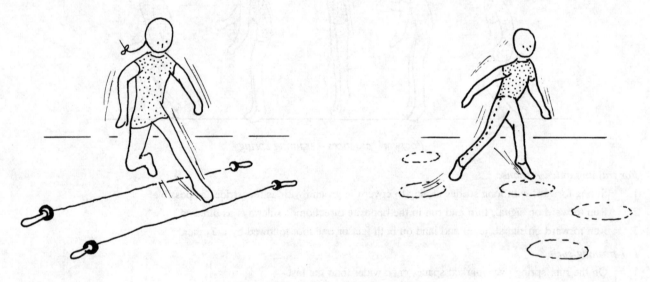

Footwork practices – training spring

Fielding Practices

A good fielder must anticipate when and where to move in order to field a ball. Watch the batsman's movements which will indicate in what direction the ball is likely to be hit. If going for a catch, fielders should move with arms stretched towards the ball; if going for a low ground drive, they should bend low, hands curved to gather it up to 'throw in'. Later, when more experienced, wide balls, whether they be in the air or on the ground, may be fielded with one hand. The skilful player will learn to gather in or catch and return the ball in one action.

In pairs

1. A pitches or rolls a ball to B and then to either left or right. B moves to cover the ball and returns it with an accurate throw without any break in the action. Later B runs forward or sideways to meet the ball, fielding it on the run.
2. Partners face each other, both with their backs to a wall or marked line. A thows a ball to bounce between them: if the ball passes B and hits the wall or passes over the chalk line, A scores a point. B aims to field the ball so as to prevent it from passing over the line or hitting the wall. Immediately B has fielded it, B pitches it trying to make it pass A. Each player counts his own score.

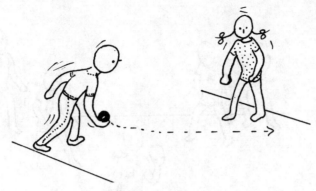

Fielding practices

In small groups

3. 4-10 players round a garden roller or other curved surface. One pitches the ball onto the roller; as it will rebound in any direction, all players must be ready and 'on their toes' to receive it. The one who has caught it then pitches it.

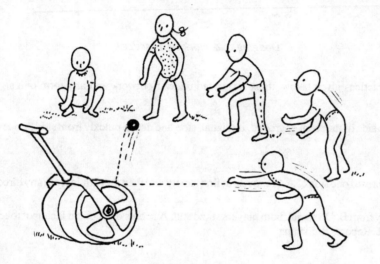

Fielding practices

4. **Pitch and Roll Relay**

Each team of 6-8 players divides into 2 files which stand facing each other, some distance apart. No. 1 holds a small ball, No. 1 pitches or throws the ball to No. 2 and then runs forward to stand behind No. 8. No. 2 keeping the feet behind the line, fields the ball, rolls it to No. 3 and runs forward to stand behind No. 7. The game continues until all are back in their original places. The ball is always pitched or thrown from one side and rolled from the other. The team to finish first is the winner.

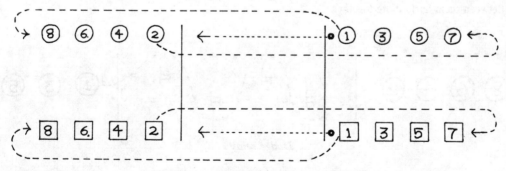

Fielding practices – pitch and roll relay

Dodging and Marking Practices

Dodging and marking are difficult techniques both to teach and to master, nevertheless attempts should be made to teach them since they are important skills for many games. Good footwork makes quick adjustment of balance possible while concentration and observation enable the player to observe the position of the ball and the whereabouts and actions of other players. Effective dodging and marking can be achieved if:

the marker is kept close to the opponent and anticipates every move;

the dodger makes every effort to outwit the marker.

Both are always ready to change from defence to attack.

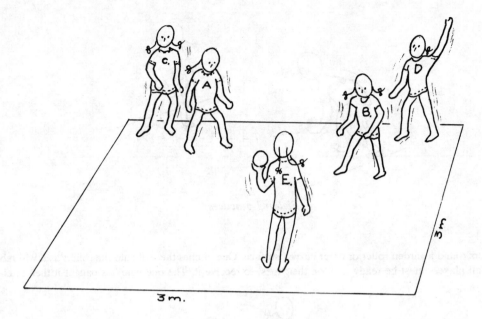

Dodging and marking practice

In addition to the practices given below, those suggested under Footwork and any form of Tag are useful.

For individuals

1. Run fast from side to side of the room or ground, on signal, stop and dodge quickly from side to side once and then continue running.

In pairs

2. B in front of and slightly to one side of A. A moves, at first slowly and then more quickly in any direction and B tries to keep close to A.

3. A dodges to get away from B. On signal, both players stand still. A scores one point if B cannot touch A. B scores one point if A can be touched. Repeat, B dodging.

In small groups

4. 3-6 players facing the teacher. The teacher dodges in any direction — the group shadow him.

5. 5 players in a space 3 x 3 metres (10 x 10′). A and B mark C and D respectively and E is the 'odd' one. E tries to tag. C or D and A and B mark closely to prevent this. When a dodger is tagged, he becomes the 'odd' one and dodgers and markers change places.

6. As (5) E holding ball. E tries to pass to C or D (no overhead passing allowed). When A or B intercept a pass, all change places and the practice continues.

7. **Dodge relay.** Each team of 4-8 players divides into 2 half files — odd numbers face even; 3 or 4 chairs are placed in the space between them fairly close together.

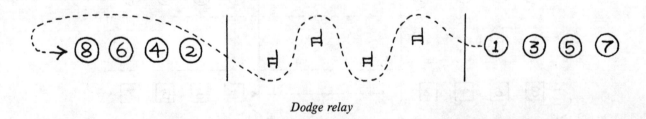

Dodge relay

No. 1 runs the course dodging the chairs, touches No. 2 and runs on to stand behind No. 8. Each player has two runs. When No. 2 is touched by No. 8 after the second turn, No. 2 holds up a hand. If any player touches a chair the whole course must be run again.

8. **Touch and hand over.** Two teams, red and blue, of 4-10 players in free formation — one football. Reds make as many passes as possible. Blues try to touch reds. If a Red, whilst holding a ball, is touched by a Blue, the Red hands over the ball to the Blue and the Blue team then passes. Running with the ball is allowed but players should pass the ball as quickly as possible, otherwise they run the risk of being touched. Team leaders count their score aloud and the team making the greater number of consecutive passes is the winner; if the ball is dropped, counting has to re-start at one.

The area of play must be adapted to the number of players. It should not be too large.

Interception Practices

When intercepting, i.e. preventing a moving object arriving to a player for whom it is intended, a fielder must anticipate the direction of its flight and accurately judge when to move, so as to outwit the opponent; try looking at the player with the ball or object you want to intercept.

In small groups

1. In threes — A and B standing in chalk circles 600 mm (2′) in diameter and 3-5 metres (10-16.5′) apart, and C at mid-point. A and B pass a ball or beanbag to each other — they may use any type of throw but must have one foot in the circle when receiving the ball. C tries to intercept: if successful, C changes places with the player who threw the ball.

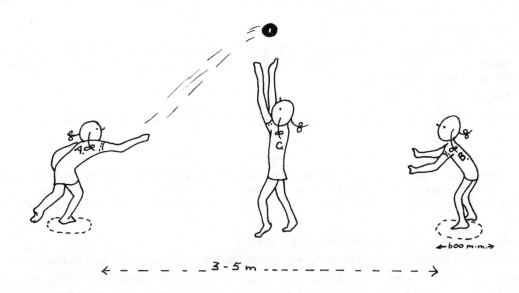

Interception practices

2. Four players stand some distance apart, A and B being partners, C and D being partners. A holding a quoit tries to throw it over a short stick held by B. C and D try to intercept the throw. If B catches the quoit, it is thrown back to A. When the quoit is intercepted the couples change over.

3. A and B stand 3-5 (10-16.5′) apart, C between them. A and B throw the object one to the other — C tries to intercept. If successful, change places as in (1).

4. As (3), but C stands back from A and B. C runs forward to intercept as the object is passed from A to B.

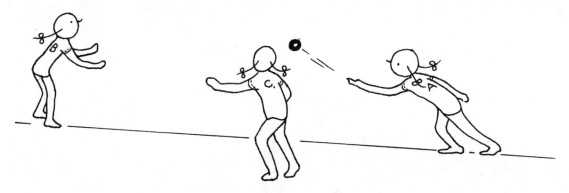

Interception practices

If successful, change places as in (1).

Hitting Practices (Bat, Racquet or Stick)

Keep the eye on the ball from the moment it has started on its flight towards the hitter until it is actually hit. Feet easily apart. Hit with the centre of the bat, racquet or stick. Keep the bat away from the body (no tucked in elbows). Stand sideways with left shoulder pointing in the direction in which the ball is to travel (right-handed hitter). Grip the hitting implement lightly at first but firmly as contact is made with the ball; the hitting implement should be regarded and felt as an extension of the arm. With a preparatory swing backward of the arm slightly bent, the weight is transferred onto the back foot, so that the weight of the body may be put into the hit, the arm and body following through in the direction in which the ball is to travel.

For training the ability to watch the ball onto the hand, bat or racquet or stick.

1. Pat bounce a small ball downward with stick or bat, left and right hands alternately: vary the height of the bounce.
2. As (1) pat ball upwards.
3. As (1) pat ball alternately upward and downward.
4. (1-3) on the move walking — running.
5. Bat ball against a wall, let it bounce and bat it back against wall.
6. As (5) without letting the ball bounce.
7. Pat bouncing between two players, at first allow ball to bounce twice and later one bounce — see which couple has the highest score of consecutive single bounces.
8. Hit ball to a partner across a net, rope or bench.
9. One ball and one bat or stick between three players: A fieldsman stands behind the hitter, the bowler 3 m away. The bowler bowls underarm — the batsman stops (not hits) the ball with the bat, stick or hand, the aim being to watch the ball right onto it. After 6 balls players change places.
10. As (9) but batsman hits the ball.

It is sometimes an advantage to hit a ball back and forward over a low net or against a wall with the hand before using an implement.

For training the adjustment of the stance so that the ball may be hit in any direction:

Stand sideways, left shoulder towards wall. Throw ball up with left hand and hit with right hand. Practise hitting the ball in different directions by altering the stance so that the left shoulder points towards the direction in which you want the ball to travel. Let ball bounce, on its rebound hit it again: progress to use a stick, bat or racquet. Aim to hit the ball accurately rather than strongly.

For training the specific batting action of the game to be played:

1. Practise the swing and follow through of the batting section with the appropriate implement — racquet, bat or stick.
2. In small groups of 4 or 5 — 1 bowler, 1 batsman, 1 fielder (backstop) behind the batsman and 2 or more deep fielders. The backstops of each group stand on the circumference of a circle — backs to the centre some distance away from each other.

Batting practice

The batsman varies the stance in order to place the hits in different directions.

SAFETY

During any hitting practice, consider the positioning of the players in relation to the flight of the ball. All practices must be carefully organised and controlled.

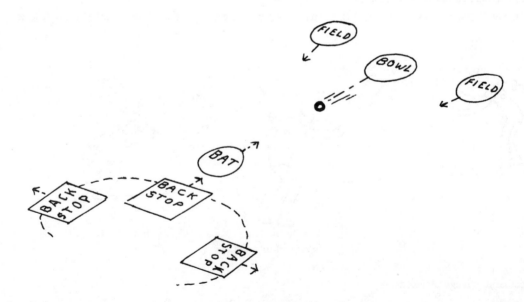

Organisation of batting practice

EXAMPLES OF MINOR GAMES

Non-Stop Cricket

Equipment: One rounders or stoolball bat, one ball (tennis, rounders or stoolball), one wicket approximately 305 mm (1') high and 229 mm (9") wide, and one base (chalk mark or object).

Formation: Two teams of 6-11 players. The base is marked or placed 3-5 m (10-15′) obliquely behind the wicket, and a bowling line is drawn 6-8 m (20-26′) in front of the wicket. The batsmen line up at the side of the playing area. No. 1 ready in front of the wicket; of the fielding team, the bowler stands towing the bowling line, the wicket-keeper stands behind the wicket, and the remainder position themselves over the pitch. See diagram.

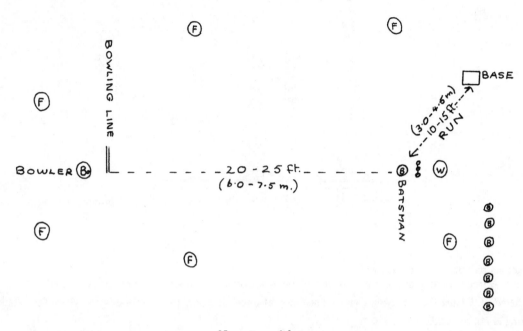

Non-stop cricket

Game: The bowler bowls the ball underarm, close to the ground. The batsman, guarding the wicket with the bat, hits at the ball; if the ball is not hit, the bowler re-bowls. When the ball is hit, the batsman turns and runs to touch the base behind the wicket and returns to the wicket, thus scoring one run. Meanwhile, the ball having been fielded is returned to the bowler who immediately bowls again, whether or not the batsman has got back to the wicket.

The batsman is 'out' by being:

1. bowled or caught;
2. playing on (knocks down the wicket);
3. obstructs a fielder;
4. hit on the leg by a bowled ball while defending the wicket — lbw.

When out the player immediately drops the bat and the No. 2 of the batting team takes over.

Whilst this change is being made, the bowler may continue to bowl at the wicket, if it is hit the new batsman is 'out'. The game continues until all players of the batting team are 'out', when the teams change over. The team making the most runs is the winner.

N.B. Leave out the lbw rule until it is understood.

Coaching points

1. The batsmen should place their hits between the fielders; backwards hits are allowed.
2. Fielders should return the ball quickly to the bowler, who should bowl immediately it is received.
3. To prevent the slowing up of the game, the following rule can be made: if a batsman fails to hit the third ball bowled the batsman is out and the next batsman runs in.

Change Hockey

Equipment: 2 Unihoc sticks, 1 air flow ball.

Formation: Two teams of 8-12 players. Two goal lines are drawn, one at each end of the playing area, and a goal 1.70 metres (6′) wide is marked by chairs/skittles in the middle of each. The players stand in twos behind their own goal line and the ball and the four sticks are placed in the centre of the pitch.

Game: The right hand couple of each team run out, pick up the sticks and try to hit the ball through their opponents' goal. When the umpire calls 'change' the playing couples drop their sticks and return to the left-hand end of their own teams, whilst the couples then standing at the right-hand ends, run to the pitch and continue the game, without waiting for a further signal. If, after the word 'change' has been called, the ball continues rolling of its own accord and passes between the goal posts before the new defending couple can prevent it, a goal is allowed. After a goal has been scored the game is re-started with the sticks and ball in the centre of the pitch. When all the players have had one (or two) turns, the teams change ends. The team scoring the most number of goals is the winner.

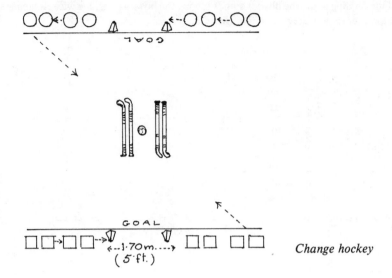

Change hockey

Rules:

1. Dangerous play must not be allowed.
   Penalty: A free shot at goal taken by one of the opposing couples from where the offence occurred.

2. On the word 'Change!' the playing couples must stop **at once,** dropping their sticks exactly where they stand.

3. Kicking is not allowed.
   Penalty: A free pass taken by one of the opposing couples, from where the offence occurred. This hit may not be taken at goal.

4. Players standing behind the base line must not interfere with play.

N.B. Too strict adherence to hockey rules will slow up the game and spoil its spirit.

Change Mat Ball

No. of players: 2 teams of 6-11 players.

Equipment: One football and two fibre mats: if mats are not available, 2 circles 1.20 m (4′) in diameter can be used.

Formation: The play area is a rectangle 21 x 12 m (70 x 40′) divided into two equal parts. A smaller area should be used for teams smaller in number, 18 x 9 m (60 x 30′). The mats (circles) are placed at each end. One player 'the catcher' stands on the mat (or in the circle). Teams play towards their own catcher. The other players position themselves as for hockey or football.

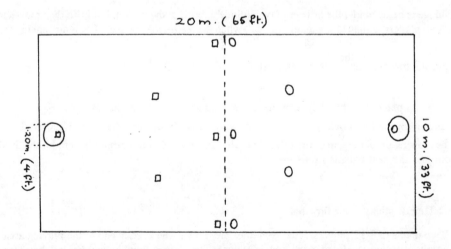

Change mat ball

Game: The ball is thrown vertically between the two centre players. Each team then passes the ball between their players until it can be thrown to their own catcher by means of a clear pass, i.e. the ball must not strike the floor in flight between the thrower and the catcher, thus scoring one point. Immediately the catcher receives the ball, he bounces it out into the field of play. Once it has touched the ground it is deemed to be in play, but it may not be touched by any player until it has bounced. The catcher, having thown the ball into the field of play, immediately changes places with the thrower and the game continues without a break.

Rules:

1. No player other than the catcher may step on to the mat (or into the circle).
   Penalty: For an offence by (i) an attacker, a free pass to the defending team, taken from the edge of the mat; (ii) a defender, a free pass taken by the catcher of the opposing team.

2. No player may run more than three steps whilst holding the ball, or hold it for longer than three seconds.
   Penalty: A free pass to the opposing team taken from where the foul occurred. This free pass may **not** be made direct to the catcher.

3. No rough play, e.g. barging or kicking is allowed.
   Penalty: A free pass to the opposing team from where the offence occurred. This pass may, if desired, be made direct to the catcher and a point scored from it.

Coaching points:

1. Players should mark their own opponents and should use the whole space available.

2. Encourage players to pass and run into a space.

Danish Rounders

Equipment: One rounders or tennis ball and a rounders stick or small bat (hand may be used in place of bat).

Formation: Two teams of 6-15 players. The playing area is a square (or rectangle) with sides of approximately 12-15m (40-50') (boundary lines need not be drawn), a base 1.80 x 1.80m (6 x 6') being marked at each corner: a bowling circle 1m (3.25') in diameter is drawn between first and fourth bases, and the batting line 1m (3.25') from the bowling circle is at right angles to the side line. The batsmen line up behind fourth base; the fielders position themselves in the square and in the deep field, the bowler standing on the side of the bowling circle further from the batting line.

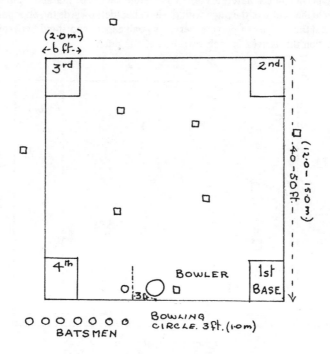

Danish rounders

Game: The bowler bowls by throwing the ball almost vertically upwards between himself and the batsman, to a height of approximately 1.80m (6'). No. 1 of the batting team, standing on the batting line, hits at the ball with his hand or closed fist and, whether or not he hits it, immediately runs to first base: he may continue running onto the other bases unless the bowler, holding the ball, touches the ground in the bowling circle and calls 'Stop!' If he is between two bases when 'stop!' is called, he is out. Batsman No. 2 takes his turn as soon as the bowler has the ball, and the game continues until all the batsmen are 'out'. The two teams then change over.

A batsman scores a rounder each time he gets to fourth base having hit the ball, and a half-rounder if he completes the course without having hit the ball. Any number of batsmen may be in the same base at one time; batsmen may also pass one another when running between the bases. The team scoring the greater number of rounders is the winner.

Rules:

1. If, from a hit, the ball is caught by a fielder, the batsman who made the hit and any other batsman running between the bases when the catch is made are 'out'.

2. All batsmen who are between the bases when the bowler shouts 'Stop' are 'out'.

3. The ball may not be hit behind the line forming fourth and first bases.
    Penalty: the batsman who made the hit is 'out'.

4. If there is no batsman waiting for his turn, the bowler throws the ball vertically upwards to a height not less than 1.80 m (6') to give one of the batsmen in the field of play a chance to get to fourth base before the ball falls to the ground: if no batsman succeeds the whole side is 'out'.

5. One ball only is bowled to a batsman unless a 'no ball' be given: a good ball is one which, if it fell to the ground, would land within the bowling circle.

Coaching points:

1. In a beginners' game, batsmen may be allowed to get to first base without being put 'out'.

2. The bowler should remain close to the bowling circle so that he is ready to receive the ball from the fielders. When players are quite new to the game, it is helpful if the teacher bowls, as he can then control the game.

3. The batsman must run outside the bowler on his way to first base.

4. Batsmen should be coached to place their hits, and fielders to make a quick return of the ball to the bowler.

Variation: The game can be adapted for use indoors. If the space is long and narrow, first and third bases only may be marked, chairs being placed where the other two bases would normally be; the runners must run round the chairs on their way to the bases, but may only stop at the bases proper. For this variation, two teams of 6 or 7 players make a good game.

Floor Handball

Equipment: One football and coloured bands (a lighter ball can be used).

Formation: Two teams of 6-10 players. The playing area is a rectangle, with a goal line 1 m (3.25') inside each of the end boundaries; the side walls may be used as side boundaries. If the playing space is very wide, or if there are not sufficient players to have more than one goalkeeper, goals of approximately 2.70 m (9') in width should be marked off in the centre of each goal line. One player from each team stands in the centre of the pitch with the left shoulder towards the opponents' goal; one, two or three, according to the size of the area and the number of players, serve as goalkeepers and stand between the goal line and the end boundary; and the remainder position themselves in their own half of the pitch.

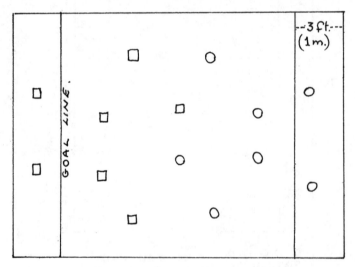

Floor handball

Game: The game is started by a 'bully off' between the two centre players, each using her right hand. The players of each team then aim to pass and dribble the ball towards their opponents' goal line. The ball must be kept on the floor; both hands may be used to stop it, but when hitting, players may use only one hand at a time. After a goal is scored i.e. when the ball passes over the goal line or between the goal posts, if marked, the game is re-started from the centre. After a given time, the two teams change ends. The team scoring the most goals is the winner.

Rules:

1. The ball may not be kicked, nor may it be propelled by any part of the body except one hand.

2. No player may pick up the ball or raise it off the ground when hitting.

3. Rough play is not permitted.
    Penalty: For an infrintement of any of the above rules, a free hit is taken by a player of the opposing team from where the offence occurred. This hit may not be made direct at goal.

4. No player, except the goalkeeper, may cross the goal line (the goalkeeper **is** allowed to move forward into the field of play).
    Penalty: For any offence by (i) a defender, a free shot at goal, taken by one of the attacking team, standing 3.65 m (12') from the goal line; (ii) an attacker, a free hit by one of the opposing goalkeepers, from where the offence occurred.

5.   No goal is allowed if the ball, when it passes over the line or between the posts, is off the ground.

Coaching points:

1.   Players in the field may move anywhere on the pitch and should be encouraged to combine.

2.   The goalkeeper may pick up the ball when it is behind his own line and place it at the point from which he wishes to hit it out into the field of play; it must be hit from between the end boundary and the goal line.

3.   When there is more than one goalkeeper, they should be encouraged to interchange and work together behind the goal line.

4.   The game is extremely energetic, especially when played in a small space and should not, therefore, be continued for too long a period.

Team Hand Tennis

   Equipment: One small ball and one rope or badminton net.

   Formation: 4-6 players. The maximum size of the court, which should be adapted to suit the play area available and the number and skill of the players, is 15 x 9 m (50 x 30'); the side and back lines may be marked with chalk, or the natural boundaries of the hall may be used. A small serving base is marked on each of the back lines and the rope or net is stretched across the centre of the court 1.20m-1.50m (4-5') from the ground. The players divide themselves equally between the two sides of the court.

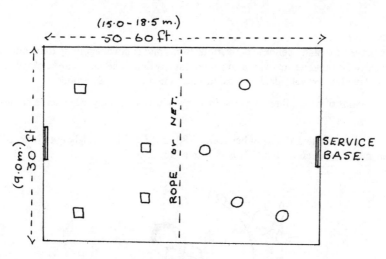

Team hand tennis

   Game: The server bounces the ball within the service base and then, with the palm of the hand, hits it over the net and into his opponents' court or, alternatively, to one of his partners who may be standing nearer to the net. After the first server has served 5 times consecutively, the service is taken by a player on the opposite side; when the first team regains the service, another player acts as server.

Rules:

1.   The ball is in play and may be returned over the net as long as it is still bouncing. It is 'dead' only when it has rolled along the ground or has been hit into or under the net.

2.   The ball may be batted with the palm of the hand, but must not be fisted or knocked. It is permissible to bat the ball up into the air to control it and then to allow another player who is better placed to bat it across the net.

3.   Only one service is allowed; if it is a faulty one, the server's opponents score one point if scoring method (ii) is being followed.

   Scoring: Two alternative methods:

1.   As in lawn tennis.

2.   The first team to reach a certain number of points, or the team making the higher score after five minutes' play on both sides of the net, is the winner.

GAMES WITH A DIFFERENCE

Batington

   General description of the game. Batington is a combination between the games of badminton and tennis, using a large table tennis or beach ball type of bat, and a badminton shuttlecock. It is played in an area similar to that of a badminton court by two or more players.

   Equipment: A bat approx. 305mm (12") long and circular in shape. A shuttlecock. A badminton net with two posts to support the net. A previously marked out course.

Game: The game can be played by the severely handicapped and the more able, consequently the rules of the game can be varied and the equipment can be made smaller or larger. The game can be played competitively or as a general fitness exercise. Two or any number can play as long as the size of the area allows enough space for the players to move safely and easily.

The game is started by the toss of a coin, the winner serves, if he misses he does not have a second try — opponents serve. If the shuttlecock falls out of the playing area or does not fall in the opponent's area, the service is lost.

In doubles, the same rules and scoring apply, apart from the service which is taken alternatively by the team. A game can consist of 11 or more points. Scoring as for table tennis is recommended in the early stages.

Coaching points:

1. Discuss the game with the trainees. Let them handle the equipment.

2. Introduce bat and shuttlecock and begin to practise. Develop co-ordination between bat and shuttlecock.

3. Introduce partner and then practise hitting over the net.

4. Gradually introduce the rules. Scoring.

It is a game for all trainees and is easy to learn. It helps to build up speed and can be played competitively or just as a fun game.

It can be played with simplified rules, inside or out, and can be played with two or any number of trainees depending on the size of the area.

The Game of Petanque

Petanque has been played for many centuries in various forms and is now beginning to be popular in Britain. The joy of petanque is that it can be played by anyone, anywhere and almost at any time. The game can be played by men, women, children, young and old. It can be played on gravel (ideal), grass, tarmac, smooth or rough ground.

No. of Players: Two teams of two or three players. In teams of two, each player has three boules; in teams of three, each player has two boules.

Equipment: Metal or plastic boules, diameter between 70-80mm (2¾-3¼"), weight not to exceed 800gm. The marker ball (cochonet) is wooden, diameter between 25mm (1") and 30mm (1⅕").

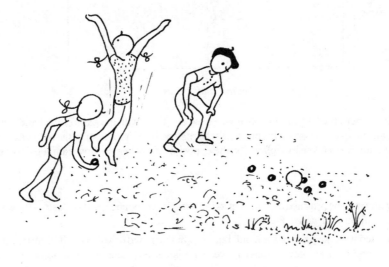

Petanque

Game: The starting team is decided by the toss of a coin.

1. The first thrower throws the cochonnet between 6m (20′) and 10m (33′) away, not nearer than 2m (6′) from any obstacle (wall, tree, etc.).

2. He then throws his first boule trying to place it as near as possible to the cochonnet.

3. A player in the other team then comes into the circle and tries to throw his boule nearer to the cochonnet, or knock away the leading boule. The boule nearest to the cochonnet leads.

4. It is then up to a player in the team not leading to throw until his team gets a leading boule, and so on . . .

5. When a team has no more boules the players of the other team throw theirs and try to place them as close as possible to the cochonnet.

6. When both teams have no more boules the points are counted. The winning team gets as many points as it has boules nearer to the cochonnet than the best of the losing team.

7. A player of the winning team throws the cochonnet from where it is, and the game starts again until one team reaches 13 points.

Unihoc

Among others, unihoc is a game which can be easily adapted to the mental and physical ability of mentally handicapped people.

Members of the Alton Adult Training Centre (among others) have played unihoc since 1977. The manager says: 'When asked to enumerate the pros and cons of unihoc, I have found it all advantages. At a cost of under £30.00 unihoc is the least expensive of the games introduced into the Centre'.

Alton found that most trainees could play unihoc successfully, but that teams must be carefully balanced. Space is not a limiting factor and the game can be played on any surface, indoors or outdoors. The sticks are not rigid and neither they, nor the ball, can hurt anyone struck accidentally.

Unihoc is not a formal game and therefore can be played 'instantly'. As it is easily set up and has immediate impact (it gets going quickly) less active and/or older staff members are just as able to organise and participate.

Presentation: Trainees who have played team games like football and netball can be talked through the rules and be taught to apply them as the game progresses. At the same time the teacher can explain how they should help the less able who may eventually be part of their team.

For the less able trainees at Alton, unihoc was broken down into its component parts:

1. hitting and stopping the ball;
2. passing the ball;
3. tackling;
4. scoring goals;
5. team and competitive play.

'This method of presentation has proved successful and there have been no injury or fear problems providing the less mobile are not indiscriminately mixed with the over active.

'Several methods of play have been devised: these range from six-a-side games in the dining hall with upturned tables used as barriers (with all non-players cheering behind them) through use of a larger space at the Sports Centre to twelve-a-side games on the sports field.

The Manager concludes: 'There are innumerable combinations and adaptations of size, abilities, speeds and settings. Such has been the spread of the game since Alton started playing, that we feel it is the most complete game available, especially in the field of physical education, for the mentally handicapped.'

Many other centres, hospitals and clubs are playing unihoc.

No. of players: Two teams of six players.

Equipment: 1 set of unihoc, twelve sticks. Air flow balls or standard size, or pucks

Formation: Any size play area from a small gymnasium to a hockey pitch, e.g. 40 x 20m, 60 x 30m. The game can be played on both smaller or larger areas by reducing or increasing the number of players. The goals should be placed 1.5m (5') from the walls allowing play to continue behind the goal as in ice hockey.

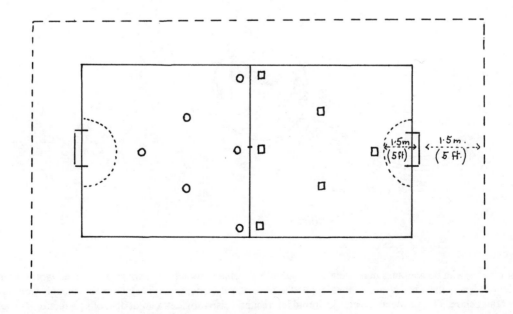

Unihoc – plan of court

Scoring: As in ice hockey or hockey each goal counts one. The team scoring the most goals is the winner.

Game: To start. Bully off or a 'centre stroke'. All players must be standing in their own half.

Bully off: The referee drops the ball between the stick heads of each team centre forward. Each player must endeavour to hit the ball into their opponents' half. Play then continues as normal.

Centre stroke: The centre forward passes the ball to a team member. Opponents should be 3m (10') from the centre spot.

Rules:
1. A player may pass and accept a pass irrespective of his own, his team mates and his opponents positions.
2. Stop or intercept the ball with any part of the body provided that the manoeuvre is to himself.
3. Shield the ball from opponents with the body and/or stick.
4. Play against the side or back walls as in ice hockey or 5-a-side football.
1. *A player may not* kick, trip, tackle, push or charge with any part of the body or stick.
2. Pass or move the ball in any way with anything other than the stick.
3. Raise the stick above the knee, nor use it to trip an opponent or throw it at either an opponent or the ball.
4. Kneel or lie on the floor in such a way that he prevents an opponent from passing or shooting.

When the rules are broken, the referee may award a free shot (or if possible play to the advantage rule).

Free shot: Where a free shot is awarded, the members of the opposing team must be 3m (10') away from the ball. When the rules are broken within a 3m (10') radius of the goal, a penalty should be awarded.

Penalty shot must be taken from a distance not less than 7m (23') from the goal. The goal must be unguarded. All players other than the player taking the penalty must be at least 2m (6½') behind the ball.

It is recommended that unihoc be played without a goalkeeper but for those who wish to play with one — the following rules are added:
1. The goal should be larger — a small size 5-a-side soccer goal.
2. The goalkeeper plays with a stick and is allowed to stop and catch the ball within the goal area using his stick or any part of his body.
3. The goalkeeper may throw the ball to the members of his team, but it must bounce at least once in his own half. Alternatively, the goalkeeper may not pass the ball out of the goal by any other means than using the Unihoc stick.
4. In the event of a penalty, the goalkeeper must remain on the line until the ball has been hit. The penalty is taken from a minimum distance of 4m (13') from the goal line.

Unihoc equipment can be purchased from: C. G. Davies & Son, The Sports People, 93 Far Gosford Street, Coventry CV1 5EA.

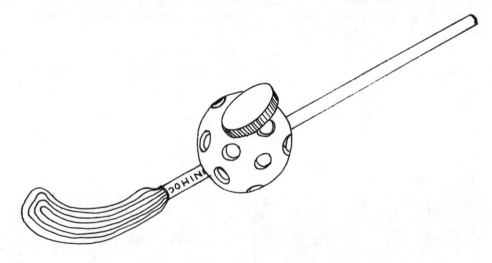

Unihoc stick, ball and puck

Boomerangs

Whilst playing with boomerangs may seem to be rather a novel activity it does have three main advantages when viewed from the point of view of the adult mentally handicapped person. Firstly, boomerangs can be made cheaply from plywood in a workshop or craft centre. This of course creates an initial interest and also provides a great deal of satisfaction — irrespective of the level of craftsmanship — when the varnished boomerang is ready to throw. Secondly, everyone learning to throw a boomerang will have to learn to judge distances, the amount of effort needed for the throw and learn the right 'feel' of the release. The third benefit is that throwing a boomerang will probably involve a considerable amount of additional physical activity in chasing and 'running away' from the curling boomerangs.

Throwing techniques: Throwing is best attempted in a large space like a park or field as boomerangs can get carried considerable distances by the wind. The thrower should be positioned so that he faces into the wind/breeze with the throwing direction at approximately 30°-45° to the right (for right handers). The best grip is the first-club grip, all fingers wrapped around one lower end of the boomerang. It can be launched with the hand forwards or backwards. Perhaps one of the best ways of launching the boomerang after the best throwing arm and grip has been sorted out is to tell the thrower to throw the boomerang straight at the top of a 1.80m (6') high stake placed in the gound about 20m (66') from the thrower. The result should be that the boomerang on nearing the upright post will turn sharply leftwards and upwards high in an arc before descending and turning and thus back towards the left side. All very theoretical of course! However, by trial and error the right angle of throw and effort can very soon be worked out.

Construction: The best way is to obtain a proto-type and copy it exactly — especially the angles on the surfaces so that the right aerodynamics will result. Also, M. J. Hanson's *The boomerang book* (see Further Reading p. 60) has excellent illustrations and ideas.

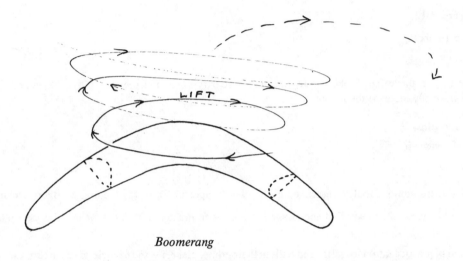

Boomerang

Frisbees

Once a new craze in the U.S.A. and now a feature of any English park scene, these colourful plastic 'saucer top' objects are particularly suitable for use in a physical education — recreation session with mentally handicapped people. They are cheap (approximately 40p), easy to store and do not break windows! Whilst they can be thrown very hard and over considerable distances their big asset is that they can also be launched with very little effort into a 10 metre (33') flight to a friend. On such occasions their relatively slow hovering speed makes them easy to monitor for the catching — fielding partner. For this reason many mentally handicapped pairs find it a very satisfying activity for a short period — twenty minutes or so.

After a degree of ability has been developed throwing a frisbee can be made into a game by:

(i)   trying to throw it so that your partner doesn't have to move to catch or touch it;

(ii)   trying to get it to land or skim through your partner's outstretched legs;

(iii) aiming at a wall target or hoop on the floor;

(iv)   or just going for distance.

Most of these games, boomeranges and frisbees can be played in a small sym or hall, but any institution or club could help those interested in the games to develop their skill by providing opportunities for them to be used in the break times throughout the day. In addition this interest could be fostered at home if a member of the family was prepared to take part in a fifteen minute activity session in the evening in the garden.

Coaching points:

1.   Hold the frisbee with the index finger along the outer edge, thumb on top, other fingers supporting underneath.

2.   Make sure the frisbee is level with the floor or ground before, and **as** it is thrown.

3.   Bend the arm and push (to start off with) the frisbee in the direction you want it to go.

4.   Follow through so your wrist and fingers point to where the frisbee is to go.

5.   Do not swing the arm too vigorously right across the body during the throwing action.

Frisbee golf

Equipment: Frisbees.

Formation: Design a course, according to space available. Map out the holes, including dog legs, hazards etc.

Directions: Using standard golf rules, each player tries to reach the hole in the least number of frisbee throws.

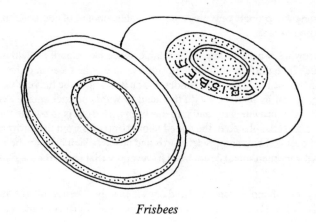

Frisbees

Circle frisbee

>**No of players:** 3-12.

>**Equipment:** Frisbees.

>**Formation:** Circle.

Directions: Players throw their frisbees to anyone in the circle trying to catch the other player 'off guard'. Start with one or two frisbees and gradually increase the number.

Skittles (Plastic ten pins)

>(See Special Events p. 86).

Snooker

>**A method of introducing snooker** (practised at the Newry Special Care Day Centre, Northern Ireland).

To introduce the game of snooker first encourage the players to practise with a few balls. Always use the white ball to pocket a red ball.

After a period of practice introduce all the red balls in their proper place, i.e. the triangle. Each in turn uses the white ball to pocket a red ball. If successful, red scores one point and another turn.
The player with the highest score is the winner.

If the players are capable of counting, the other balls can be introduced in their places with their score values printed on them with chalk of felt pen. The aim is to pocket a red ball which scores one point and the 'free' shot can be taken at a coloured ball with a higher score value. At the Newry Centre no points penalty was imposed for pocketing a white ball as this often resulted in a minus score. However, when the players become skilled at the game the full rules can be implemented.

TRAMPOLINING

The trampoline can be used in two quite different contexts.

1. For mentally handicapped people with minimal physical handicap where the aim is to develop a wide range of trampolining skills.

2. For the multiple handicapped where the aim is usually to provide stimulus and to create a feeling of movement where they are unable to initiate it themselves.

In the first case trampolining is being undertaken as a sport which means all normal safety precautions must be observed, e.g. four spotters in position, one on each side of the trampoline. In the second case the fact that there is a one to one relationship and the activity should always be taken under the supervision of an experienced member of staff ensures safety.

Trampolining as a sport — fundamental skills

1. Mounting and dismounting.
2. Feet bouncing.
3. Seat drop.
4. Knee drop.
5. Hand and knees bounce.
6. Front drop.
7. Back drop.
8. Swivel hips.

Teaching points

1. To kill the bounce (stop bouncing) land with the feet flat, slightly apart, and with knees bent.

2. The fingers should point forward in a seat drop since this bends the arms and prevents any possible jar to locked elbows.

3. Never arch the back in a knee drop.

4. The legs are carried backward in a front drop.

5. The hips are carried forward in a back drop.

6. In swivel hips the arms swing up and the legs swing under the body.

Safety precautions

1. Check the trampoline before use to see that it has been put up correctly and is safe.

2. Make sure there is sufficient headroom from floor to lowest overhanging obstacle.

3. Never jump from the trampoline direct to the ground.

4. See that the four spotters are in position and **never jump alone.**

5. Jump for a short period only — 45 seconds is enough. This ensures maximum control because fatigue is avoided. It is also more fun for those taking part because there is a quick rotation of turns.

6. Make sure that the trampoline is checked and serviced regularly by the manufacturers.

The use of trampettes

Under supervision, a trampette is a valuable piece of gymnastic apparatus. The landing area must be both spacious and resilient.

Elementary skills

1. Bouncing and making a controlled stop while remaining on the trampette.

2. Bouncing and jumping off with a soft landing. It is essential to train those being taught to hold their heads in an erect position at this stage.

3. Bouncing and jumping off making a specific leg movement pattern in flight, e.g. legs straight and together, legs astride.

4. Bouncing and jumping off facing in another direction.

These skills develop the enjoyment of flight. They all start **on** the trampette and therefore avoid the problem of the trampette shifting.

Longer sequences which might include a running start should only be considered when trainees are thoroughly proficient in the above skills.

GYMNASTICS

Simple gymnastic exercises are used in some hospitals and adult training centres. In Gogarburn Hospital, Edinburgh, and the Attleborough Adult Training Centre, Norfolk, residents and trainees take the Sunday Times British Amateur Gymnastic Association awards.

From Gogarburn Hospital 12 male adolescent residents attend the Heriot Watt University Sports Centre once each week for a class arranged by the Physical Education department. The programme includes floor agilities, vaulting using the buck and the horse, trampette and, finally, the favourite activity, 3 full-size trampolines.

These young men have taken the British Amateur Gymnastic Association 4th Grade Test and are preparing for the 3rd Test. At the Attleborough Adult Training Centre, Norfolk, some 25 trainees — 12 women, 13 men — are training for the awards. All have gained the 4th Test and are now working for the 3rd and 2nd grades.

The routine practice seen by the author while visiting the Centre was impressive — the enjoyment was obvious and the sense of achievement rewarding to the trainees and staff alike.

The British Amateur Gymnastic Association may be approached for help and advice. The Association make the following comments.

Standards of Performance

The Sunday Times/BAGA Awards Scheme may be adapted to enable mentally handicapped young adults to take part in the Scheme. The exercises in the Scheme may be modified to suit them and the standards of performance to be achieved may be at the discretion of the instructor, who should be aware of each individual's physical capabilities and limitations and readiness to perform the exercises in a satisfactory manner. Clearly it is neither practicable nor desirable to lay down hard and fast rules regarding such standards to be achieved.

Safety Precautions

It is stressed that, for safety reasons, every exercise must be carried out under strict supervision of a qualified teacher of physical education, coach or member of staff who must accept responsibility for the safety of each gymnast while catching, supporting or standing-in for each individual. No exercises should be practised or attempted without adequate supervision.

Modifications and special exercises

1. It would be quite acceptable, for example, to select any six exercises from the Charts 4 and 3 together in order to qualify for the Award 4 badge and subsequently, if taken to a higher standard at the Physical Education instructor's discretion, for Award 3.

2.   Similarly, if the instructor further considers that the individuals are able to take any six exercises to a higher standard of proficiency in accordance with their physical capabilities, he may consider that they have qualified for Award 2.

FURTHER READING   GAMES AND SPORTS

MINISTRY OF DEFENCE: ARMY SPORT CONTROL BOARD. *Small side team games and potted sports.* Ministry of Defence: Army Sport Control Board, Clayton Barracks, Aldershot.

DIAGRAM GROUP. *Enjoying racquet sports.* Paddington Press, London, 1978.

KNOW THE GAME SERIES. A series of seventy titles covering every major sport and pastime. E.P. Publishing Ltd., Wakefield. (Books printed in collaboration with governing bodies of sport which give rules and basic skills).

FRITH, J. R. and LOBLEY, R. *Playground games and skills.* A. & C. Black, London, 1971.

HANSON, M. J. *The boomerang book.* Kestrel Books, Penguin Books, Harmondsworth, 1974.

LENEL, R. M. *Games in the primary school.* University of London Press, 1969.

SPORTS COUNCIL. *The handbook of sport and recreation building design* (see sections on dimensions and specifications for sports and on swimming pools). Architectural Press and Sports Council, 1980. (A condensed version — data sheets — on dimensions is available from the Technical Unit for Sport, Sports Council).

WISE, W. *Games and sports.* Heinemann Educational, London, 1969.

NOTE: Coaching manuals, rules, wall charts and posters, films and videotapes of the major games and sports are available from the governing bodies of sport (see Appendix 3) and sports shops and large booksellers. The latter will order books not in stock.

CHAPTER SEVEN

Athletics

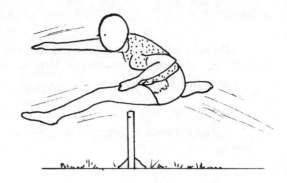

Considerations prior to training – Track events – Sprinting nd Staggered middle distance – Relays including baton changing – Field events – Throws (soft ball, medicine ball, small ball, beanbag) – Jumps – Standing long (broad) jump – Long jump – High jump – Safety

Athletics, both track and field events, are part of many hospital, adult training centre and gateway club programmes.

1. The emphasis in one type of programme can be geared to the more able who may in time work alongside athletes in the wider community.

2. An alternative programme may be geared to maximum participation regardless of ability, emphasising the value of social relationships and fun through shared activity.

In the first programme the rules and methods of training recommended by the National Governing Bodies of Athletics — the Amateur Athletic Association (AAA) and the Women's Amateur Athletic Association (WAAA) — should be observed. In the second programme there should be flexibility.

The following programme is predominantly based on the methods of training athletics for a sports day by the instructor at the Stonebridge Adult Training Centre in Brent, but takes into account the experience of other hospitals, adult training centres and clubs.

CONSIDERATIONS PRIOR TO TRAINING

1. Know the people you are working with:

    their: (i)   medical history

    (ii)   handicap (s)

    (iii) personal interest in particular events

    (iv)   initial standard of performance.

2. Regular fitness training is desirable. If this cannot be arranged, then it is important to gradually build up physical fitness as early as possible before the sports day itself. If possible, practise the events throughout the year.

3. Discuss each event, procedure and visit the sports centre.

4. Interest and incentives are very important and must be offered to the group to get the best out of them. This will help the instructor to discover which trainee is most suitable for individual events, and to work closely with the individual interest of the trainees.

5. Personal involvement is very important, always in a non-competitive way, by pacing, etc. If trainees see the instructor involved in the sport they themselves derive more satisfaction and consequently are encouraged to work harder.

6. Bearing in mind that a field day or athletics meeting usually takes place only once a year, the concept of athletics will take a longer period of time to develop. Older trainees who have known several sports days get more pleasure from the work involved and the waiting for the big event, in fact the waiting and this 'build up' have possibly been learnt and accepted as part of the event. This is not always true of the younger competitors whose acceptance of the sports may only last for a short time and what they have previously learnt can be forgotten on the day.

7. Develop a certain competitiveness among the group but make sure that this is done in a constructive way, i.e. only relating to one particular event. Like most athletes, trainees may often develop their own particular event and this becomes their special part of the day.

8. Correct dress and shoes should be worn both on and off the track and a track suit should be put on after and while waiting for an event.

TRACK EVENTS

Sprinting

1. In the early stages the use of blocks is not advised. If the handicapped person feels that it is difficult to learn to use blocks or if it is too involved he can be very awkward, delay the progress of others, or may be put off altogether. Introduce blocks at a later stage.

2. While practising, use a short run to restore energy, say 50 m.

3. Discuss the starting orders, keep as far as possible to the right sequence.

Take your marks — on this command the competitors walk forward to the starting line and take up the position behind the nearer edge. All should be motionless — then the starter will command 'SET'.

Set — competitors get into their final position and when all are still:

Go or gun — run.

4.   Discuss and practise keeping in lanes. Get the group to walk up the track within the lines if necessary.

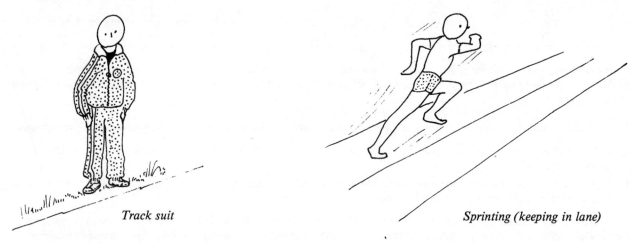

Track suit   *Sprinting (keeping in lane)*

5.   If there is time, use the pre-draw system — this can add to the excitement and avoid any argument as to lane advantage.

6.   During and after each run, go across and discuss with the trainees what took place —
        (i)   breathing
        (ii)   use of legs, arms, hands, head.

7.   Make contact with the respective Athletic Associations.

        In the first instance, run with the trainees to encourage them.

Staggered middle distance

        Always make sure that, on the day of the meeting, starting procedure has been agreed upon. Use 'Take your Marks – Set – Gun'.

        Take your marks. On this command the competitors will walk forward and assume their starting position behind the line and when all are still – Set – Gun or Go.

        False starts. Competitors must not move a foot or arm over the line.
At first allow three false starts per competitor.
Watch for dangerous jostling crossing lanes.

        The finish. The one who crosses the finishing line first is the winner.

        In training, discuss and show how to maintain a steady pace and restore energy for the final sprint. This concept is often difficult to convey to mentally handicapped people, who tend always to want to set one pace and try to maintain this for the full distance.

Relays including baton changing

        Baton changing is difficult to teach and will take much practice to perfect.

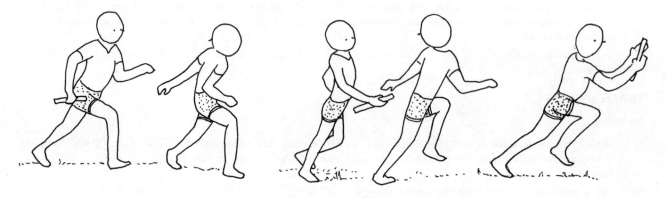

Baton changing

1. Discuss the race with the group. Explain it with the use of a blackboard and diagram.
2. Let them handle the baton.
3. Teach how to hold it, support the baton between the thumb and first two fingers and hold with the third and fourth.
4. Practice with two, then with the four, placing it in the hand of the person in front. The person in front will probably need to look at first, in order to get the feel of it being placed in the hand and to grasp it fully. Gradually speed and accuracy will improve.
5. Later take the group on to the track and explain the marking on the field. The start and finishing line, and the 20m (66') box.
6. Use a short run at first then gradually build up to a longer, faster run. Check times with a stop watch.

Rules. The first man holding the baton must not hold the baton or any part of it over the starting line.
Starting procedure will take the form of the middle distance races.
The baton must change hands within the 20m (66') area.
No pushing. No throwing of the baton.
If dropped, the runner who dropped it must pick it up.
After the change-over, the runners should remain within their own lanes.

There is no easy way of gaining this efficiency apart from repeated practice. If the stages are taught correctly and slowly enough, there will be a gradual build up of experience.

FIELD EVENTS

Throws

Throws can play a significant part in the physical development of the chest and should always be included in the programme — the non-ambulant can also take part. If the discus, javelin or shot are considered to be appropriate the rules, techniques and safety precautions recommended by the AAA and WAAA (see p. 183) should be followed. Coaches with experience in these events should be invited to assist.

For many mentally handicapped people, easier equipment requiring simpler rules will encourage a greater number of competitors to train and thereby improve their technique, e.g. soft ball, medicine ball, small ball, bean bag.

Training Techniques

1. Overarm throw (see Chapter 6).
2. Double handed overhead throw as in football or any other adaptation which assists participation.

    Rule: Both feet must be behind the throwing line throughout the throwing action.

    Scoring: Three attempts and record the furthest throw for each competitor.

Jumps

Jumps requiring a running start can give rise to difficulties of co-ordination and overstepping the starting line, therefore standing long (broad) jump is a good starting point.

Standing long (broad) jump

Training techniques

1. Place feet a little way apart with toes pointing forwards behind the take off line.
2. Bend and stretch knees several times with relaxed arm swinging forward and back.
3. Push off vigorously from the take off with strong arm swing forwards and upwards to provide lift.
4. Look forwards.
5. Land with feet parallel carrying body weight forward.

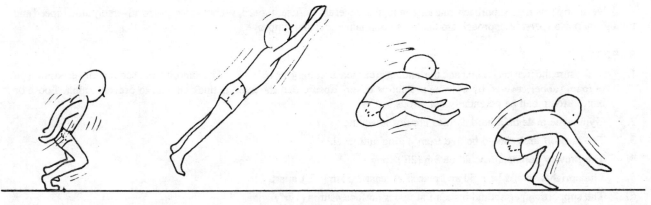

Standing long (broad) jump

Rules

1. Toes must be behind the take-off line.
2. A two-footed take off must be used.
3. Jumps are measured from the take-off line to the nearest contact point on the ground. Ideally this should be the heels but faulty techniques may mean it is the seat or hands.

   Scoring: Three attempts and record the furthest jump.

Long jump

Make sure that the take off board is stationary and in the correct position— placed at least 1 m (3¼′) from the nearest edge of the landing pit. The runway should be in good condition, the sand moistened and clean to allow for accurate measuring. A long run up is needed.

Training techniques

1. Begin the jump with a steady run building up to the maximum speed towards the latter part of the runway.
2. Practise the timing of the run so that the landing is correctly on the right foot on the take off board. This will only be achieved by constant practice and patient instruction.
3. Remind the jumpers to take a vigorous jump into the air and encourage them to be aware of the use of the arms for balance and extra distance.
4. Help the jumper to throw both legs forward for added distance before landing.

High jump

Experience has shown that very few mentally handicapped people have the ability to do this jump competitively. Where the ability is present then the rules and guidance of the AAA or WAAA should be followed.

Fun and confidence can be experienced by a less competitive approach to this event providing there is a good resilient landing area. In the early stages a rope may be preferred to a bar.

Training techniques

1. Establish confidence by letting each individual run jump and arrive in the landing area with or without a very low bar in position.
2. *Centre jump.* Indicate the starting point, continue as in (1) and jump taking off with one foot. Note which foot each individual uses for take off. Repeat several times to make sure the same take off foot is used consistently.
3. *Side jump.* Divide jumpers so that those who take off from the right foot go to the right side of the take off area and those who take off from the left foot go to the left side.
4. *Jump and twist.* Perform the same jumping movements as in a side jump — while in mid air twist or turn to land facing the original starting point.

   The twisting of the body after take off is the most difficult part to learn. The landing takes place almost naturally holding the head forward with the arms offering further support. Arms should always be in a supporting position for landing.

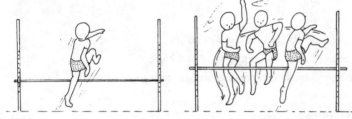

High jumps

Develop a seven step approach, one long enough to generate sufficient speed, yet not so long as to adversely affect speed and timing. Increase speed of approach gradually as confidence and skill improve.

SAFETY

1. Make sure the runway is clear and the landing area measures 5 x 4 m (16′ x 13′). The material most commonly used is a type of foam rubber covered by a strong protective cover. Ensure that the foam is thick enough to prevent injury. Loose or bagged foam can be potentially dangerous.
2. Gymnastic mats on a hard surface are **not** adequate.
3. The take off area should be free from pitting and level.
4. The runway approach should be 8m (26′) long.
5. The uprights should be rigid and placed at least 3.55m (12′) apart.
6. The supporting peg should have a flat upper surface 40mm (1¾″) wide.
7. The crossbars are usually triangular — 30mm (1″) diameter and approximately 4m (13′) long.

FURTHER READING

DIAGRAM GROUP. *Enjoying track and field sports.* Paddington Press, London, 1979.
KNOW THE GAME SERIES. *Athletics.* E.P. Publishing, Wakefield.
EDMUNDSON J. AND BURNUP, C. R. E. *Basic athletics,* (4th ed.). Bell & Hyman, London, 1979.

For booklets and wall charts on individual events apply to the Amateur Athletic Association and Women's Amateur Athletic Association (see Appendix 3).

Chapter Eight

Swimming

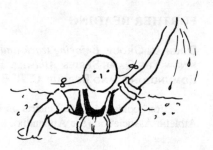

Introduction – ASA coach's method – The Halliwick method – General hints on the organisation of swimming sessions – Personal hygiene – Tips before going into the pool – Water confidence – Water games – Discipline and safety – Competition – Hints on the organisation of swimming galas – A swimming club for 'any swimmer' – the fromation of an ATC swimming club and the advantages of affiliation to the Amateur Swimming Association – Swimming at Craig Phadrig Hospital, Inverness – ASA awards scheme and certificates.

Swimming is very high on the list of popular activities available to mentally handicapped people. It offers everything — training in discipline, hygiene, stamina, perseverance. It develops courage and self reliance and is in fact a total social exercise.

The ability to swim and be water safe enables mentally handicapped people to enjoy water sports such as canoeing, sailing and angling where local facilities exist or at outdoor pursuits centres, holiday camps, field study centres and youth hostels which are often situated near sea or inland waters.

Practically all hospitals and training centres make every effort to provide an opportunity for some residents and trainees to swim. Rarely are facilities available on the spot, but good use is made of those in sports leisure centres, schools, universities and public and private pools.

Sadly, because of transport problems, high maintenance costs of hospital and private pools, shortage of staff qualified to teach swimming, and of helpers, only a relatively small percentage have the opportunity to swim regularly. Yet the general feeling is that it is one of, if not the most beneficial physical activity for mentally handicapped people and has perhaps the greatest spin-off — educationally and socially.

It is important that any coach in charge of swimming, whether a nurse teacher or instructor, should have **a recognised swimming teacher's life-saving qualification.** The minimum qualification is the Royal Life Saving Society Bronze Medallion.

Naturally many coaches evolve their own methods of teaching swimming in the light of experience. Two methods of teaching swimming to mentally handicapped people are included in this Chapter, one in which swimming aids are used, e.g. arm bands, rings and floats, and the other in which swimmers are taught on a one-to-one ratio of instructor to swimmer (the Halliwick Method).

ASA COACH'S METHOD

A swimming coach holding the Amateur Swimming Association's (ASA) Advanced Teachers' Certificate and the ASA Club Coaches' Award, who is the Senior Swimming Coach at the Gloucester Leisure Centre, uses this method. He was closely involved with the selection and coaching of the mentally handicapped team of swimmers who took part in the Special Olympics in New York in 1979.

In his experience mentally handicapped young children learn to swim much more quickly than the mentally handicapped adult.

A swimming lesson should be structured according to the needs of each individual. Ideally, it is a time when play is a way of learning; when people speak of work in a swimming lesson they should mean putting away the equipment after it is over!

The aim is to encourage the swimmer with many activities involving physical and mental effort.

Remember that people differ, both in their physical and mental capabilities; they therefore require the freedom to explore for themselves and to discover their own natural abilities.

Artificial aids enable the swimmer to feel the sensation of moving in water in a horizontal position as soon as possible. Early success will stimulate enthusiasm to come again.

Stages in teaching the mentally handicapped adult to swim

STAGE ONE

Aids Each individual is equipped with:

1. inflatable arm bands (the double or single chambered type can be used and should have safety valves);
2. inflatable rubber rings. Check that aids are sound and worn correctly.

Entry Down steps if available. For mentally handicapped people it is best to avoid traditional swivel entry because some have problems of balance.

Allow swimmers to discover:

1.   balance and orientation;
2.   Walking — heel, toe, fairly big steps, with the shoulders under water to avoid slipping — if the head and shoulders are out of the water they move faster than the hips because there is no water resistance.

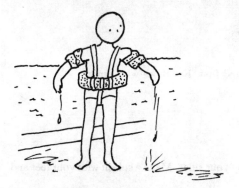

Buoyancy aids

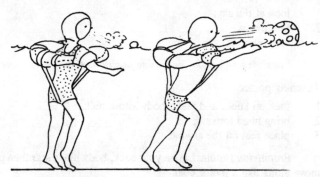

Walking — blowing ball

Bring in direction

    (i)   forwards
    (ii)   sideways
    (iii) backwards
    (iv) turning.

Bring in space

    (i)   circles
    (ii)   squares
    (iii) triangles.

Sometimes guess what pattern the swimmer is making and also point in the direction for the individual to walk. This can be great fun when you change directions.

Walk, blowing a ball (e.g. table tennis ball).

STAGE TWO

Buoyancy and propulsion prone

Prone position. Shoulders down, tuck up your knees and spin like a ball, using your hands to pull you around (teacher spins a ball on the water).

Prone floating. Spread arms like an aeroplane and lie down on the water and pretend you are an aeroplane in the sky.

Teaching points:

1.   stretch arms and legs;
2.   chin down on water.

Regaining feet from prone float. Just ask the swimmer to stand up on the ground.

Teaching points:

1.   tuck up knees and make body into a ball;
2.   bring head back;
3.   place feet on ground.

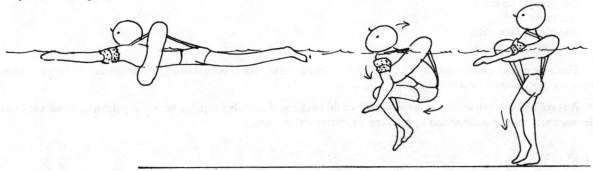

Regaining feet from prone floating

Propulsion prone. Lie down on the water again, arms like an aeroplane, legs out straight. Now make a big splash with your feet. Now you are moving like a motor boat.

Ask swimmers to use all of pool, then move from A to B.

Next bring in the arms. Pull the water with your hands. Show how a dog swims.

STAGE THREE

Buoyancy and propulsion supine

Supine floating. Lie down on the water on your back, spread your arms and legs and make your body like a star in the sky.

Teaching points:

1.   look at the sky;
2.   tummy up;
3.   toes pointed.

Regaining feet from the supine position. Ask the swimmer to try and stand first. For those who can't-

Teaching points:

1.   tuck up knees and make body into a ball;
2.   bring head forward;
3.   place feet on the ground.

Propulsion supine. Lie on your back, body like a star then put your arms by your sides. Make a splash with your feet and move along like a motor boat.

Teaching points:

1.   toes pointed;
2.   hips, tummy up;
3.   look at sky.

Some may find this difficult; sometimes a pair of flippers may be of help in gaining propulsion. If the swimmer is frightened to go on the back then stay on the front.

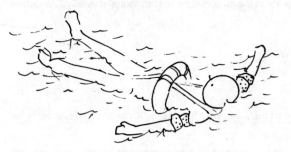

Supine floating

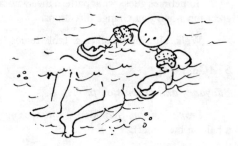

Approach to breast stroke

STAGE FOUR

Approach to the breast stroke. Simply ask the swimmer to pull with the hands under the water. If the swimmer pulls with a symmetrical action, his legs will often automatically follow the same pattern.

The swimmer can try the kick on the back or the teacher can sit on a chair and demonstrate the leg action, or even give manual guidance. Kick like a frog!

Teaching points:

1.   feet brought up together;
2.   feet turned out;
3.   feet part draw a circle;
4.   feet then stretch back.

Those swimmers who are best suited to this type of stroke can be seen at once. Usually it is the ones with very good dorsal flexion, and poor plantar flexion of the feet.

An excellent way to learn the leg action is to lie on the back and kick while watching the feet. A polystyrene float can be used under each arm to help balance and so promote a symmetrical leg action.

STAGE FIVE

Combination of strokes

Swimmers should be encouraged to try a combination of leg and arm action e.g. Breast stroke arms, crawl legs; Dolphin legs, breast stroke arms.

Remember the aim at first is to get them swimming any stroke, any way, then learn the basic strokes.

The use of flippers. A swimmer who cannot manage either of these kicks is given a pair of flippers to aid propulsion. Usually the swimmer is taught to make use of them on his back.

Teaching points:
1. keep flippers under water;
2. kick from hips. Sometimes manual guidance is needed.

The flippers can be used to teach all strokes.

Flippers must be the shoe type and flexible.

When to get rid of the aids. It is surprising the number of people who ask to swim without aids. This is sometimes an indication that they are ready.

Gradually let the air out of the aids until the person is swimming.

Always tell them the air is being let out of the aids.

When the swimmer first tries without aids always swim towards the rail of the pool. The distance from where he stands to the rail is 'the river'; ask the swimmers to name 'the river', they then swim across it — progress by 'widening the river'.

Water play. Use incentives like 'Who can swim from A to B without putting their feet on the bottom?'

Coloured hoops partly submerged, represent tunnels. The swimmers are the trains going through the tunnel. They are encouraged to make train noises as they swim. This helps breath control. It is fun when each swimmer gets through the tunnel (hoop) and the rest clap.

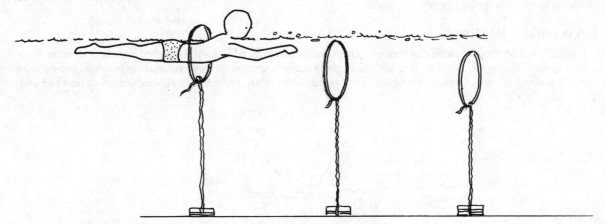

Swimming through hoops (tunnels)

Swimmers hold inflatable toys and kick — e.g. Dolphins, Donald Duck.

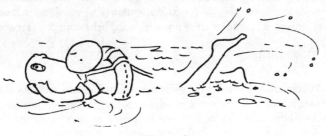

Water play

There is a special toy to encourage swimmers to go under water, called 'Sammy the Magic Star Fish' — a coloured plastic star fish which floats partly submerged. The swimmer goes under water and retrieves it.

With small children, puppets are used successfully: a puppet called 'Swim Tim' can be made to do a kind of breast stroke and can illustrate various ways of floating.

Puppets have not been tried with the handicapped adults but an inflatable Dolphin held by a teacher was the means of attracting a reluctant mentally handicapped adult into the pool.

Praise and encouragement. Give lots of praise for effort as well as for progress.

Incentives

Phase 1 — With aids
1. Walk across the pool
2. Blow a ping pong ball across pool
3. Face in water blow bubbles
4. Swim 10m (33') on front
5. Swim 10m on back.

Phase 2 — Without aids

As Phase 1 (1-5).

Phase 3 — Without aids

1. Push and glide — face in water
2. Push and glide — kick on front
3. Push and glide — kick on back
4. Swim 10m recognised front stroke
5. Swim 10m recognised back stroke.

Phase 4 — Without aids

1. Swim 25m deep to shallow water
2. Tread water for 30 seconds in deep water
3. Jump into deep water
4. When swimmer jumps confidently diving from the side can be taught.

Notes

1. When swimming the 25m deep to shallow end, keep the swimmer close to the side and carry a pole for swimmer to grasp if he tires — until he is confident.
2. Jump into deep water near to the side (have a pole handy)
3. Diving should always be taught in deep water.

THE HALLIWICK METHOD

The Halliwick Method of teaching swimming was devised by James McMillan who began the work in 1949 at the Halliwick School for Girls in Southgate, London. It is from this school that the method takes its name. It is based on known scientific principles of hydrodynamics and body mechanics. It has proved to be safely applicable to all varieties of handicapped and non-handicapped people of all ages.

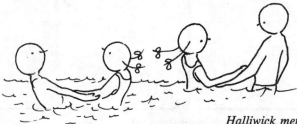

Halliwick method — one to one — no aids

Swimmers are taught on a one-to-one ratio of instructor to swimmer until the time when complete independence is achieved. The swimmer-instructor pair become a unit within a group activity so that the swimmer gains the advantages of social interaction with his peers whilst at the same time enjoying unobtrusive but constant attention of an individual instructor. Through the medium of games appropriate to age and ability, groups are made aware of properties and behaviour of water and how to control their own particular imbalance problems.

Handling

Correct handling on the part of the instructor enables the swimmer to experience a mobility unknown on land. After the initial mental adjustments to water are made and balance control principles are learned the swimmers reach a stage where they are prepared to do without instructor contact. Now, often for the first time in their lives, they experience complete independence of movement.

The method teaches swimming as a developmental programme, teaching the mental adjustment to the water, balance and control in the water, and later facilitates controlled activity by the swimmer, and produces a functional swimming stroke. In addition, a carefully thought out system of checks or tests enables the teacher to assess the reliability of the swimmers' reactions and the degree of learning achieved.

Swimmers are taught how to maintain a safe breathing position with the face clear of the surface; how to regain such a position from any other given position, and how to control exhalation whenever the face is immersed in water.

They are made familiar with all conceivable body rotation and learn how to initiate, control and arrest such rotations at will.

Waters powers of upthrust, turbulence, independence to movement are studied, together with metacentric effects. The end product is a secure swimmer whose confidence is based upon sound knowledge of water and his own movement controls.

Halliwick method used by a physiotherapist

A tutor at St. Thomas' Hospital Physiotherapy School and a member of the National Education Committee of the Association of Swimming Therapy, has used the Halliwick Method for more than fifteen years with mentally handicapped children and adults. She says 'I have found that it is applicable to all degrees of incapacity, and believe that it is beneficial to their development. It stimulates the most inactive to some degree of response which appears to be ongoing, and enables the over-active or hyperkinetic swimmer to gain considerable control.

A further great advantage of the method is that it is able to take account of, and accommodate, any physical disability that may be present concurrently with the mental disability.

The degree of safety that is achieved by the method is remarkable, almost entirely, I believe, due to the lack of apparatus used: it allows for no swimming aids such as floats, rings, arm bands etc., so there is no danger teaching a swimmer dependence on this kind of support, which in the unreliable person may be inadvertantly discarded. Equally, the supervision of the swimmer prevents problems arising from fits etc. in that they are coped with in a safe manner if they arise.

The process of learning whilst seriously and objectively being controlled is essentially recreational. The swimmers do have fun; they are taught to enjoy themselves and most skills are acquired through participation in group games and activities in the water'.

Anyone who is thinking of undertaking this type of tuition should consider the care and safety of the mentally handicapped on the bath side. In addition to the team of instructors, a back up team is required to care for them on the bath side, to:
1. help with dressing and undressing
2. provide refreshments
3. supervise activity and bath side behaviour
4. organise transport if necessary.

Those interested in learning about this method of teaching swimming should contact the Secretary of the Association of Swimming Therapy, Education Committee — Mr. D. Mahoney, 85 Bartholomew Road, London, NW5., who can put them in touch with clubs in their area who would teach the Halliwick Method and be able to give information of further courses that are organised in all parts of the country from time to time.

GENERAL HINTS ON THE ORGANISATION OF SWIMMING SESSIONS

When organising swimming sessions consider:

Water temperature

It is generally recognised that the temperture of the water should be 82-84° Farhenheit (28-29°C) when teaching mentally handicapped people. For physically active mentally handicapped people 80°F (27°C) is adequate — this is the average temperature of most public swimming pools.

Size of group

Ideally each mentally handicapped swimmer should be partnered by a non-handicapped helper (ref. Halliwick Method). When this is impossible, a ratio of two instructors to six swimmers is generally accepted.

Frequency of sessions

Obviously, the more frequent the sessions, the quicker the trainees or residents will be able to swim. A swimming period every day or even three time a week is better than once each week.

Ability in group

In classes of mixed ability some form of grouping is advisable.

Equipment (miscellaneous swimming aids)

Check that aids, floats, armbands when used are suitable, serviceable and available at the start of the session. Inflatable rubber rings can be used: a safety tape over the shoulders should be used to prevent the rings slipping downwards. A tape between the legs would prevent the tape riding upwards.
1. Balls, hoops, ducks, buoys, coffee-jar tops; any intriguing object to challenge the swimmer both above and under water should be used. Colour, texture and shape can be important.
2. Flippers help those who can already swim to achieve a more effective leg kick.
3. Rubber bricks, or coffee jar tops can be used for retrieval from the bottom of the pool.
4. Courlene rope. Rope can be used to divide the pool lengthways and widthways — it can also be used to set targets for swimmers to go underneath.
5. Drum. A clear basic rhythm can be set — it is valuable for sculling and change of direction exercises.
6. Rubber mattresses and towels — these are useful for entry and exit from the pool and protection of the skin for the multiply handicapped.

Facilities

Be familiar with the layout and procedures.

Staff and helpers

Make sure that everyone knows exactly what is expected of them.

Swimmers

Be sure to get any medical and/or parental permission required, well in advance. Be aware of any special disabilities, e. g. epilepsy.

PERSONAL HYGIENE

1. Where it is required for technical reasons, e.g. filter plant, swimmers should always co-operate by wearing bathing caps.

2. Men should wash oil from hair and keep it short.

3. The use of tissues, the toilet, showers and footbath are an essential part of preparation.

4. Swimmers suffering from catarrh, sore throat, skin or foot infection, or open sores should not be taken swimming.

5. Wash costumes out after use. Do not wring out costumes into the pool after use.

6. On completion of swim, have a brisk rub down. Dry hair, ears and feet thoroughly.

7. Get changed quickly or there is a risk of catching a cold.

TIPS BEFORE GOING INTO THE POOL

1. Let prospective swimmers come along to watch for just as long as they like, leaving the individual to make the first step into the water.

2. Practise getting the face wet in a bowl of tepid water with a mirror at the bottom to encourage them to open their eyes.

3. Blow bubbles under the water.

WATER CONFIDENCE

First and foremost it is essential for swimmers to gain confidence in the water and in the teacher by doing what **they** want to do with the teacher; sometimes walking, sitting or just talking in the water.

It may take some time to establish this relationship and for the swimmers to be able to move around with or without aids in shallow water without fear.

Encourage jumping up and down — 'washing face', blowing bubbles and holding hands to walk across the pool.

Pull and push the water with the hands.

Touch head, shoulders, knees, feet etc: make shapes with hands, arms, knees and legs.

WATER GAMES

The learner's pool is an ideal place for water games as the depth is 1 m (3.25′) — as an alternative use the shallow end of a large pool roped off. An occasional game introduced into a swimming session often maintains enthusiasm and interest. The following are examples of water games:

1. *Fishing Net*
   Trainees standing in 1 metre area of the pool. Two trainees join hands and the others spread out anywhere in the area. On hearing a given signal the two holding hands begin to chase the others. Anyone whom they touch joins them and the game continues until all the trainees are in the chain with their hands joined.

2. *Team passing*
   Equipment: Floats and plastic ball.
   Trainees divided into two equal teams. One team stands on one side of the trhee foot pool and the other team opposite. Floats can be used for goalposts and left on each side of the pool about four metres apart. A light plastic ball is thrown up between two centre swimmers to start the game and team passing begins until a score of ten is reached by either side. Team scores a point when ball is hit or thrown between the two floats.

3. *The retrievers*
   Equipment: Two rubber rings.
   Trainees are divided into two teams. Two rubber rings are placed in the centre of the roped off area of the pool. The teams line up on opposite sides. On a signal a member from each team retrieves the ring either by walking, swimming or running, and hands it to the next swimmer who replaces it in the centre again. This is continued until the first team with the ring over the first swimmer and in a straight line, shouts 'stop'.

4. *Relay race*
   Equipment: Floats.
   Swimmers are divided into two teams. Half of each team on one side and the other half on the other side of the pool. First swimmer of each team, with float, jumps or climbs in to the pool and swims or walks to the other side, gets out and hands the float to his team mate who repeats this until one team wins by finishing the relay and all team members are gathered together on one side in the pool in a straight line.

5. *Push partner*
   Equipment: Floats.
   Swimmers are paired off with a float between them at arms length in a prone position. They hold tightly to the float and do a leg kick and try to push each other to the side of the pool. A good game for balance and equilibrium.

DISCIPLINE AND SAFETY

A swimming bath is an obvious source of potential danger and therefore a teacher or instructor must take all the necessary safety measures. Discipline is essential. Certain rules which must be obeyed, together with an acceptable code of behaviour will ensure a happy, relaxed atmosphere and minimum risk.

1. No trainee may enter the water until instructed to do so.

2. No running along the bathside or pushing each other into the water.

3. Signals by hand or whistle should be promptly obeyed, especially those indicating stopping and getting out of the pool.

4. Diving only permitted under supervision.

5. Long poles should be placed at the side of the pool to be used in case of emergency.

6. If not in the 1m pool, a rope should show the limit of shallow water appropriate for the class lesson.

7. All must leave the water immediately when instructed to do so.

8. Supervision is important in the changing room. Make sure an enthusiastic swimmer does not wander back into the pool. If aids are put on **in** the changing room, safety on the pool side is ensured.

9. Never swim without a qualified life saver with a whistle on the pool side whose sole job is to watch every individual and to blow the whistle in the case of an emergency to stop all activity — use of the whistle should be practised from time to time.

10. The teacher or instructor with the swimmers should be aware of all the safety apparatus available and be acquainted with the necessary and normal emergency arrangements provided at the pool.

11. The teacher should be qualified in methods of resuscitation and first aid.

12. When bathing or swimming in inland waters or in the sea, special attention should be paid to all safety precautions, especially those laid down locally. The teacher/parent should know about the local tides, dangerous currents, depth of water- weirs, rocks and any other hazards.
If you have any doubt — don't!

COMPETITION

Many mentally handicapped people once they have learned to swim like to test their ability in competition. This is arranged in clubs and at regional, national and international level by many organisations. There are various methods of competition. Some Inter-Adult Training Centre annual swimming sports and galas are run under the Amateur Swimming Association rules and with the help of ASA officials.

Awards

These can be devised locally or by a national organisation e.g. Scottish Amateur Swimming Association. These awards provide an incentive to both swimmer and teacher.

HINTS ON THE ORGANISATION OF SWIMMING GALAS

The following officials should be appointed:

Gala Co-ordinator	Starter	One or more
Referee	One timekeeper for	Placing Judges
Chief Whip	each lane in use	Chief Judge
Pool Supervisor	Recorder	Chief Timekeeper
Life saver		Announcer

The responsibilities of the officials shall be:

Gala Co-ordinator — shall be responsible for the overall efficient conduct of the Gala and shall appoint such further assistants as required. He shall have overriding authority in all matters.

Referee — shall give a decision where the opinion of the Chief Judge and Chief Timekeeper differ. If in the opinion of the Referee a competitor has been fouled to a degree that endangers his or her chance of success, he shall have the power to re-run that race or enable that competitor to compete in the next round or final. He may disqualify any competitor he considers guilty of wilfully obstructing another competitor.

Chief Whip — shall ensure that all competitors are at the starting point at a reasonable time prior to the commencement of their race.

Starter — shall satisfy himself that timekeepers and judges are at their appropriate stations and are aware that the race is about to start. He shall start the race by giving a preliminary command 'take your mark' followed by a starting signal.

Timekeepers — shall start their watches at the starting signal and shall stop their watches when the swimmer in the allocated lane completes the appropriate distance. The time recorded shall be made known to the Chief Timekeeper.

Place Judge —|shall note the order of finish and advise the Chief Judge accordingly.

Chief Timekeeper — shall resolve any timing dispute and enter each swimmer's time on appropriate form for submission to the Recorder.

Chief Judge — shall resolve any dispute between Placing Judges and shall enter the placings on the appropriate form for submission to the Recorder.

Pool Supervisor — shall ensure that suitable arrangements are made for competitors to enter and leave the water and that helpers in the water are properly instructed in their duties in that they neither impede, physically assist, or swim directly in front of any competitor. He shall ensure that free passage is maintained at the bathside.

Recorder — shall have a record of all times and placings as submitted by the Chief Judge and Chief Timekeeper. He shall prepare a list of award winners for use at the time of presentation.

Note — The presence of a lifesaver on the pool side and lane ropes are desirable at all times.

A SWIMMING CLUB FOR 'ANY SWIMMER'

'Sport for all', the Sports Council's slogan triggered off a member of the staff of the Birkbeck Adult Training Centre in Leytonstone, Essex, in 1977 to form a swimming club for 'any swimmer'. Club members include mentally handicapped and physically handicapped people as well as other swimmers — a good example of integration.

Affiliation

Affiliation to the amateur Swimming Association was accepted and consequently opportunities to take part in competitions — water polo — diving and swimming awards have been provided. Some members are now training for their ASA Bronze personal survival awards.

Club grades

For those members who are less able swimmers an easier set of swimming grades has been compiled. These are proving to be an invaluable asset to members in achieving some form of self confidence not only in themselves as swimmers but as people.

The conditions of each of the five grades are:

Elementary: Swim 25 yds.

Intermediate: Jump (or dive) in and swim 35 yds.

GRADE I

1. Jump in and swim 25 yds of a recognised stroke.
2. Tread water for 3 minutes.
3. Swim 50 yds of a recognised stroke without touching the sides or bottom.
4. Get out of the baths unaided without using the steps.

GRADE II

1. Jump (or dive) in and swim 50 yds of a recognised stroke.
2. Tread water for 5 minutes.
3. Swim 75 yds of **ONE** of the following strokes without touching the sides or bottom of the bath:
   (i)   Front crawl
   (ii) Back stroke
   (iii) Breast stroke.
4. Do one surface dive during the 75 yds swimming.
5. Get out of the baths unaided, without using the steps.

GRADE III

«. Dive in with a pair of pyjamas (top and bottom) over swim suit.
2. Swim 100 yds within a set time of 10 minutes.
3. Tread water for 5 minutes, whilst discarding pyjamas.
4. Swim for 300 yds of **ONE** of the following strokes without touching the sides or bottom of the baths:
   (i)   Front crawl
   (ii) Back stroke
   (iii) Breast stroke.
5. Do 2 surface dives in the 100 yds swimming.
6. Get out of the baths unaided without using the steps.

Safety. When undressing in water, all discarded clothing must be removed from the pool immediately.

SWIMMING AT CRAIG PHADRIG HOSPITAL, INVERNESS

This hospital is fortunate in having an excellent pool, purpose-built, opened in 1970. Three full-time qualified instructors with the Royal Life Saving Society's Teachers' Award are employed, two men and one woman.

All residents swim unless they are excused on medical grounds. There is an excellent standard of personal hygiene with special care for incontinent patients who wear rubber pants. Everyone showers both before and after swimming. Epileptics swim, but wear red costumes for quick identification.

Small groups

Residents swim in small groups with a one-to-one helper-swimmer ratio when paraplegics are in the water and with other when possible. The helpers are nursing staff who are encouraged to attend the instructors' class and to go into the water with the residents. Voluntary help is given from boys from the Inverness Academy as part of their community service training.

New residents

New residents start in a very warm paddling pool and progress to the big pool as confidence increases and they feel they want to.

Programme

The daytime programme has an educational bias and groups are graded where possible. Recreational groups swim during the evenings and at weekends. Anyone can join in whatever age or ability, but must have nursing staff with them.

Competitive swimming events

These are run within the hospital. The size of the teaching group varies. Paraplegics have two lessons a week and other residents who can swim use the pool during recreational hours provided there are instructors present. Some other active patients are able to swim every day and this is of great benefit to them.

The pool is not open to the public, but children from a nearby school for physically handicapped people use it.

The pool is used a great deal for teaching purposes and residents who can swim are given the opportunity to do so at any time during recreational hours.

ASA AWARDS SCHEME AND CERTIFICATES

The Amateur Swimming Association has an award scheme starting with a badge for 10 metres to survival awards. Details from Miss L. V. Cook, 12 King's Avenue, Woodford Green, Essex.

The ASA has pilot conditions for two certificates:

(i)   pilot conditions for the ASA Teacher of Disabled Swimmers Certificate;

(ii)   pilot conditions for the ASA Instructor – Aide Certificate of Disabled Swimmers.

These certificates should be of interest to all those who are teaching or contemplating teaching swimming to mentally handicapped people of all ages.

NOTE: Some Gateway Clubs include swimming as part of their programme (see Chapter 14 p. 166).

FURTHER READING

AMATEUR SWIMMING ASSOCIATION *The teaching of swimming.* Amateur Swimming Association, Loughborough, 1974.
ELKINGTON, HELEN. *Swimming.* Cambridge University Press, 1978.
LOVESEY, J. *Swimming a lifelong activity.* World's Work, Tadworth, 1980.
ROYAL LIFE SAVING SOCIETY. *Life saving.* Royal Life Saving Society, London, 1975.
WILSON, C. *Swimming.* Barrie & Jenkins, London, 1977.
DIAGRAM GROUP. *Enjoying swimming and diving.* Paddington Press, London, 1979.

CHAPTER NINE

Special Events in Sport and Physical Activities

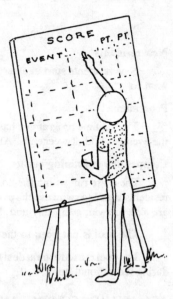

Displays – Tournaments: American or League; Knockout tournament; Progressive games tournament – Ladder and 'house' competitions – Matches – Athletic sports – Tabloid or potted sports – 'Mob sports' – Swimming sports or galas – 'It's a Knockout' – Miscellaneous events: Indoor or outdoor 'Have a Go' sports meeting – League finals day – Inter-hospital skittles competition.

Several types of events are suitable for single players, couples, teams or a number of teams from one establishment — some competitive some not. Providing the players have practised the necessary skills to an adequate standard, competition can be challenging and fun for participants and spectators alike. Some events such as displays, sports days and swimming galas, give parents and friends the opportunity to see for themselves just how high the standard of performance can be reached. It is possible to organise many types of events, and the rest of this section contains suggestions as to how such events can be organised.

DISPLAYS

Displays promote enthusiasm and a better standard of performance; they inspire confidence and help the social training of those taking part.

Displays can be of one or a series of items according to the purpose of the display.

The venue. This can be indoors or outdoors, on a stage or at ground level with the audience seated round or in rows. Entrances, exits and dressing room accommodation should be taken into consideration.

Music. If music is required check the availability of piano or other instruments and sound equipment.

Lighting. Check what lights can be used if required and what additional lights are necessary.

Programme

1. Decide on the length of the programme including intervals.
2. Select items which ensure variety and in which as many as possible can take part. The inclusion of a guest item such as a gymnastic or dance group can add interest, introduce a new activity and bring in more spectators. This special item can be professional or amateur.

Commentary

A good compere can 'make' a display. The audience should be given some information about the performers and the purpose of the display both verbally and in writing (programme) to ensure maximum and accurate publicity.

Organisation

Detailed organisation will, of course, vary but helpers will be required to –
look after performers
costumes
equipment
audience
programmes
first aid etc.
press and radio coverage (if applicable).

Sources of help. Other members of staff, students, sixth formers, members of voluntary organisations, local sports council, regional officers of the BSAD (see Appendix 2), parents and friends.

Invitations. Written invitations should be sent to civic dignitaries, local and hospital authorities, sports councils and any notable sports personality in the area.

Rehearsals. Performers should be rehearsed sufficiently to give them confidence and a feeling of achievement, but not to such an extent that they lose interest and sponteneity.

The compère

The compère is the key person at the performance itself. Select someone with a good voice and a sense of humour who will ensure the continuity of the performance and keep the audience informed; someone who will talk enough, but **not** too much.

TOURNAMENTS

American Tournament — League System

	Team 1	Team 2	Team 3	Team 4	Won	Lost	Draw	Points	Place
Team No. 1		Won 3–1	Lost 1–3	Draw 1–1	1	1	1	3	2nd
Team No. 2	Lost 1–2		Lost 2–4	Draw 2–2	0	2	1	1	4th
Team No. 3	Won 2–1	Won 1–0		Won 3–1	3	0	0	6	1st
Team No. 4	Draw 0–0	Draw 3–3	Lost 1–3		0	1	2	2	3rd

Suitable for Soccer, Cricket, Hockey, Basketball, Netball etc.

Points Win = 2 points. Draw = 1 point. Lose = 0 points.

Tie In the case of a tie, the position is decided on goal average.

Knockout tournament (How to conduct the draw)

The number of entries in the competition, if not already a power of 2, i.e. 4 - 8 - 16 - 32 etc. must be made so by means of 'byes' — if there are 5 entries in a competition, the number must be brought to 8 by giving byes to three competitors. All byes are decided in the first round. The best means of drawing is to put the names of all entries in a box.

An example: 12 entries — there must be 4 byes to bring the total to 16. The first 4 names drawn will be byes while the remaining 8 play:

1st Round	Semi Final	Final	
1. Bye			
2. Bye			
3. Bye			
4. Bye			
5.			Winner
6.			
7.			
8.			
9.			
10.			
11			
12.			

Some examples:

Number of entries		Number of byes	Number of matches in 1st round
9	7 short of 16	7	1
15	1 short of 16	1	7
24	8 short of 32	8	8
29	3 short of 32	3	13

Progressive Games Tournament

A well organised tournament of this type can provide vigorous exercise for many at the same time. As with all mass events, success depends on thoughtful preparation and good organisation.

Layout of ground: draw a plan of the ground — the positioning of the various games is important. Make sure that there is plenty of space between pitches so that there is no danger of competitors from one game getting in the way of those in another, of colliding or of being hit with a ball. Pitches should be numbered (see diagram). Mark out pitches before players arrive and see that all fixed equipment, goal posts, wickets, etc., are readily available and safe.

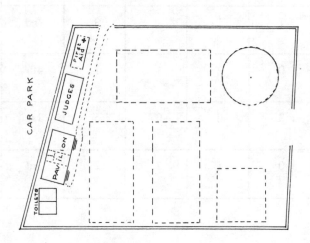
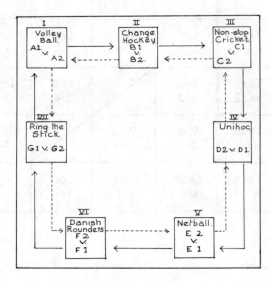

Layout for Progressive Games Tournament

Choice of games: choose games suitable for those taking part — this particular example is a tournament for men and women (mixed play) — and ones which do not require lengthy explanation and involve specialised techniques.

Alternate very energetic games with less vigorous ones. As each team plays all the others, the number of games should be **uneven.**

Course officials: appoint a competent leader/referee to be in charge of each game. When the teams move on to the next game, these referees should stay on their own pitches and be responsible for teaching, umpiring and scoring. Also appoint a controller whose job it is to ring a bell or blow a whistle at the start, half-time and at the end of each round of matches.

Each team should have a leader/helper to see that players progress quickly to the next game.

Competitors: divide players into an even number of teams with the two sexes in the same ratio in each, not more than twelve players in all, then arrange for the election or appointment of a team captain. Number each team A1, A2; B1, B2 and so on. By the end of the tournament all the 'one' teams will have played against all the 'two' teams. When the teams are ready, explain the organisation of the tournament, how the teams change, the time allowed for each match and the method of scoring.

Order and time of play: in the first period of play, A1 will compete against A2 at game No. 1.

B1 will compete against B2 at game No. 2 and so on.

At the end of the first round, all the 'one' teams move clockwise and the 'two' teams counter-clockwise on to the next game.

At the start of the next round, allow five to ten minutes for the leader/referee in charge of each game to check that the players understand the rules before the match begins. The time allowed for each match will vary according to the time available for the whole tournament; 5-7 minutes each way is suggested.

Scoring: at the end of each round the captain or leader of each team takes the result to the controller (helper) who enters the score on the scoreboard:

a win scores 2 points

a draw scores 1 point.

At the end of the tournament, gather teams together at the scoreboard, total the points and announce the winner. If two or more teams tie, arrange a simple relay to decide the winner.

	1	2	3	4	5	6	7	Total Points			1	2	3	4	5	6	7	Total Points
A1										A2								
B1										B2								
C1										C2								
D1										D2								
E1										E2								
F1										F2								
G1										G2								
	Section Total										Section Total								

Scoreboard for Progressive Games Tournament

LADDER AND 'HOUSE' COMPETITIONS

Ladder

Ladder competitions are a useful means of maintaining interest over a period of weeks. Individual couples or teams can compete in such games as:

badminton   quoit tennis
table tennis   team hand tennis
padder tennis   volley ball,

and many other minor and major games.

Each competitor (individual couple or team) is given a number. The draw is then made and the competitors are listed in the order in which they are drawn.

Any competition may challenge the one immediately above on the list (ladder). If the challenger wins, he moves one step up the ladder; if he loses, there is no change in the order. All matches must be played according to agreed rules. It is often necessary to encourage players to challenge the player above. The ladder should be made so that the name tabs can be pulled out and slotted in the new order.

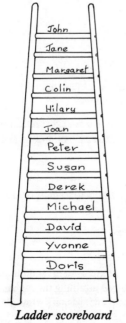

Ladder scoreboard

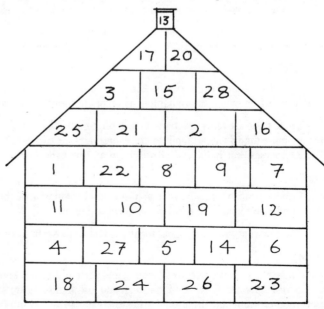

'House' scoreboard

House

The principle of this type of competition is the same as for the ladder competition, but it allows more scope for challenging. Starting at the chimney of the 'house', position all the competitors according to the order of the draw (see diagram).

A competitor may challenge any other in the same row of bricks. If he wins, he may then challenge anyone in the row above; if he wins agains, he then takes the place of the competitor he has beaten.

MATCHES

Matches can be arranged in almost every game between groups from hospitals, adult training centres, gateway clubs, hostels, wards, etc., and against school and youth clubs. Matches against schools and youth clubs provide an opportunity for integration and the subsequent social training.

ATHLETIC SPORTS DAYS

These should be run as near to the Amateur Athletic Association rules as possible (see p. 183 for address).

TABLOID OR POTTED SPORTS (For men, women or mixed teams)

Tabloid or Potted Sports, played indoors or out-of-doors, can provide a considerable number of people with varied, objective and enjoyable exercise. Events can be of different types involving the skills of throwing, aiming, running, dexterity and balance.

Each competitor is competing against a high or a low standard and scores points towards a team total at each event.

The events selected should vary according to the standard and interests of those taking part, the space and equipment available, and the occasion — for instance, at a social function, the aim is not so much to test physical ability as to provide the maximum amount of fun. No miniature sports meeting will be enjoyed unless it is well organised.

Preparation

Know the exact position of each event in relation to the surroundings. Take any hazards into consideration. Make a plan of the space available. Be sure that all the apparatus is to hand before the start of the meeting. If possible, find a few reliable volunteers to make the ground markings, to set up the events before the rest of the competitors arrive, and to help with judging, scoring, assisting competitors etc.

Selection of events

In selecting events, remember that they must be suitable for the competitors and that they should call for different forms of skill and effort, e.g. speed, accuracy in aiming at target, balance, endurance, skill in handling, spring. Arrange the course so that the less vigorous events alternate with the strenuous ones.

Competitors

Divide the competitors into teams of not more than ten players in all; no one should be left out. If a team is one short, player No. 1 can have two turns at the first event, player No. 2 at the second, etc.

Collect the competitors together to explain the general organisation of the meeting. When all are in their places at the first event, the judges explain the events and make the scoring clear.

Organisation

Start team A at the first event, team B at the second and so on. When all the members in every team have completed their turns at their first event, the signal for the teams to move on to their next event will be given.

Try to choose events which will take approximately the same time; otherwise some teams may get restless while waiting. If there are more than 8 teams, duplicate the events, and run two parallel meetings. Thus, teams A-E and F-J will be working round different courses, but in the end all will have a turn at the same events.

Officials

Provide a judge for each event, and a recorder to summarise the scores. Get each team to appoint its own leader, and make him responsible for moving it from one event to the next.

The recorder gives the signal for the teams to move from one event to the other.

Scoring

There are various methods of scoring, but perhaps the best known is the double standard system (sometimes referred to as the A and B standard system). In this, high and low standards are set for each event; those attaining the higher standard win 2 points for their team, and those gaining the lower standard, 1 point. In order to decide the standards, ask a few players of average ability to try out the various events before the start of the meeting.

At the same meeting double and single standard systems can be used for different events. To remind all competitors of the standards, display them on small cards, or chalk them on the floor at each event. As each event is finished, the judge fills in a score card, signs it, and gets one of the team members to take it to the recorder. A specimen card might read:

TEAM:	A.	
EVENT:	Throwing a ball for distance	
Points scored:	High standard — 6 players	12
	2 points	
	Low standard — 4 players	4
	1 point	
		———
		16

Judge's signature ....

The recorder places the teams in their correct order of merit and enters on his summary (see plan below) the number of the place gained. In each event the winners score 1 point, the second team 2, and so on. If two or more teams tie for a place they are awarded the average of the places tied for, e.g. two teams tying for a second place score 2½ points each. At the end of the meeting, the 'place points' for each event are totalled, including those awarded for the relay, and the team with the **lowest** number of points wins. It is a good idea for the recorder to use a blackboard, so that the teams may see their progress.

An alternative method of scoring — which can be used when all the events are being judged on the single standard system — is to count the actual points gained. This is a simpler method for inexperienced leaders. and competitors sometimes find it less confusing and more stimulating; when looking at the scoreboard they can easily see how their team stands. It may not give, however, a completely true result, particularly if there is a wide range between the number of points which can be scored for the various events. The actual points won at each event are entered on the scoreboard and at the end of the meeting the team with the **greatest** number of points is the winner.

Final relay

If, when the points are finally added, two or more teams have tied, arrange a simple relay to decide the winners of the whole meeting. Such a relay can be run, in any case, as a grand finale. Award points to each team according to its place in the race, the winners gaining 1, the second team 2 and so on. (If the alternative method of scoring mentioned above is used, the winning team will score the highest number of points and the last 1.)

An ingenious leader will be able to think out a great variety of events, and competitors will enjoy making them up for themselves. Those suggested below are merely samples. Although the standard given may be said to be average, remember that standards vary considerably, according not only to the ability of the competitors but also to the conditions, e.g. outdoors, indoors, grass or asphalt.

TEAM	Speed POINTS	Speed PLACE	Spring POINTS	Spring PLACE	Balance POINTS	Balance PLACE	Aiming POINTS	Aiming PLACE	Skills POINTS	Skills PLACE	Relay PLACE	TOTAL PLACE POINTS	FINAL PLACE
A	8	2	6	1	4	5	10	1	6	1½	2	12½	1st
B	2	5	1	5	10	1	7	4	6	1½	4	20½	5th
C	4	3	5	2	6	4	9	2	4	4	5	20	4th
D	10	1	4	3	7	3	6	5	2	5	1	18	2nd
E	3	4	3	4	9	2	8	3	5	3	3	19	3rd

Potted Sports scoreboard

Examples of events

		Average standards	
		High	Low
Aiming			
1.	12 throws of a tennis ball into an inclined bucket, from a distance of 2-3m (6-10'). The ball must remain in the bucket. Score 1 point for each successful throw.	4 or more points	2 or 3 points
2.	12 throws of a rubber or rope quoit to ring a peg 450mm (18") high, from a distance of 2-3m (6-10'). Score 1 point for each successful throw.	2 or more	1 point
3.	6 single-handed overarm throws of a football at a netball ring, from a distance of 4.9m (16') i.e. edge of circle. Score 1 point for each successful throw. Throwing points within the circle area can be selected.	2 or more points	1 point
4.	10 underarm bowls with a cricket ball towards two skittles 300mm (12') apart, from a distance of 7-8m (23-26'). Score 1 point when the ball passes between the skittles without touching them.	5 or more points	2 to 4 points
5.	4 throws of a football to knock down a skittle, from a distance of 6m (20'). Score 1 point for each successful throw.	2 or more points	1 point
Speed			
1.	Dribbling with a unihoc stick and ball over a course of 20m (22yds), with three obstacles (poles, chairs or medicine balls) separated by 5m (16.5'), the first being 5m (16.5') from the start.	32 seconds	36 seconds
2.	Circular potato race. A circle of 6m (20') diameter is drawn and 8 potatoes are placed at regular intervals round its circumference. A bucket is placed in the centre of the circle and a starting line is drawn 1.8m (6') from the circumference of the circle. Starting from the line, run and pick up each potato separately and put it into the bucket; then run with the bucket to the starting line.	32 seconds	36 seconds
Spring			
1.	Hop, step and a jump, from a stationary start.	6m (20')	3m (10')
2.	Three consecutive forward jumps with feet together. No hesitation allowed between jumps.	4m (13'2")	3m (10')
3.	'Haphazard hops'. 8 circles (300mm (1') in diameter) are drawn in zigzag formation and numbered 1-8. Stand on one foot in circle 1 and hop to circle 2, then to circle 3 and so on to circle 8. Hopping must be continuous, the feet must not be changed and the ground between the circles must not be touched. Two turns, one with either foot. Score 1 point for each successful round.	2 points	1 point
Balance			
1.	Balance walk along a bench (narrow side up) or a plank supported at both ends, balancing a book or beanbag on the head without touching it with the hand.	full distance	half but not full distance
2.	Mount and dismount three chairs in a line, balancing a book or beanbag on the head without touching it with the hand. Score 2 points if successful with three chairs and 1 point if successful with two.	2 points	1 point
3.	Flower-pot walking. Stand on two flower-pots (or bricks), balance on one and move the other forward with the hand. Walk forward in this way for 6m (20'), turn and walk back to the starting point. Dismounting is not allowed. Score 2 points for the double journey and 1 point for a single journey.	2 points	1 point
Miscellaneous			
1.	'Juggling' with two small bats (a) both hands (b) one hand	10 or more continuous changes	6-10 continuous changes
2.	Balance a pole on the fingers of one hand and change it to the other without the hands touching.	4 or more continuous changes	2 or 3 continuous changes
3.	Blow a table tennis ball along the ground between parallel lines 200mm (9") apart with **one** breath. (Only suitable for indoors).	6m (20')	4m (13'2")
4.	Reaction. Two judges (or competitors) hold a stick, 600-900mm (2'-3') long, at hip height. When the competitor is ready he says 'Go!' At any time after this signal, those holding the stick release it and the competitor tries to catch it before it touches the ground. When waiting for the stick to be released, the competitor may hold his hand over it but must not touch it. Six attempts. Score 1 point for each success.	3 or more points	2 points

'MOB SPORTS' (A variation of Potted Sports)

Arena:

> 30 - 40 - 50m long according to ability.

Formation:

> 2 competing teams A and B divided into two streams each. Two against two in each heat. (3 teams A, B, C can compete.)

X X X X X X X X X X X X X X X X	'A' Team ⟶	
X X X X X X X X X X X X X X X X	'B' Team ⟶	

Heats

8 7 6 5 4 3 2 1

A race is a complete series of heats in one event.

> **1st race** (Each heat). Players run and remain at the far end in heat places — points awarded 1 - 2 - 3 - 4.

> **2nd race** (Each heat). Players race back but with some variation in the race. Continue ad infinitum.

> **Note:** (1) The 2nd heat can be started before the 1st heat has passed the winning line and so on. (2) It is possible to run 120 heats in 45-50 minutes.

Variations

1. Straight sprint
2. Jump over balance bench at halfway stage
3. Run to a hoop. Pass it over head, step out and run on.
4. 2 hoops on the ground, throw 'objects' e.g. bean bag, from 1 hoop to the other and run on.
5. Erect a deck chair
6. Crawl under a net
7. As 3, but with 2 hoops instead of one.

Scoring

1. Points are totalled at the end of each race or at the end of the meeting.
2. Have separate score cards for each race, 'A race' 'B race' etc.
3. The team with the **lowest** total is the winning team.
4. Scorers only use Team Initials 'A' and 'B'. No names should be taken.

Races	1	2	3	4	Points 'A'	Points 'B'
	A	B	B	A	5	5
	B	A	A	B	5	5
	A	A	B	B	3	7
Total Points					13	17

Team 'A' has the **lowest** number of points and is the winner.

Indoor events

1. Bouncing a ball into a bucket - box - bin (5 times).
2. Quoits (5) throw quoit over post — turn
3. Deck Quoits (5) use a soft broom to push them into circles, each circle a different number of points in value.
4. Tossing shuttlecocks (5 old ones), into a hoop or circle on the ground from a given distance.
5. Standing broad jump.

> The principle in all these sports is to have maximum participation. In the 'Mob Sports', nobody should be barred — a team could consist of 40 players.

SWIMMING SPORTS OR GALAS (For details of the organisation see Swimming, Chapter 8 p. 73).

'IT'S A KNOCKOUT'

The staff of the Chelmsford Training Centre believe that healthy competition and inter-action between trainees should be encouraged. Therefore with three other centres — Braintree, Colchester and Little Clacton — they have formed themselves into the North Essex Training Centre Sports Association. The Association, which has been in existence for little more than two years, has already organised football, netball, skittle and darts leagues, an annual sports day and, in 1978, organised an 'It's a Knockout'. The Deputy Manager, says: 'We believe that **every** trainee within the centre should be given the opportunity and encouragement to participate in the activities of the centre and with this aim in mind, the 'knockout' was devised. Sports Days are usually an occasion of happiness for a small team of athletes, but maybe of boredom, or of little interest for the spectators. We wanted to change this, certainly for our centre'.

The Sports Association, when drawing up its programme, suggested that the Chelmsford Centre should promote a 'Knockout' for the four centres. The staff agreed, and immediately applied to Chelmsford District Council for the use of their Sports Stadium, which afforded a certain amount of weather protection and also uninterrupted viewing for the spectators. Staff were then asked to suggest games. A colleague in another centre knew someone who ran a disco and he agreed to take a day off work, organise all the public addressing and also run a disco during the lunchtime break for spectators and competitors alike. After some weeks the Council agreed to the hire of the stadium at a reduced rate of £5, leaving the organisers only two months to prepare.

The determining factor in the choice of games was the suitability of the idea, the ease with which props could be borrowed, or made, and the ease with which they could then be transported to the site. A printed schedule was sent to the competing centres six weeks before the competition date so that they could practise the chosen games.

Games were selected specifically for more severely handicapped people, and this was noted on the schedule. The **rules** were fairly **flexible,** the most important being that each competitor was limited to one game only, ensuring that a large number of people competed. In fact, the teams numbered about 48 members each. A suitable backscene was procured — a castle wall — a part of one of the floats from a local carnival procession.

The deputy manager says:
'All the props were moved to the site in our transit van during the previous three days, hurriedly erected on the morning of the competition, and suddenly everything took shape. I must admit that I had some doubts that it would. We had bunting that we had made, some borrowed from other centres, and other authorities, and colourful props which had been made by us and other centres, together with the local hostel. We had music, the stands crowded with about 500 spectators and a good atmosphere. The National Westminster Bank presented us with a splendid trophy'.

The games were all fairly simple, designed to be enjoyed by competitors and spectators alike as they are in the BBC's 'It's a Knockout' — each one revolved around any one of maybe a dozen ideas. It is the 'props' and the theme that differ.

Programme of events

1. Raising the flag.
2. City gent game.
3. Crown and balloon game.
4. Coronation obstacle race.
5. Roll o'cloth.
6. Royal yacht race.
7. Royal banquet.
8. Royal wine cellar.
9. The King is in his counting house.

Raising the flag

Team: 10 members.

Object: To pass a given number of flags along the line, putting them into a holder. The first team to complete the event wins.

Method: Each team member stands within an arm's length of the next, and passes flags along the line from one end to the other. Final team member inserts flags in holder, the final one in the top of the holder.

City gent game

Team: 2 members.

Object: To complete in the quickest time. It is a two runner relay race.

Method: Each team member at the start is dressed in shorts, T-shirt and plimsolls for convenience. The first member starts off with brief-case, runs to first point, picks up bowler hat, puts it on head, runs to second point, puts on trousers, to third point, puts on jacket, to fourth point and picks up umbrella. This he must put up. He then races back to the start, drops the brief-case there, and then deposits the other articles back where they came from. He finally races back to the start for team member No. 2 to start.

Crown and balloon game

Team: 2 members.

Object: To burst the balloons that are hanging from the team members crowns without using hands. First team with all balloons burst wins.

Method: Each team member wears on his head a crown from which is suspended by string a number of balloons. Both team members take part together and either burst their own balloons or help their partner. They may use any part of their body except their hands.

Coronation obstacle race

Team: 4 members.

Object: For each team members to paint a recognisable picture of a given subject, in a given time. The resulting four pictures will be judged; on that the points will be awarded.

Method: Each competitor needs the costume of an artist, i.e. a smock and a beret. The area to be painted by each competitor will be approximately 2′ square. The first team member is given a pallette, with paint, and brushes, at the word 'go' he will have to quickly, but recognisably, paint his subject. When time up is signalled, he must pass his pallette and brushes to team member 2, then hang his painting up in the gallery. This procedure is repeated until all four pictures have been hung. They will then be judged and points awarded. The four subjects to be painted are:

Royal Yacht Britannia
The Queen's corgi
Windsor Castle
The Queen's crown

They should be painted in that order, i.e. team member 1 to paint the yacht, number 2 to paint the corgi, etc.

Roll o'cloth

Team: 4 members.

Object: To burst all the balloons on the course in the fastest time.

Method: Two members stand facing each other within a 'hoop' of cloth. They must move the hoop forward bursting balloons anchored to the ground. It is a relay race, with the swap over at the halfway point.

Royal yacht race

Team: 4 members.

Object: To propel each team member in turn from Tower Bridge to Hampton Court in the shortest time.

Method: A boat is mounted onto a trolley. Team member 1 pushes boat across 'water' from Hampton Court to Tower Bridge.
Team member 1 climbs into boat, pushed back by team member 2
Team member 2 climbs into boat, pushed back by team member 3
Team member 3 climbs into boat, pushed back by team member 4
The first boat to complete the last leg, wins.

Royal banquet

Team: 6 members.

Object: To set table for banquet.

Method: Each team has a table and six chairs at far end of course.
Team member 1 puts cloth on table and returns to the start line
Team member 2 sets six places with cutlery and returns to the start line
Team member 3 places six cups and saucers and returns to the start line
Team member 4 places six plates and returns to the start line
Team member 5 places a serviette on each plate and returns to the start line
Team member 6 places a vase of flowers on middle of table and sits down. The other team embers then run back to the table and sit down. The first team with their table correctly set and their team seated wins.

Royal wine celler

Team: 6 members.

Object: To fill large wine bottle with as much 'wine' as possible. First full one placed onto banquet table wins.

Method: Each team member in turn fills empty bottles from water in a container, places bottles on tray and on arrival at the table at the other end of the course, transfers water to large wine bottles. When this is full, the bottle is transferred to the banquet table.

The King is in his counting house

Team: 5 members.

Object: To stack as many 'coins' onto the counting table as possible within the given time, 'coins' are made of hardboard, 8″ in diameter.

Method: One team member stands behind a large picture of a king. He is wearing wicket keeper's gloves, partly for protection, partly for hindrance. Putting his hands through cutouts in the picture he attempts to catch and stack coins that have been flicked towards him by the other team members. He has a table in front on which to stack them. He is only able to stack those coins that have landed on the table. There will be small holes cut in the king to enable him to see the coins being flicked. No coins can be retrieved from the ground inside the throwing area.

At the end of the programme for the day at Chelmsford the following notes appear:

The list of events as supplied to each of the team will be adhered to as much as possible, but Chelmsford Training Centre (the organisers) reserve the right to alter the games if this becomes necessary. Should this eventuality arise, the teams will be notified immediately. One competitor may compete in one event only (the marathon, although played twice by each team, counts as one event). This will enable more people to compete.

On the day of the event, it is the responsibility of the team manager (or staff) to supply the competition control area with a list of competitors together with those staff who will be managing the team. Team Managers of staff (two from each team) will be allowed into the competition area during the events to advise only. They will not be allowed to handle equipment unless otherwise directed to do so by the referee.

It is desired that each centre supplies all its spectators and competitors with rosettes in the correct colour of their designated country.

The referee will have the final say in any dispute.

The scoring on each game will be as follows:

> 1st place — 4 points
> 2nd place — 3 points
> 3rd place — 2 points
> 4th place — 1 point

When a joker is played (on any one game by any team, except the marathon) that team has its score doubled on that game. The scoring on the marathon is as follows:

> 1st place — 8 points
> 2nd place — 6 points
> 3rd place — 4 points
> 4th place — 2 points

MISCELLANEOUS EVENTS

Indoor or outdoor 'Have a Go' sports meeting

The purpose of an indoor or outdoor sports evening is to give mentally retarded people an opportunity to 'have a go' at various games and activities. If some young people who already take part in these activities, together with trained coaches, teachers, instructors, nurses, leaders etc., offer to coach the games, referee and take part, mentally handicapped people will have a chance to see and join in a selection of activities from which they can make a choice. Also those planning a continuing programme of sports and physical activities will have an opportunity to discover which activities are most enjoyed by the clients.

The organisation of a 'Have a go' meeting is similar to a Progressive games tournament (see p. 78) but without the competitive element. Refreshments at half time will, of course, add to the enjoyment and give people a chance to get to know one another.

League finals day (Indoors or out-of-doors)

Out-of-doors: In some counties the season is ended with a League finals day to which parents and friends are invited, together with mayors, councillors and officers of the various authorities, voluntary and sports organisations. These usually take place on a football ground, hospital or industrial sports ground or park.

During the day the final matches between the sections of the various games such as football, netball, volleyball and unihoc etc. are played off. Usually a buffet lunch is provided and there is a prize-giving ceremony at the end of the day. Such a day encourages healthy competition and enables parents and all others present to realise the standard of play which can be reached with patient coaching and practice.

Indoors. A similar event held in a sports leisure centre differs only in the games played — for example: basketball, unihoc, trampolining, badminton, volleyball, archery, table tennis, etc. Games such as netball, basketball, archery etc. can be played as part of an outdoor or indoor finals day.

Inter-hospitals skittles (plastic ten pins) competition

As played in the Inter-hospital Sports Association South of the Thames. 23 hospitals play to these rules.

Apparatus: A set of plastic ten pins (skittles). 2 balls.

Formation: Arrange 10 pins in a shallow triangle, sufficiently far apart to allow a ball to pass through without touching any skittle.
2 Teams of 5 players.

Game: No. 1 bowls 1 ball — any skittles knocked down are removed. No. 1 then bowls a second ball. The total number of skittles knocked down are scored.

NOTE: If **all** the skittles are knocked down by the first ball, they are replaced before the second ball is bowled.

Scoring: Each team plays 3 rounds to complete a game. The total number of skittles knocked down in the 3 rounds are scored, the highest number wins the game. Games points are awarded: 2 points for a win; 1 point for a draw.

A match consists of 3 games (15 players from each side). At the end of a match, all games points are totalled and compared:

	A team	B team
1st game	2	0
2nd game	1	1
3rd game	2	0
	5	1

The A team win by 5 points to 1.

FURTHER READING

MINISTRY OF DEFENCE: ARMY SPORT CONTROL BOARD. *Small side team games and potted sports.* Ministry of Defence: Army Sport Control Board, Clayton Barracks, Aldershot, Hants.

CHAPTER TEN

Movement and Fitness Training

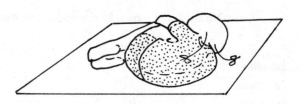

1. Movement training – Laban's principles – An example of a basic movement lesson – Examples of movements with emphasis on different body parts – Musical accompaniment and selection of music for movement – Two lessons based on Medau Rhythmic Movement – Sequences of movements using balls, hoops, scarves or ribbons – A Keep Fit lesson including hand apparatus – Two examples of Keep Fit in hospitals (i) Keep Fit at Manor House Hospital, Aylesbury (demonstration team) (ii) Keep Fit at Harperbury Hospital
2. Fitness training – Fitness training exercises – National fitness training schemes – Other methods of fitness training – Trim tracking (Trim trails) – Weight training and weight lifting – Kung Foo and Karate exercises – Yoga – Regular daily fitness training sessions – Examples of two daily dozens with and without chairs – Weight watching with mentally handicapped people – Assessment

Movement and fitness training is a general term used to cover the many different systems of training which aim, to a greater or lesser degree, to:

improve general health and maintain a high degree of fitness;

teach management of the body;

preserve normal movement in all the joints;

maintain all muscles and organs in a healthy condition;

improve stamina by increasing the power of the heart and the capacity of the lungs (circulation and respiration);

increase mobility and strength;

facilitate the learning of specific skills;

give each individual an opportunity for creative physical activity;

encourage communication of feelings and ideas;

increase the span of concentration.

(See also Chapter 1, p. 2).

Some form of movement training is important for both men and women and most activities can be enjoyed by and be beneficial to all. Although movement training particularly when it is accompanied by music could be said to be more suitable for and popular with women, there is evidence that groups of men and women working together benefit providing the movements are selected carefully.

All the different systems of movement training can be successfully adapted to meet the needs of mentally handicapped people. There is no 'one way' but a choice which depends on a number of factors — on the knowledge and experience of the nurse, instructor, club leader and teacher, the availability of experienced teachers of movement in the area, what facilities exist within the hospital, centre or club and in the community, and on how much time can be allocated to movement training within the framework of the daily or weekly programme. This section includes information about the different types of movement training and good practice being carried out in hospitals, adult training centres and clubs. For the sake of clarity, the activities involved in movement and fitness training are divided into two sections.

MOVEMENT TRAINING

Most of the movement training lessons are based on Laban's Principles: Educational Rhythmics, Keep Fit, Medau Rhythmic Movement or a simple 'Daily Dozen'.

On whatever system the lesson is based, all parts of the body need to be thoroughly exercised. There should be a balanmce between movements which emphasise stretching to counteract the all too common 'slouch' posture and relaxing movements to relieve tension.

The content of the lesson, which should be lively, interesting and enjoyable, may have to be adapted not only to the ability of the group members, but to far from ideal conditions. The teacher may have to use her ingenuity. Versatility will ensure that interest is maintained and that the training effect is comprehensive. There must be a sound purpose behind all that is selected and taught.

LABAN'S PRINCIPLES

One method of movement training which is being taught increasingly in special schools is that based on Laban's principles.

Veronica Sherborne, Senior Lecturer in the Faculty of Education at Bristol Polytechnic, who has for twenty years been training teachers of mentally handicapped children, has developed ways of using these principles for such children and is now introducing them in a sub-normality hospital and an adult training centre. Briefly, her aims, which are equally valid for mentally handicapped adults, are to help develop mentally retarded children to experience ways of moving which they have missed and which are necessary if they are to acquire sensory awareness of their bodies and the ability to be aware of other people and form relationships.

'Feeding in' body awareness

The parts of the body which it is most important that the retarded person should become aware of are those which bear weight, particularly the knees, and the centre of the body, the trunk. Initially, much of the work involves using the floor, or mats, as a surface against which the retarded can experience the body in such activities as rolling and sliding. Many ways of 'feeding in' bodily experiences, both of parts of the body and the body as a whole, are described in *Physical and creative activities for mentally handicapped children* (see Further Reading, p. 112).

Development of relationships

The different kinds of relationship play include ways of giving support and of being supported; the use of free flow experiences such as sliding, rocking and swinging; containing and being contained; and a variety of ways of experiencing the control of strength through pushing against or pushing a partner.

Relationship play can be adjusted to the individual, ranging from work with the severely retarded — who appear to make no response to activities — to those who can take responsibility for the care of a partner. Finally, many adults and children can collaborate in groups of three or more. This aspect of movement teaching is described in detail in *Physical education for children with special needs* (see Further Reading, p. 112).

The movement activities are presented in an enjoyable way, and the movement teacher, and any helpers, should join in the sessions. Veronica Sherborne's methods can be adapted to the needs of hyperactive people, to those with autistic tendencies, and to those who are multiply handicapped.

It is essential for the teacher using these methods to have had personal experience of developing his or her own bodily awareness and of building relationships. Although Veronica Sherborne's approach is essentially very simple, it requires intelligence, intuition and considerable powers of observation as well as experience in working with mentally handicapped children or adults.

New developments

In the sub-normality hospital Veronica Sherborne is working with a multi-disciplinary group of nurses, physiotherapists, occupational therapists, speech therapists, aides and teachers from the hospital school. Movement plays an important part in the school programme, and nurses and therapists, working together, are experimenting in using movement with some of their patients.

In the Adult Training Centre it is the deputy manager, trained under her, who is responsible for the movement training, and the results are already most encouraging. These developments under Veronica Sherborne's guidance are proving valuable in linking the work in special schools with the adult training centre and hospital programme (Groves and Upton p. 112).

Although the plan of a lesson will vary with the principles of the particular system of movement and fitness training followed, the following outline of a lesson and examples of movements may be helpful to those with little specialist knowledge and experience.

AN EXAMPLE OF A BASIC MOVEMENT LESSON

Since the length of lessons, the ability of class members and other factors will vary (whether they take place in hospitals, adult training centres and clubs) the content must be flexible, but should include:

Movements

1. **A warming up activity** to prepare the group members for the lesson.
2. **General body movement** i.e. movement of the whole body with emphasis on one or more body parts.
3. **Movements** designed to strengthen the muscle groups — (a) extending the joints (particularly those of the spine); (b) of the abdominal wall.
4. **Group activities**

NOTE: (2) and (3) can be performed in standing, sitting or lying positions. Foot and hand movements can be included in any part of the lesson. More time should be spent on (3) and (4) than on (1) and (2).

A lesson can be varied by including: the use of hand apparatus — hoops, balls, clubs, scarves, ribbons; the use of fixed or portable gymnastic apparatus — benches, ladders, beams, box, climbing apparatus and agility activities using mats; a national or other form of dance at the end; training ending with a game or relay; the movement training principles of one of the organisations listed in Appendix 3 (see pp. 184-185).

EXAMPLES OF MOVEMENTS WITH EMPHASIS ON DIFFERENT BODY PARTS

Warming up activities

1. Run a little way and stop still
   Run further, stop and curl up small near the floor.
   Run again, stop. Arms stretched high — V-shape — wide stretch.
2. Stand with feet a little way aprt — knees easy
   See how many parts of the body you can slap lightly — knees, thight, back, chest, shoulders, head, toes, ankles, backs of legs, neck.
   Variation: use a light springy touch instead of a slap.

3. Stand or sit, rub the arms, hands, thighs, shoulders, legs, feet.

4. Shrug shoulders up and hold, down and hold, up down, up down. Circle shoulders singly and together vigorously.

Movements with emphasis on the shoulder girdle

1. In any starting position, trace various patterns with the hand in front of the body, e.g. '0', 2, 3, and to the side. **Variation:** lead with the elbow instead of the hand.

2. In any starting position, clap the hands lightly in any direction round the body, concentrating on the outward movement after the clap, and varying the levels above the shoulder.

3. Sitting or sitting on heels: beat a strong rhythm with the fists on the floor in a wide circle, then stretch both arms slowly in any direction. Gradually change the level of movement by reaching higher during each stretch.

Movements with emphasis on hip girdle

1. Standing, with one knee leading, circle it towards the supporting leg and outward — draw a circle with the knee.

2. Step with wide steps in different directions across, behind, sideways, cross behind, diagonally forward and back; each leg in turn and then alternately. Trace a variety of shapes on the floor.

3. In various kneeling, sitting and lying positions, draw one knee up to the chin then stretch it away from the body in various directions. Vary the speed of the movement, changing legs and starting positions.

4. Standing in lines or pairs (hold hands lightly for support) swing left leg forward and back — keep the body upright and the supporting knee straight. Change legs — change to swing back and forward.
   Variation: Swing right leg forward and back — repeat (1-4). Step right, left, right, lift left leg behind ready to swing (5-8). Repeat, swinging left leg — repeat 1-8 continuously. This can be performed moving up the room.

5. **'Walking'** Sit upright, legs stretched in front, hands relaxed on knees. 'Walk' forwards and backwards from the hip joint, bouncing off the seat. Lift and push right leg forward past the right. Repeat these 'walking' steps rhythmically with the music.
   16 forwards and 16 backwards, then cut down to shorter phases of 8 or even 4.
   Note: The effort of sitting upright is often difficult; give a short rest in between turns.

6. **Rocking**
   Sit upright, the palms of the hands resting on the floor at the sides. Rock rhythmically from side to side, taking weight alternately on each side.

Movements with emphasis on the whole spine and abdominal muscles

1. Sitting with legs apart, knees slightly bent, turn to the right, left arm reaching forward and downward to touch the floor as far outside the right foot as possible (1), return to sitting position (2). 'Stretch up tall', repeat 3 times (3-8), repeat turning to the opposite side (9-16).
   Variations: (i) 2 turns to each side; (ii) alternately right and left.

2. Lying, draw one knee up and stretch it out. Repeat with alternate legs, with both legs together. Vary direction and level.

3. Sitting with one leg straight and one leg bent up, change the position of legs at different speeds — lift the legs as they change. Use hands as support; later repeat exercise without support of hands.

4. In any starting position, draw circles with the arms in all directions round the body; small quick circles, large slow circles, circular floor patterns, arms singly and arms together. Facing a partner, shadow the other's movement with variations of speed, strength and levels. Other shapes can be invented.

5. Lying on the back, with the arms stretched out in a low V, palms upwards, slowly stretch arms up to a high V, keeping backs of hands on the floor, stretch the legs, and point the toes. Hold this position for 8 counts. Slowly curl up onto one side into as small and round a shape as possible for 8 counts.

Foot movements

Foot movements can be introduced at any stage in the lesson except immediately before or after movements involving strong use of the feet.

1. Move each joint in the feet separately: (i) lift heel and lower — keep toes on the floor; (ii) lift heel, then the whole foot to stretch the toes, but keep contact with the floor; (iii) lift the whole foot off the floor through stages (i) and (ii) 'peeling off'. Repeat each stage several times; develop into running on the spot.

2. (i) Sitting down, bend and stretch the ankles alternately and together — pull the toes up — stretch them down; (ii) cross one leg over the other at the ankle, ankle circling outwards; repeat with other foot — repeat circling inwards — encourage the drawing of a large 'O' with the big toe.

3. Sitting — open and close the toes.

   Different combinations of the last three movements can be made into short sequences.

4. Suggest simple movements involving changing the weight from one foot to the other in various directions, forwards — backwards, diagonally forwards and backwards — sideways — across in front and behind.

5. Walk on toes.

6. Walk quickly, slowly, quietly, loudly, with short and long steps, stamp. Combine any two, e.g.: (i) 4 long steps followed by 8 short steps; (ii) stamp (1-4) walk quietly (1-4); (iii) walk on toes (1-4), walk with short steps (5-8); (iv) walk quietly (1-4). Stamp on the spot (5-8).

7.   Practise dance steps, e.g. skip, polka, slip.

Hand movements

1.   Clench fingers tightly. Open hands sharply and fully. Repeat, slowly clenching the fingers and slowly stretching them apart.

2.   Shake the hands freely in different directions and levels, encourage relaxation in the wrist.

3.   Sit on the floor — play on imaginary instrument, encouraging individual use of the fingers.

4.   Kneel or sit — pretend to 'glue' the palms of the hands onto the floor. Slowly peel the hands off and away, lifting the wrist and palms first then the fingers. Chant: 'Stick, lift, stick lift.'
     Repeat this movement but 'glue' the hands together or to parts of the body, e.g. to the legs, sides. Chant: 'Push it away'.

5.   Sit or stand, stretch hands: (i) move first finger to thumb, repeat with the other three fingers; (ii) play a five finger exercise in the air or on the floor. Repeat (i) but when each finger in turn is touching the thumb, press together gently. Chant: 'Touch and press', 'touch and press'. Can the thumb touch all the fingers together?

6.   Circle the wrist outwards and inwards, keeping the elbows to the sides. Stretch arms forwards, palms turned to face the floor. Turn palms up and down continuously.

7.   Sit or stand, pretend there is a door in front, push it open. Encourage the palms and fingers to be stretched before pushing.

   Composite lesson. A short warming up period of general exercise selected for example from the above movements — one or two from each section — can be followed by a dance(s), game(s), movements using balls, hoops or scarves or simple gymnastic agilities.

MUSICAL ACCOMPANIMENT AND SELECTION OF MUSIC FOR MOVEMENT TRAINING

Accompaniment

   Accompaniment can either be provided by the teacher's voice, piano, recorded music (record and tapes) or by a percussion instrument. A steady pulsating rhythmic beat will help the trainee develop more feeling for movement. In creative work, it will enhance movement, quality and expression. The music so 'reinforces' the movement that, as soon as a particular tune is played, the trainee may well perform a specific movement automatically. Include where possible music selected by class members; perhpas some members could produce their favourite tune to which a special movement sequence could be devised for all to perform. Music should help the class to improve their performance as well as providing enjoyment. It should help them to move more lightly on their feet, swing their limbs more freely and give them a feeling of stretch or poise where necessary. To achieve this, suitable tunes must be chosen to fit the movement: i.e. for their rhythm — smooth, dotted or swinging, pattern — rise and fall of melody, number of phrases — and for their character — heavy or light, sharp, flowing.

Voice

   The teacher's voice is all-important: by giving clear explanations and indicating the rhythm, speed and quality of the movement, both to the class members and to a pianist, when one is available, the teacher can create the right atmosphere in the class. The teacher can use words to encourage, prompt and coach by chanting them in time with the music.

Piano

   Played by a good pianist who can improvise for different movements, the piano accompaniment is perhaps the ideal. The advantages of using a pianist are:

(i)   the continuity of the lesson is more easily maintained since the teacher is not involved with records and tapes;

(ii)   the speed of the music can be varied, the quality of movement enhanced;

(iii) a greater variety of tunes can be used;

(iv)   adaptations can be made on the spot.

Percussion

   The most useful percussion instruments include clappers, cymbals, tambourines, drums, triangles and a tunable tambour with a round headed beater. Simple percussion instruments can be improvised and made quite cheaply. A beat can be indicated by tapping two sticks together.

Recorded music — Tapes and records

   Recorded music is less suitable because the speed cannot be varied and the phrasing is often not consistent throughout the record. Non-vocal records are generally more suitable since the rhythm is clearer. It is also difficult to teach the component parts of the movement using the music as the teacher cannot be continually putting the record on and off in order to correct and coach details. With the help of a good pianist, tapes can be made of a selection of suitable music for simple movement sequences including pauses during which the teacher can prompt and coach. After a pause, the music can be repeated at a slower or quicker speed as necessary; in fact, a tape can be 'tailor-made'.

   If a pianist or musician who can improvise is not available, well known tunes can be used but only if they are simple and their tempo is suitable to the movement; complicated music will tend to dominate the movement.

Music for movements of different types

   Skipping — 6/8: for skipping, galloping, pas-de-bas steps and jumps, e.g. '100 Pipers', 'The Lancashire Poacher'.

   Walking — 4/4: many familiar marches, provided they are played without too marked an accent, e.g. 'Waltzing Matilda'.

Running — 2/4: 2 runs to a bar, e.g. 'Bobby Shaftoe'.

Swinging — 6/8: continuous rhythm, e.g. 'Skye Boat Song'.

Swinging — 6/8: with accent, e.g. 'My Bonnie Lies Over the ocean'.

Swinging — 3/4: triple runs — lilts, e.g. Many Chopin waltzes.

Sharp, light — 2/4: e.g. 'This Old Man' — 6/8 e.g. 'Bonnie Dundee' 'Little Brown Jug'.

Smooth, flowing — 4/4: e.g. 'All Through the Night', 3/4 'The Ash Grove'.

Strong sustained — 4/4: e.g. 'The Volga Boat Song', 'Old Man River'.

Beaten, accented — 4/4: e.g. 'John Brown's Body'.

Combined swinging and stretching — e.g. 6/8 'Blow the Man Down', 'Rio Grande'.

Combined beating and lifting — 6/8 e.g. 'Girls and Boys Come out to Play'.

Polka — 'See me Dance the Polka'.

Waltz — Strauss waltzes.

Mazurka — Mazurka from Coppelia.

Rope skipping — syncopated 4/4: e.g. 'Scatterbrain'.

TWO LESSONS BASED ON MEDAU RHYTHMIC MOVEMENT

Two lessons based on Medau Rhythmic Movement are included for the following reasons:

to show the simple stages through which movements are built up over a period of time;

to show how hand apparatus, balls, hoops and scarves can be used to aid the movement and to add variety and interest.

The following sequences using a ball, hoop or scarf can be memorised and used for a display or be introduced into the ordinary lesson.

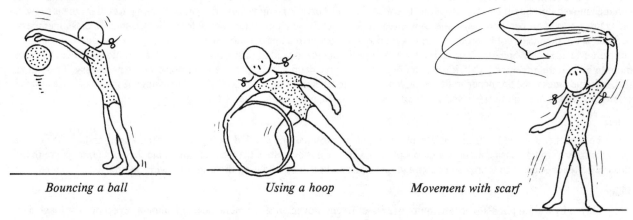

Bouncing a ball   Using a hoop   Movement with scarf

Lesson 1.

Opening activities

1. Clapping and stamping.
   Stand in a space. Clap hands in any direction e.g. towards the ceiling, the windows, the floor. Clap hands 4 times moving arms to full stretch followed by 4 claps on the knees.
   Repeat No. 2. 4 claps in any direction and 4 claps touching either knees, calves, ankles. Repeat clapping upwards with 3 claps and stretch higher on the 4th beat, bend to clap over the knees 3 times. Stamp feet 8 times lifting the knees up high.
   Repeat clapping as in No. 4, then 4 stamps facing front, 4 stamps to turn around on the spot.

2. Transfer of weight with body swings and partner work. Stand with feet apart, weight on the right foot, swing body and arms to the left, right and left, and clap out to the left side. Repeat to the right.
   Partners face each other, with one hand joined and weight to the same side, swing arms to transfer the weight from side to side with a swinging action in the legs and hips. Repeat all with the other hand joined. Partners face each other as in 7, swing across and out, swing across and run forward with partner side by side. At the end of the phrase change hands and repeat.

3. Walking and running.
   Following a leader, walk and run according to the rhythm of the music.

   Main section (with a ball, 17.8 cm (7″) diameter, 0.5 kg (1 lb) weight).
Aim: To exercise the whole body rhythmically, encouraging a stretch through the body.

1. Sit on the floor in a circle, with legs wide apart and the ball between them. Hit the top of the ball with the palm of the hand using alternate hands to a given rhythm.
   Repeat making a fist with the hand on the slow beats and using fingers on the quick beats.
   Repeat making a fist with the hand on the slow beats and rolling ball away from the body and back on the quick beats.
   Repeat above movement with the ball by the side of one hip keeping a hand on the ball; roll it as far sideways as possible and back again. Repeat to the other side.

Sit with the legs apart, the ball by the right hip. Roll the ball down outside of right leg round the feet, and up the inside of the right leg. Then roll down the inside of the left leg around the foot and up the outside of the left leg to finish by the left hip. Repeat in reverse.

Repeat No. 4 but as ball reaches the left hip, continue to roll it behind the back and change hands behind the back, finish with the ball by right hip.

2.   Sit with legs wide apart, bounce the ball — a continuous movement keeping hands on top of the ball.
Repeat, bouncing the ball with both hands, also 1 hand at a time.
Bounce ball 4 times, followed by one strong bounce, stretch up towards the ball and catch.
Bounce the ball, gradually changing to standing whilst bouncing. If this is too difficult, stand up and then start to bounce.
Bounce, roll and catch with partner.

3.   Stand with a ball facing a partner, bounce the ball for the partner to catch. Encourage a good stretch through body.
Face partner. Strong bounce across to partner, who catches the ball, and bounces it back to partner. Bend down and roll the ball across to partner who picks it up.
Face partner — a little distance away. One partner rolls the ball across to the other who bends the knees to pick it up and throw it upwards and across to partner. Repeat the movement with the other partner starting the roll.
One ball each, start from the end of the hall. Bend and roll ball forward, run by the side of the ball as it rolls, overtake it to come in front of the ball, bend and pick it up into a throw, stretch and catch. Repeat movement to continue rolling ball down the hall.

4.   Walking — bouncing a ball continuously.
Collect the balls by throwing them into a large bag held open by 2 class members.

Final Section. Aim: To encourage mobility in hip joints and a feeling of spring.

1.   Stand in a circle with hands joined. Stand on left leg, swing right leg forward and back, 3 times, stamp right, left, right. Repeat leg swinging on right leg.

2.   Step forward on right leg, swing left knee up high, and step back on left leg, back on right leg. Repeat on left leg.
Repeat 2, swinging the knee out to the side.

3.   In a circle, a wide step to the right, close left foot to right; repeat to the right 3 times; repeat all to the left.

4.   Gallop to the right for 8, repeat to the left.

5.   Facing a partner, hands joined, repeat gallop step sideways, adding a variety of claps or stamps.

Teaching. When **bouncing the ball,** follow the bounce with the body to give a feeling of resilience or elasticity. Keep the hands on top of the ball to give a feeling of drawing the ball up like a yo-yo.

When **throwing the ball,** stretch towards it with arms and body before catching.

When **rolling the ball,** bend the knees, keep the seat down, with a long back.

Lesson 2. Using a hoop. 61cm-76.2cm (24-30′) diameter.

Opening activity (warm-up). Stand with hands joined in a circle.

1.   12 walking steps to the right. 4 stamps with alternate feet, and on the spot turning to face the opposite direction.
12 walking steps to the left. 4 stamps on the spot. Repeat taking longer steps to the right, 12 steps. Stamp alternate feet 3 times — rhythm: quick, quick, slow.
Repeat walking to the right.
Repeat this phrase walking and stamping to the left.
Practise the rhythm with hand clapping and stamping separately — quick, quick, slow.
Repeat to the left: finish facing the centre of the circle.
6 walks forward to the centre of the circle, clap hands — quick, quick, slow.
6 walks backwards, clap hands — quick,quick, slow.

2.   Combine the two movements as follows:
In a circle with hands joined.
6 walks to the right and 3 stamps — quick, quick, slow. Repeat to the left.
6 walks into the centre, 3 claps — quick, quick, slow.
6 walks away from the centre, 3 claps — quick, quick, slow.

3.   Repeat 2 with running steps.

Main section (with a hoop). Aim: Work with a hoop to increase the mobility of the spine, to twist, stretch and curl it.
Stand inside the hoop holding it with one hand on each side, with straight arms.

1.   Turn the hoop so that one hand comes forward and the other back, the body twisting at the same time, twist back to the starting position. Repeat in the opposite direction.
Repeat so that it is a continuous twisting first to one side then the other — twist and a twist and a twist

2.   Repeat twist 4 times.
Lift hoop vertically up to stretch to the ceiling. Lower hoop over the body to the starting position. Repeat.

3.   Repeat twist 4 times.
Lower hoop to put it onto the floor, slowly. Stand up without hoop and stretch both arms to the ceiling.
Bending knees and keeping back long, pick up the hoop and return to original starting position.

4.   Repeat twist 4 times.
      Lift hoop down over the body and bend to lower the hoop to within a few inches of the floor. Return to original starting position.

5.   Partners standing side by side with one hoop; one partner holding the top of the hoop in a vertical position with the lower edge of it on the floor. The partner without the hoop bends down to crawl through it, returning to standing position to take the hoop for the other partner to crawl through. The movement could be done to a set rhythm, add rhythmical clapping after crawling through the hoop and before holding it for the partner to repeat the movement.

6.   One partner holds the hoop as in 5, with feet apart and weight to one side, with a swinging action through the legs and hips, gently roll the hoop from side to side 4 times.
      Hold the hoop still whilst the partner bends to crawl through it and to take the hoop for the other partner to repeat the rolling from side to side.

7.   Each person with a hoop. Start from one end of the hall. Roll the hoop from side to side with a swinging action in the legs, as in 6, 4 times, followed by rolling the hoop forward. Run with it to catch it — 'roll — roll — roll — roll run — run — run and catch'. Repeat continuously.

8.   Roll hoop running with it, clap a short rhythm before catching it and repeating the movement.

Floor section. Aim: to encourage mobility of the spine.

1.   Hoop flat on floor. Sit in it with feet outside, with alternate hands, reach out to touch the hoop in different places, so twisting the body e.g. touch in front, at the side, behind, sitting as before. With right hand, touch in front, twist and touch on left side, twist further and touch towards the back and come back to original position.
      Tap the floor with a simple rhythm.
      Repeat with the other hand.

2.   Sit behind the hoop — flat on floor — reach to touch different parts of the hoop. With alternate hands, stretch 4 times and tap a simple rhythm on the floor, with hands in the middle of the hoop to end of phrase. Repeat, stretching alternate legs so that the foot touches different parts of the hoop, then tap a simple rhythm with the feet.

3.   Sit slightly sideways to the hoop with legs to one side. Trace the shape of the hoop using one foot, repeat with the other foot. Continue to trace the shape of the hoop, using the hand and arm or foot and leg as if painting the hoop.

Final section Standing in a circle.

1.   Stand on the right leg in a circle with hands joined, tap the floor in front with the left heel, then left toe twice, feet together and pause. Repeat with the right heel and toe.

2.   Heel and toe with right foot stamp right, stamp left, stamp right — quick, quick, slow. Repeat left.

3.   Stand on right leg with left leg stretched forward. Make a large 'pawing' movement with the left leg twice and stamp, stamp, stamp, — quick, quick, slow. Repeat with the other leg.

4.   Partners side by side travel up the hall. Repeat 3 once with right leg and walk forward for 8 steps. Repeat movement with the left leg.

5.   Walking, either following a leader or with a partner, change to a phrase of running and return to a phrase of walking — change to a phrase of skipping and return to a phrase of walking.

SEQUENCES OF MOVEMENTS USING BALLS, HOOPS, SCARVES OR RIBBONS

Movement sequences are only suitable for more able trainees/residents. Teach each movement separately and then combine them in any order, gradually working towards a sequence of all the movements.

1.   Music of 'Eye Level' or a similar rhythm. Bounce ball 8 times, followed by strong bounce, stretch catch, strong bounce, stretch catch.
      Repeat 3 times.

2.   Hold the ball in both hands, feet abpart and weight to one side.
      Swing changing weight from one side to the other 4 times; swing the ball into a large circle and swing.
      Swing the ball into a large circle and swing.
      Repeat.

3.   With feet together: throw ball up, stretch and catch
      bend to put ball on the floor
      clap hands upwards towards ceiling (clap, clap, clap)
      bend to pick up ball.
      Repeat.

4.   Repeat the 1st movement again.

A sequence of movements with a hoop. Music: 3/4 e.g. 'Edelweiss'.

1.   In two's face partner, partners hold hoop horizontally between them, with hands under the hoop and at the sides. Weight to one side, swing, changing the weight from side to side, 6 times then slowly swing and lift the hoop up high, turning under it as if to turn the hoop right over — pancake turn.
      Repeat. Finish holding the hoop horizontally with right hand.

2. Waltz steps (1, 2, 3) round each other in a clockwise direction, slightly pulling away from the hoop, then change hands. Repeat waltz steps in an anti-clockwise direction. Repeat.

   Finish with one of the partners holding the hoop in a vertical position with the edge of the hoop on the floor.

3. Twist and spin the hoop in a vertical position, both partners run round the spinning hoop — finish in original places. While one catches the hoop, replaces it on the floor and spins it again, the other partner claps hands to the rhythm of the music. Repeat, the other partner catching the hoop.

   Finish holding the hoop flat between partners as in 1, ready to repeat the sequence.

Movements with scarves or ribbons

These movements are suitable for and enjoyed by mentally handicapped people. Scarves — one metre square. **Big** scarf movements can increase the range of movement. Holding the scarf by the corner, make the following movements:

1. swing it from side to side or back and forward;

2. make circles in front, at the side and around the body, also above the head;

3. run, trailing the scarf;

4. for dexterity: fold the scarf with both hands, or one hand only;

   screw it up in one hand and throw it high;

   watch it as it floats down;

5. use it as an obstacle for stepping over;

6. dance with the scarf (own interpretation) while a pianist plays various styles of music, e.g. Spanish, Ballet, Can-Can, gypsy.

A KEEP FIT LESSON INCLUDING HAND APPARATUS

The Keep Fit lesson at the Chelmsford Adult Training Centre is taken by a member of the centre staff who is also a keep fit teacher. Through the experience of working in two centres, she has found that the following type of lesson is both educationally and socially beneficial.

Part 1

General warming up and intermingling using lively music to stimulate and setting the mood for the lesson.

1. Walking in any direction using the whole space. Sixteen walking steps, finish with feet apart, sway right, left — feet apart. Four slip steps to right, sway left, sway right. Four slip steps to the left, sway right, sway left.

   Repeat.

2. Walk 16 steps to meet a partner, finish with feet apart, side by side holding inside hand.

   Sway right, left — feet apart (1-4). Repeat 6 times (5-16).

   Repeat to meet another partner.

   Variation: (a) Sway facing partner with both hands joined. (b) Substitute slipping steps sideways for swaying.

Part 2

Using small apparatus.

Hoops

1. Standing with feet together, hoop held undergrasp in right hand and out to the side.

   Swing hoop in front to the left and to right continuously, repeat with left hand.

   Variation: (i) Repeat swing with right hand (1-6), pass hoop into left hand and out to the left side (7-8). (ii) Repeat exchanging the hoop overhead (7-8). (iii) Repeat with feet apart and swaying from foot to foot.

2. Standing with feet apart, holding hoop in front and parallel to the ground with both hands.

   Swing hoop across body to left, swaying from right to left foot, repeat to right repeat continuously left and right — increase the width of the swing.

3. Sitting on floor with feet on right hand side. Holding hoop on floor in front — palms facing upwards. Lift hoop in fornt and high towards ceiling. Lower hoop over head to touch floor behind. Return slowly, pausing overhead, with a high stretch and lowering hoop to floor in front.

Balls

1. Stand with feet apart holding ball in right hand. Throw ball from right hand into left hand and back, continuously.

2. With feet together, throw ball up and catch four times (1-8).

   Pass ball at waist level around body, twice (9-16).

   Repeat throw and catch (1-8).

   Repeat passing ball round body in the opposite direction (9-16) 4 times. Suggested tune 'Eye Level'.

Streamers (made from short dowelling rods 250mm (10″) long with streamers of ribbon or crepe paper 50mm (2″) and 1.5 m (60″) long). This part of the lesson encourages class members to make up their own movement patterns, the only instruction being a verbal reminder that there are different 'levels' to move in, i.e. low, medium and high, and that one can balance on different parts of the body, e.g. left or right side, left or right knee, both knees, sitting, lying, using both hands in turn to manipulate the streamer. Each member should decide on their own starting and finishing positions.

Suggested music: Slow waltz-time.

Part 3

Calming down, relaxing period.

Suggested music: waltz-time.

8 waltz steps anywhere in the room — 8 bars (1 step to 1 bar).

Raise both arms to shoulder level — 2 bars.

Lower to sides — 2 bars.

Relax head and shoulders forwards — 2 bars.

Stretch to standing position — 2 bars.

Repeat several times.

Variation: Single or double arm raising sideways, forwards or upwards, downwards in any combination of directions.

TWO EXAMPLES OF KEEP FIT IN HOSPITALS

Keep Fit at Manor Hospital, Aylesbury (demonstration team)

In 1971 the Manor House Hospital in Aylesbury approached the Buckinghamshire Keep Fit Association for a teacher to take a keep fit class with a group of young women resident in the hostel attached to the hospital. Two teachers volunteered They started with a group of 8 young women termed moderately and severely mentally handicapped, their ages ranging from 22 to 37 years. From the beginning all wore white shorts, yellow cotton shirts and white plimsoles.

Progress. At first only very simple movements were taught in a circle formation and singing action games. After some weeks, 6 young men joined the group and the lesson was adapted to include not only keep fit exercises but country dancing which provided opportunity for social training. Gradually hand apparatus was introduced — hoops, clubs, scarves and ropes. Later, special attention was given to freedom of expression at one stage in the lesson. The teachers were surprised to see how the class remembered what had been taught, and how well they were able to make up movements of their own. Later the boys were involved in outside rehabilitation training, and were too late back to join in. More young women joined the class bringing the numbers up to 12. They responded well to the music and greatly enjoyed moving. After a visit to one of the Keep Fit Association functions, they asked to wear leotards. The hospital fitted them out with black ones, which they wore with their ordinary tights and plimsoles. They were not yet prepared to work with bare feet.

Demonstrations. The group have given demonstrations at various functions with great enjoyment. Their latest demonstration is performed with scarves 1 metre square in all shades of blue green. Not only does this group demonstrate the pathway or pattern of the movements but also strength and lightness and other qualities of movement. (Details of this scarf sequence re. end of section). Each member of the group was a member of the Buckinghamshire Keep Fit Association.

Integration. Members of the teachers' other keep fit classes have shown interest by helping to teach the young women health care and the art of make-up and grooming. Each summer the teacher invites the group to a country party in her cottage, and at Christmas the other teacher arranges a party for them in Aylesbury.

Co-operation. Much can be achieved when there is co-operation between the hospital and hostel staff and the outside world; a second class has now started for a group of overweight young women. This is being taken by 2 members of a keep fit class (one a teacher) under guidance. Being more severely handicapped they need greater persuasion to join in but progress is being made.

The teachers say: 'After 7 years we are delighted with the results, and really enjoy the work. If others could help in the same way elsewhere, they would find it most rewarding and interesting'.

Spin-offs. These women have acquired poise, walk well, become more sociable, outgoing and friendly, and have made friends in the community. They have been stretched to demonstration standard, enabling them to show their enthusiasm and achievement to others. There has been improvement in their health and fitness and in their appearance — considerable loss of weight was a must for most of them if they were to wear leotards and tights.

A number of people in the community understand more about mental handicap and that mentally handicapped people **can** keep fit and, given time and patient teaching, **can** achieve a good standard.

Demonstration Using Scarves

Music: 'Love can make you happy' or a tune like 'Somewhere over the Rainbow' (Record MER 313 - 'Cocktail Piano'). Once through was found to be insufficient therefore a repetition of this music minus the introduction was added to the tape.

Scarves: 1 yard square nylon material in shades of blue green, from light to dark. The women wear black leotards and tights.

Formation: In a circle all facing anti-clockwise.

Starting position: Hold scarf square on with both hands, left hand to centre waist and right arm extended to right side — weight on the right foot. After 4 bars of introductory music has been played:

1. Swing right arm round and across to left — transferring the weight on to the left foot (bars 1-2). Repeat swing in the opposite direction (bars 3-4). Repeat twice more, 3 times in all (bars 5-12). Turn on the spot to the left and finish facing the centre of the circle (bars 13-16).

2. With right hand hold the scarf by one corner. Run into the centre of circle throwing scarf up high (flames) (bars 1-2). Run out backwards dragging scarf low (bars 3-4). Repeat in and out three times, running to finish (bars 5-16) in a space.

3. Throw scarf overhead from right to left slowly to touch floor 3 times (bars 1-16). Finish sitting or kneeling in various ways on the floor.

4. Each performer improvises with slow scarf movements e.g. swing scarf round head. All forms of stretching in various directions, with various scarf holds. At the end of the phrase run into groups, i.e. lines of 4 or 5 holding scarf by one corner with righ hand giving opposite corner to the performer on the right, joining into a line (bars 1-16). The number of bars of music used becomes flexible here, allowing time to get a strong feeling in the stretch.

5. Each line runs in an open circle, stop. The leader threads a little way through an arch made by the last two in the line, all stretch strongly in various directions keeping hold of the scarf. Return to open circle. Repeat starting from the opposite end of the line. Repeat both threading sequences again.
   Having opened out, all join up in one single circle linked to one another by scarves.

6. Walk into the cente of the circle raising arms up high. Turn on the spot to face out lowering arms overhead to end with them crossed low in front. Lift arms and scarves up to face centre again, opening arms up and out.
   Repeat.
   Leader drops right hand hold and runs to lead into a 'maze'. Unwind 'maze' and run off. Music is 'faded out', as last person exits.

NOTE: Illustrate directions to aid memory e.g. 'flames' of a fire, when running in, 'over the moon' for alternate side bends, 'flowers growing in the garden' when sitting down, go to 'Jennifer's house', 'Sylvia's house' to indicate to which line to run.

Keep Fit at Harperbury Hospital

In 1960, at the instigation of a parent of one of the long-term patients, a keep fit class came into being at Harperbury Hospital, Hertfordshire. The mother was not only concerned for her own daughter, now too handicapped to move, but for the many others becoming more apathetic and immobile each day. At first she took the class herself, doing everything to encourage and stimulate the patients in her daughter's ward. She realised that someone with 'knowledge of movement' should take the class and she consequently approached a keep fit teacher.

A challenge. The teacher accepted the challenge, although she had never had any previous contact with mentally handicapped people. After the first lesson she knew she wanted to continue and for three years she took the class single-handed with the help of a 78-year-old pianist. she says: 'It was hard going but I won the patients' affection and when I achieved, through coaxing, some movement from them, they were as happy with themselves as I was with them. I knew by then that this could go on throughout the hospital if I could first gain the co-operation of the staff and, secondly, gather in some of my keep fit colleagues. I managed to find a team of 16. We covered all the wards in the female wing and a few of the children's wards. The sisters of the wards did not accept the scheme very easily, but with the Matron's support, most of the sisters soon became our friends'.

More involvement. For another four years the teachers visited the hospital every Wednesday, the residents eagerly awaiting the visits. The teachers packed and delivered Christmas parcels for all the female patients in the hospital; this has continued each year with the support of hundreds of members of the Middlesex Keep Fit Association and has now been extended to some of the male wards.

Educational rhythmics. In 1969 the teacher attended a course in Educational Rhythmics for Mentally and Physically Handicapped People, under Ferris and Jennet Robins. She came away with many new ideas but needing equipment and records with which to implement them. The Lions gave £25, and with this the records and small apparatus, such as tambourines, were bought; the teacher made her own coloured flags and a large wooden clock. HMV provided a record player. The patients responded well to this different approach — over a period of time they were able to move and sing a rhythm at the same time — pick out colours and use their arms as the hands of a clock.
'By now our reward was tremendous — I say 'our' as I encouraged my colleagues to take my class and to work on the new method'.
She herself then worked in the wards where the patients were more severely handicapped.

Co-ordinator of voluntary services. During the past few years a 'Co-ordinator of voluntary services' has joined the hospital staff and now all voluntary workers are welcomed and directed. The classes continue with as much enthusiasm as ever, as do the Christmas parcels and entertainment by the Middlesex Keep Fit Association each year.

FITNESS TRAINING
FITNESS TRAINING EXERCISES

These exercises generally include training techniques for specific sports. If the training programmes are carefully prepared according to the likes and dislikes and the ability of the group members, it can be enjoyed equally by men, women and men and women together.

A lesson

Limbering and warming up exercises. Before taking part in any exercise, particularly of a strenuous nature, the body should be 'warmed up' to prevent unnecessary strain. Limbering exercises are often seen being practised by athletes, footballers, gymnasts and dancers on television. The trainees or residents like to associate themselves with the 'stars' and as a result more willingly take part in these movements without too much explanation.

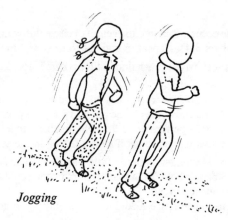

Jogging

1. **Jogging.** Run on the spot, lifting the knees high using the arms in a natural way — jog in different directions — once the beat can be maintained, introduce a simple pattern: 8 forwards, 8 backwards, 8 turning or chalk a pattern on the ground e.g. letters of their names — diamonds — triangles — squares and circles. This will enable the class to jog for a longer period and add interest. At the end of the jogging, pause for breathing to be restored to normal.

Those who cannot jog can sit or stand and lift alternate knees up and down or, if they are mobile, walk along the patterns and, if necessary, be given help to change direction.

2. **Galloping** (slip steps). Galloping develops spring, speed and quick change of direction, e.g.
8 gallops to right — repeat left
4 gallops to right — repeat left
2 gallops to right — repeat left
Gallops combined with jogging or springs; e.g.
(i)   8 jogs forwards — 8 jogs backwards
(ii)   4 gallops right — 4 gallops left repeat
(iii) 8 gallops right followed by 8 low springs on the spot with feet together.

3. **Stride jumps.** Stride jumps develop spring, co-ordination and balance; e.g.
continuous stride jumping, slowly and quickly.
Chant: Out rebound — in rebound — slow
            Out in — out in — quick.
Jumps can alternate with clapping in different directions on the spot.

Body movements

1. **Back rocks.** Sit on a mat with knees bent up, arms round the knees with fingers interlinked. Rock backwards onto the mat, uncurling the spine (head last), push up and rock forward. If the swing is broken and the momentum is lost it is difficult to rock forwards again. Take the movement slowly at first, then gradually quicken it.

2. **Side rocks.** Lie on the mat with knees bent onto the chest and elbows in at the waist with hands clasped on the chest. Rock onto right side maintaining a curled up position. As soon as the right side is in contact with the floor, push off and roll over onto the left side. This movement should be taken smoothly as many people are disorientated when lying down. It is helpful to chant instructions such as: 'to the door, to the clock' or 'right side, left side'. If the arms remain on the chest there is no chance of them being squashed.

N.B. These movements are necessary, particularly if simple vaulting or forward rolls are to be attempted, with a relaxed landing.

3. **Sit ups.** This is an easy introduction to a series of movements designed to strengthen the abdominal muscles. Work with partners suitably matched. A is the worker, B is the helper. A lies on his back with hands on the floor at the side. B, firmly but without squeezing, holds A's ankles to prevent him raising his legs whilst he is moving. A lifts his head forward and gradually sits up, keeping his legs in contact with the floor. He uncurls gently to lying position, being careful not to bang his head. Repeat with B working and A helping.

Note: Those with possible heart or respiratory problems should not attempt this movement!

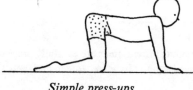

Simple press-ups

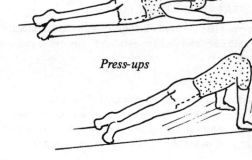

Press-ups

4. **Simplified press-ups.** Kneel with hands on the floor, right angles at hip and shoulder, keeping the hands still, move the head and body forward by bending the elbows. Return to the original position by straightening the elbows.

5. **Press-ups.** Lie on the front on the floor, hands under shoulders, fingers facing forwards, elbows bent and toes curled under. Gently push the body up, by straightening the arms. Return to starting position and repeat continuously. It is important not to repeat this movement for too long.

Agilities

A great number of agilities both with and without hand apparatus moveable and fixed equipment can be included in a movement and fitness training lesson with a gymnastic bias.

e.g. Moving through, under or over obstacles, climbing up and along and through wall bars, ladders and climbing frames.
Moving along benches — various methods e.g. walking, running, bunny hop, side to side, on and off.
Jumping to touch obstacles at various heights.
Forward and backward rolls.
Cartwheels.
Jumping off the box at various heights onto a mat into a forward roll.

Movement interpretation

In some instances fitness training can be introduced through movement interpretation of —
Indians, stalking, preparing to fight
Cowboys, cracking whips, rounding up the cattle
Pirates, hauling ropes, rowing, fighting, looting
Shipwrecked, waves striking and beating, floating, rescue
Astronauts, walking on the moon, take off
Machine, punching, rolling, swinging, turning movements
Energetic tasks, chopping wood, hammering, digging, pneumatic drilling, painting, hauling a heavy load.
Negro spirituals or Afro/Caribean Musicals provide suitable music for the above.

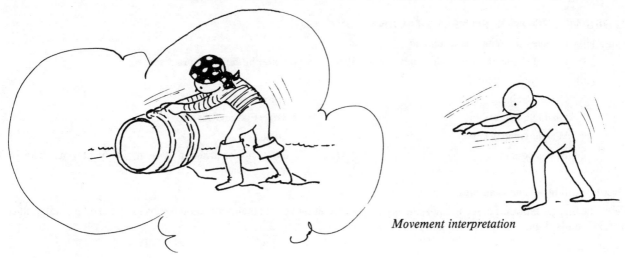

Movement interpretation

Simple gymnastic exercises

The following gymnastic activites — successfully taught in Muckamore Abbey Hospital, Northern Ireland — should be kept **very simple** unless the instructor has had some training in teaching gymnastics.

Activities with ropes

Climbing ropes with
(i)   crossed legs
(ii) hands only (warn them not to slide down rope)
travelling sideways from rope to rope
upward circle (using two ropes)
heave vault (using one rope)
heave vault (using two ropes)

Activities with beam

Crossing beam with hands
(i)   travelling sideways
(ii) travelling sideways with rotation
Downward circle
Face vault
Side vault
Heave vault between two beams
Balancing on inverted beam.

Activities with benches

Climb an inclined bench — using feet and hands
Pull self up inclined bench — using hands only
Circle round raised bench
Balancing activities on inverted bench:
(i)   walk along
(ii) roll ball along
(iii) walk along avoiding obstacles.

Activities with box

Face vault on vertical box
Through vault on vertical box
Overswing vault on horizontal box
Forward roll on horizontal box.

Activities with wall bars

Vertical climb
Horizontal climb
Vertical twist (upwards)
Horizontal twist
Diagonal twist (upwards)
Diagonal twist (downwards)
Hanging
(i)   knee lifting
(ii) leg lifting
(iii) reverse hanging.

Floor work

Forward roll
Backward roll
Head stand
Cartwheel
Handstand.

NATIONAL FITNESS TRAINING SCHEMES

Various national fitness training schemes can be introduced into the physical recreation programme.

Feeling Great	The Health Education Council
Look After Yourself (Helping you to better health)	The Health Education Council
Come Alive	England
Fitness to Live	Scotland
Shape Up	Wales
Sport for All — Exercise and Health	Northern Ireland

Schedules and detailed information obtainable from:
The Health Education Council, and
The Sports Councils of England, Scotland, Wales and Northern Ireland (See Appendix 2).

OTHER METHODS OF FITNESS TRAINING

Aims: (i)   to develop strength and stamina

(ii) to help participants to realise and develop their own potential in the skills practised.

(iii) to stimulate interest

Circuit training	Trim Tracks (trails)
Obstacle courses	Kung Foo and Karate
Weight training (men)	Yoga
Ropes courses	Daily fitness training session. Daily Dozens, with or without chairs.

Circuit training — two examples

The first example, practised in a hospital is a simple circuit for which obtainable equipment is used, the other, practised at an ATC, utilised more sophisticated equipment.

Simple Circuit

Muckamore Abbey Hospital, Northern Ireland, has devised this circuit, suitable for active young men.

Equipment: benches, skittles, canes and skipping ropes.

(i)	step ups	(iv)	press ups
(ii)	sit ups	(v)	jumping and running zig-zag
(iii)	jump ups	(vi)	skipping

If fixed apparatus is available, the following could be included in the circuit:

(i)	chin ups	(iii)	bench lifts
(ii)	rope swings	(iv)	rope climbs

Circuit using more sophisticated equipment

Hornbeams Adult Training Centre, Welwyn Garden City, Hertfordshire, has gradually acquired some interesting apparatus and equipment. The instructor says 'experience has shown that advancement has been made and there is no doubt in his mind that it is noticeably demonstrated in the workshops and many other activities'.

Equipment:

chair	footballs
rowing maching	logs — 2½ m (7') long
cycling equipment	sliding strengthening equipment
punchball stand	mats
medicine balls	

This programme starts with ground work and ground exercises, chair work coupled with brain stimulators, followed by standing activities e.g. catching and throwing using medium and heavy balls from varying distances — these can be organised as team work and on a competitive basis.

The trainees are first shown how the equipment should be used. A time target is set.

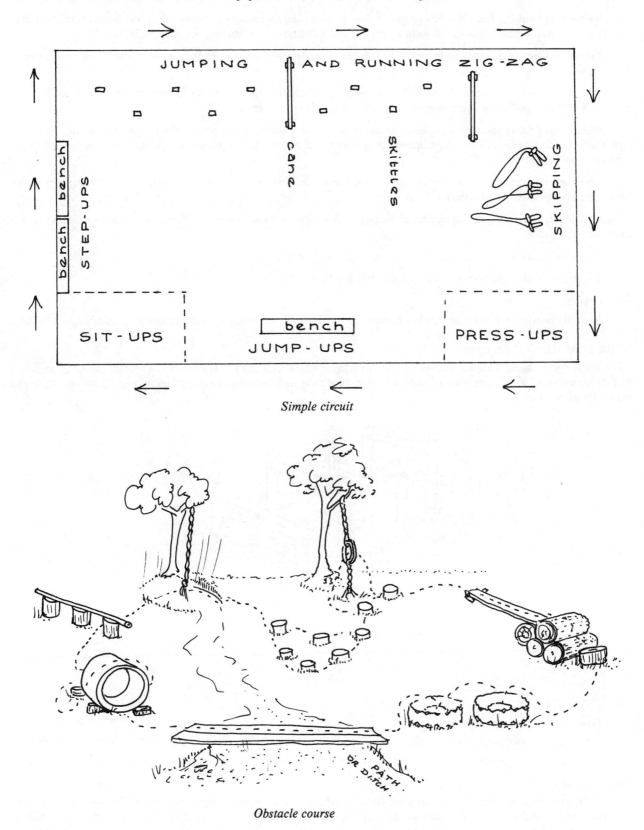

Simple circuit

Obstacle course

Obstacle course

The obstacle course is an activity especially effective for mentally handicapped people as it contains equipment requiring a variety of movement, responses and skills. Different obstacle courses can be set up both indoors and out of doors.

Arm and shoulder strength development. Hanging or climbing obstacle — Climbing and swinging obstacle — Obstacle for developing arm and shoulder strength.

Total body development. Climbing ladder — Vertical climbing obstacle — Apparatus for climbing over and through — Large tractor tyre mounted for crawling and climbing.

Balance and agility. Balancing beams and logs — Ladder used for balancing tasks — Stepping stones made from tree stumps — Balance obstacles made with inclined logs or discarded tyres — Climbing obstacle made from logs.

Indoor equipment. Balance equipment — Balance beam and support constructed from strong timber — Balance board — Rocking board.

The teacher must be aware of each trainee's disability. Each must develop as an individual aiming to reach his own maximum potential and at the same time work together with others in a team.

Sturdy, imaginative equipment can easily be made as long as it serves the purpose of the programme. A wide variety of equipment that complements a well development programme will provide adventure, social play and the development of co-ordination and manipulative skills.

An example of a simple obstacle course. 20 chairs in a line. Trainees crawl under all chairs one following on after the other. Repeat this, pushing a football in front.

Fix square pieces of cardboard together in various shapes. Arrange these shapes in different positions for trainees to climb over and step across.

Logs can be tied together to jump over and to use for balancing.

The programme starts from ground level and finishes in standing.

Ropes course

A course consisting of ropes attached to trees or other stable supports which are used for swinging, climbing and hauling.

TRIM TRACKING (Trim trails)

The Trim (meaning 'fitness') concept was first developed on the Continent. It is applied to a specific physical recreation facility known as a Trim Course, built of 'stations' of logs, specially designed to make general exercise as 'easy, enjoyable and beneficial as possible'.

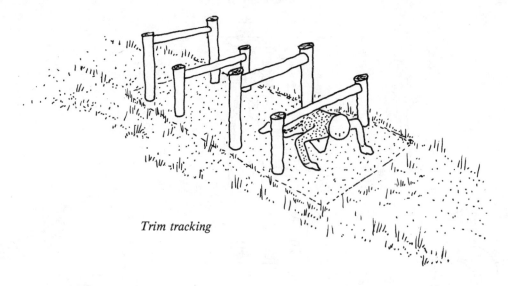

Trim tracking

Aims

Trim courses have two main aims:-

1.   to encourage those not normally engaged in active physical recreation to enjoy it at a level which suits them, and

2.   to provide additional and more intensive fitness training for those already in regular training for competitive sport.

Trim courses

A Trim course can vary in length, shape and content and can be individually designed to make the best use of the grounds available and to suit the needs of the potential users. It can be a simple training path requiring simple route marking, a kind of jogging course. Most courses, however, incorporate carefully planned exercise stations at intervals along the pathway.

The pathway design

The length of the pathway varies with the space available, 400-1500 metres. The start and finish of the route should be at the same place. A figure of 8 or clover-leaf shaped route is particularly suitable for longer courses as it provides intermediate finishing points, coinciding with the start for those who do not wish to cover the full distance.

Exercise stations

There is no set ratio of number of stations to the length of the course but experience shows that users are comfortable with 1 station to 50m over shorter courses and 1 to 75m over longer courses, i.e. a 400m course would have 8 exercise stations and 1500m course might have 20. When designing the stations follow a sequence which avoids exercising the same muscle groups at consecutive stations, e.g. the stations might be designed to exercise the whole body, then the arms, then the trunk, then the legs and so on. Stations, usually constructed of timber and logs embedded in concrete may be simple in design yet still attractive. Many hospital grounds lend themselves to trim courses as do some of the smaller spaces nearby or surrounding some adult training centres, particularly those in the country areas. The diagrams on page 102 and below of exercise stations and their use may inspire those with space available to construct a Trim course. Before embarking on a project, consult the Regional or local Sports Council.

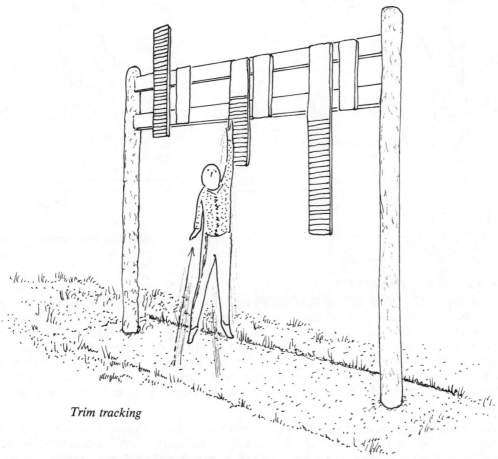

Trim tracking

WEIGHT TRAINING AND WEIGHT LIFTING

Weight training can be a valuable method of building up a reasonable degree of strength and energy. It is essential for the teacher to have expertise in this activity in order to set the right target for each individual.

It is also necessary to seek expert advice and medical sanction. If the handicapped person has any degree of spacticity care must be taken to ensure that the extended wrist grip is used.

The well planned programme must be aimed at a gradual increase over a period, it must not be an unplanned exercise destined to discover who can lift the heaviest weight.

Weight training is being practised in a few centres and hospitals, often included in a programme of circuit training. Equipment consists of barbells and weights which are fairly inexpensive and practically indestructible.

Carefully selected young men can benefit by weight training as an aid to fitness and weight lifting as a sport. Huw Price, a member of the British Weight Lifters Association, has experimented with mentally handicapped boys. He says, 'These boys had a record of failure in everything and it was necessary to find something to give them success of a deep satisfying nature so that they could improve educationally and socially'.

He already had the simple equipment necessary. The exercises taught can be easily learned and to improve all that is necessary is repetition. The boys enjoy doing this once the exercise is mastered. As weight lifting is a very individual sport, they are only competing against themselves, and soon see that there is almost daily improvement. As Huw Price says 'They can see that they are getting stronger and are aware that strength is a quality to be admired. In this way they achieve standing in the eyes of their peers'.

Spin off. Soon these boys wanted to read about weight lifting — in many cases they were non-readers — they wanted to write about the sport and even draw themselves performing. At the same time their attitude to their mates and adults improved dramatically.

Adults. 'In the same way weights can be used as successfully with mentally handicapped young adults. In no way do the rules or apparatus have to be altered or adapted to cater for them. Once they have learned the exercises they would be sympathetically welcomed into adult clubs, and this could do much to ameliorate their lives'. Huw Price is certain that weight training and weight lifting can be used to enable some to live a more normal life.

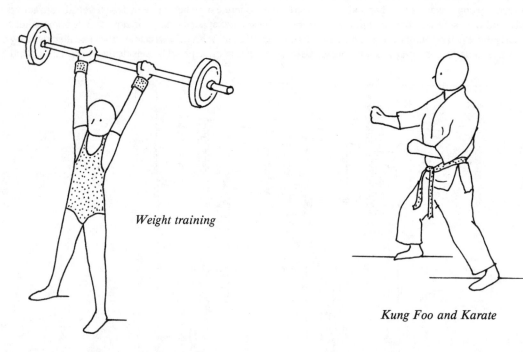

Weight training

Kung Foo and Karate

KUNG FOO AND KARATE EXERCISES

These exercises are included since they are successfully practised in a few Centres. Strong, active young men seem to derive benefit from the vigorous exercise entailed and the discipline involved. At first the men work individually copying the teacher's movement. Most respond well as they have seen the movements on television and in films. The kicks and spin involve movements requiring balance and control, the deep knee bends and jumps with feet apart develop a feeling of sustaining a movement. The strong, sharp blows and positions with the arms, use up a great deal of energy. These movements are equally successful when the men work in twos, the only rule being that they are not allowed to actually touch each other. The men infact put so much effort into the movements, that they are happy to rest at the end of the exercise, and, contrary to general opinion, do not become over-excited.

The movements include: jumps with feet apart, into a strong knee bend — free kicks, to the front and the side, and the back — short run, kick and spin — strong slicing movements with the arms, with the fingers stretched, and palms facing the floor which can be taken in different directions. — forward and backward rolls happen naturally and spontaneously.

YOGA

Yoga has been taught to mentally handicapped young people at the Kingsway College of Further Education, London, where mentally handicapped adults joined a Yoga class. The results were enlightening and it was found to be quite practical to integrate mentally handicapped people with ordinary class members who were made aware that the main attention would be given to those who were handicapped. In this way, handicapped people have other people to copy and this makes the class easier to handle.

Each week one of the young people is chosen to stand in front of the class to act as a demonstrator. This works well and there is keen competiton to take this role.

It is surprising how quickly handicapped people pick up the different postures — in this respect they differ in no way from the ordinary class members. Some of the postures involve balance, standing on one leg, these are enjoyed so much that it has been easy to progress to the more advanced stages. The work is based on stretching and strengthening the body, at the same time increasing stamina. 'We aim to get the body back to its correct shape'. This system of Yoga is designed to act on the internal organs — each posture tends to have a stimulating effect on one or two parts of the body. Yoga is an activity which gradually refines the body and there is no reason why mentally handicapped people should not reap the benefits.

Stiffness is a major problem. Young people, unlike older people, do not have the same endurance. Progress is, therefore, bound to be slower and the teacher needs to encourage the students more than usual and to devise routines which will keep their interest.

The teacher is trained by B. K. S. Iyengar and he recommends that any hospitals/training centres wishing to introduce Yoga to their residents or trainees should investigate the Iyengar method. This system is now widely accepted throughout the world by many educational authorities as the safest and most comprehensive. The teachers are meticulously trained before they can gain a qualification.

REGULAR DAILY FITNESS TRAINING SESSION

Experience has shown that daily fitness training sessions benefit all those attending hospitals and ATCs. One centre in the London Borough of Havering has successfully introduced such sessions.

Fitness training at Havering ATC

Members of the Havering staff, having decided that most of the students did not get enough physical exercise while attending the centre, devised a programme to involve as many of the students as possible in a fitness programme. Attendance was voluntary but as many students as possible were encouraged to take part, particularly the less able, who tend to miss out on exercise provided by the other organised sporting activities.

The keep fit fitness training session commences shortly after the trainees arrive at the centre, and lasts for about 45 minutes. Initially the Health Education Council's recommended exercises were used, omitting those which were too difficult. Shortly afterwards, music was introduced to vary the programme. This was a great success and added to the students' enjoyment. The Music and Motion L.P. 'Popmobility' record which involves exercising to pop music was also used, and it was found that the trainees follow the instructions more easily on the record and that this allows the staff more time to spend helping individual trainees.

Special clothing for the 'Keep Fit' Club is optional, most women wear leotards and plimsoles; the majority of men wear shorts or jeans, T-shirts and gym shoes. The objectives in providing the keep fit club are to improve health, mobility, stamina, strength and posture. It has also helped to establish a group relationship with staff from various departments within the centre and, of course, the students benefit from the team work involved in performing the various sequences of exercises.

EXAMPLES OF TWO DAILY DOZENS

1. Without chairs

Warming up. Running on the spot. Keeping the feet near to the ground gradually increase the height of the knee lift, decrease the height of the knee lift, repeat continuously higher and lower.

'Beating'. Stand with feet apart, fists clenched loosely. Beat the thighs, e.g. front, side, back, continue beating other parts of the body — arms, knees, shoulders, chest, ankles, legs, back. Move the body as much as possible, e.g. to beat behind, so twisting the body. Combine 1 and 2 until everyone is warm.

Punch and twist. Stand with feet apart fists clenched. Alternate arm punching forward with a body twist. Repeat punching to one side — across the body — repeat in different directions — upwards, downwards, obliquely.

Hip swing. Standing, shoulder grasp with partner or holding on the back of a chair for balance. Swing the right leg across the left leg to the left. Swing out to the right (1-2), repeat twice more, 'across and out, across and out' (3-6). Stand still (7) lift the left leg low sideways (8), ready to repeat the swing with the left leg. Repeat right and left continuously.

Hands. Standing or sitting. Various hand movements e.g. opening, closing, spread fingers out, circle the wrists in and out, wrist bend up and down, clap hands, shake hands. Take any two or three hand movements and make up sequences, e.g. 'open and close, open and close', wrist circle outwards and inwards (1-8).

Stretching. Stand with feet a little apart. Slow stretching alternate arms in any direction above shoulder level and out to the side. Stretch through the body to the end of the fingers.

Bend and twist. Standing with feet apart, arms relaxed. (i) Body bending sideways to left and right continuously. (ii) Body turning — twist to look behind — left and right continuously. Combine (i) and (ii) e.g. bend right, left, right and up (1-4) followed by body turning right, left, right and forwards (5-8). Repeat starting to left.

Brisk walking. If space allows (1) walk briskly in different formations, e.g. round the room — in circles — files — pairs or freely. (11) using the whole space, walk freely (1-16) find a partner, link arms or join hands and walk round on the spot (1-16).

2. Using chairs

Ordinary chairs with or without arms. Be sure that the chairs are in good repair. Move chairs quietly and in a controlled way. Teach class members to sit with thighs supported on the seat of the chair but with the whole foot firmly on the floor, feet forward. The back should be erect but not stiff — 'lift out of the waist'. 'Sit tall'.

Warming up. Clap hands with big circular arm movement — in front of the face — out to the side — below knees — towards the back with a body twist. Clap in one direction several times at first — gradually clap in other directions e.g. 2 claps forwards 2 claps to one side, repeat to the other side, 2 claps high — 8 claps.

Marking time. Marking time, slow beats followed by quick beats; finish by accelerating the speed.

Hip and back. Hold the side edges of the chair seat or chair arms firmly throughout, keep the elbows straight. Lift 'seat' off the chair swaying slightly forward. Lower 'seat' on to the chair swaying back. Increase the range of movement so that the feet are lifted off the floor on the back sway.

Variation: (i) move the 'seat' forward over the feet and back. (ii) lift 'seat' up, keep feet firm — swing knees to right and left alternately in the lifted position.

Hands. See Daily Dozen No. 1.

Stretching. Raise arms sideways and upwards to put hands lightly on head. Keeping the back erect lower arms slowly to sides — keep the whole movement slow and sustained.

Variation: as above but stretch arms to touch hands high above head. Combine the two movements.

Wriggling. Wriggle the spine, shoulder girdle and head. Slowly at first — gradually increase the movement and the speed.

Knee lifting. Grasp one knee with both hands. Pull it up as near to the chest as possible and put it down. Repeat with the other leg.

Circles or lines. Hold hands lightly round a circle or in lines — sway from side to side with as much body movement as possible — repeat swaying forward and back.

Relax. At any point in the lesson the following movement can be introduced. Bend forward slowly to put forehead on knees slowly uncurl to erect position — let the arms hang easily to the side.

The teacher can devise many variations of the above movements for warming up and giving general exercise. **All movements should be repeated a number of times to be effective.** If music is used the tempo should be slow enough to allow full range of movement. Use 4/4, 6/8, and 3/4 rhythms. See Music pp. 91, 92.

Everyone should feel thoroughly warmed up at the end of 15 minutes continuous exercise.

Note: Where there are ambulant and non-ambulant people in the same class — exercises can be selected from 1 and 2 to make a daily dozen suitable for both.

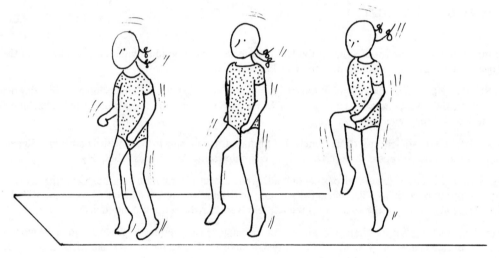

Warming up

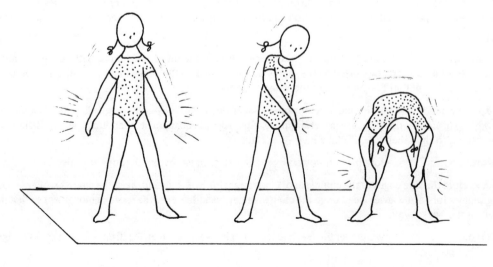

Beating

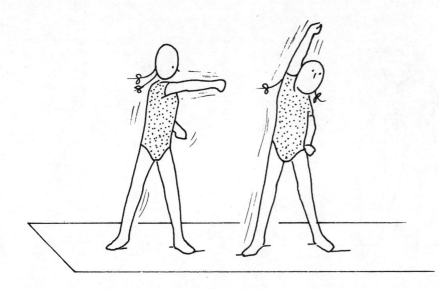

Punch and twist

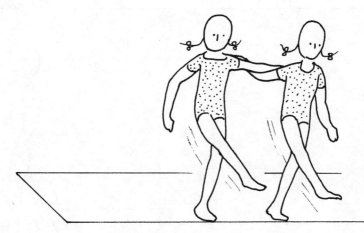

Hip swing

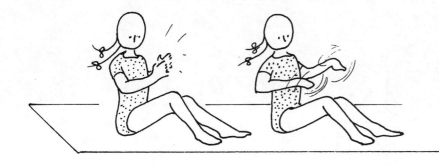

Hands

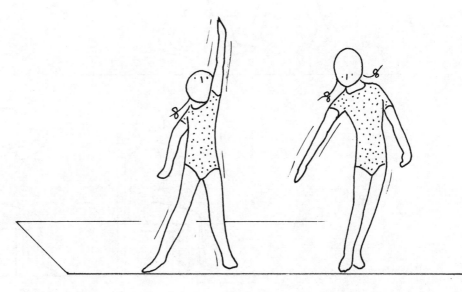

Stretching

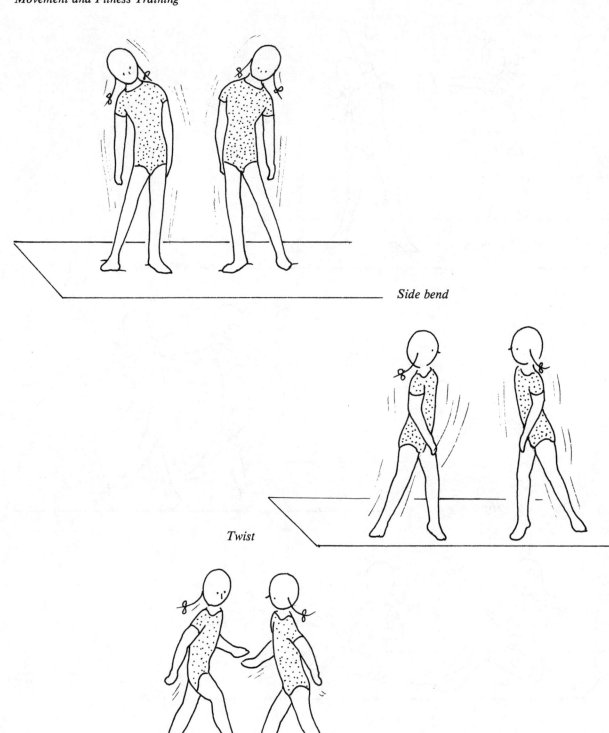

Side bend

Twist

Brisk walking

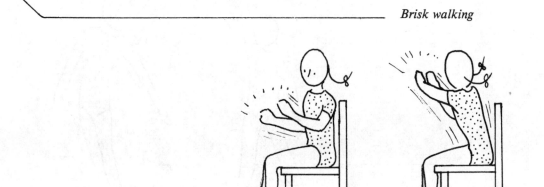

Warming up (clapping)

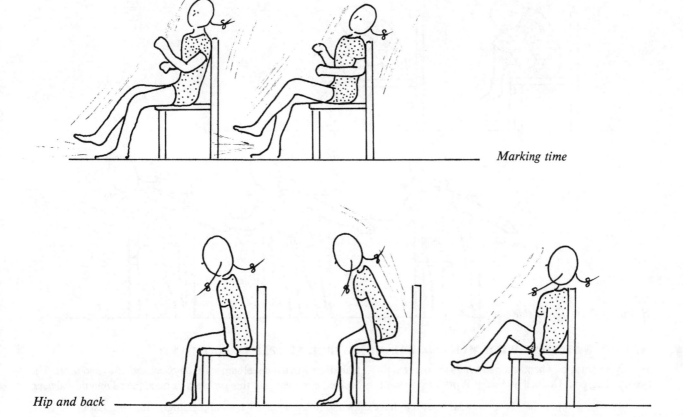

Marking time

Hip and back

Stretching

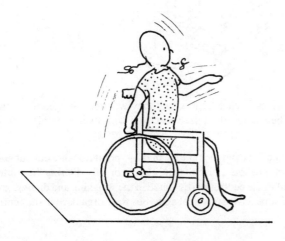

Wriggling

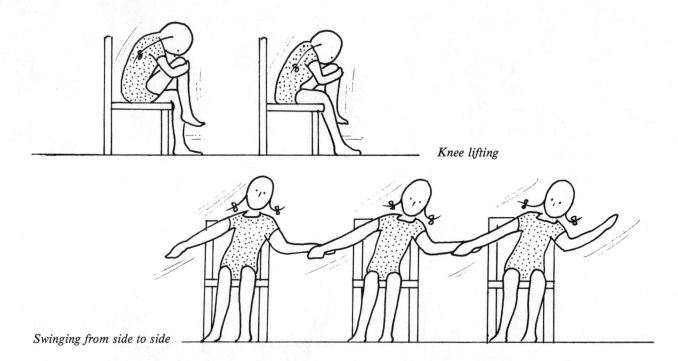

Knee lifting

Swinging from side to side

WEIGHT WATCHING WITH MENTALLY HANDICAPPED PEOPLE IN SCOTLAND

Many mentally handicapped adults are overweight — a hindrance in the development of physical activities and sport. The Lothian Regional Council — Social Work Department — decided to investigate this problem through their Diatetic Adviser.

Firstly, mentally handicapped adults seem to have difficulty in knowing when to stop eating — the appestat in the brain which controls intake seems to have impaired efficiency. Secondly, they usually have few dislikes and consiequently eat anything and everything offered. The consequence of inactive leisure pursuits is both a cause and an effect of overweight. This cycle can be broken if relatives and friends encourage physical and mental activity during leisure time rather than allowing passive pursuits such as watching television.

The risks linked with obesity include heart disease, strokes, diabetes, respiratory disorders, arthritis, piles, flat feet, and also an increased rate of accidents in the home and in the street due to decreased mobility. Apart from these medical reasons for losing weight, weight loss also has social benefits — improved looks and improved choice of clothes. These latter are more immediate advantages and can be used to inspire will-power.

Since many members of the Adult Training Centres in the Lothian Region had weight problems, Weight Watchers Clubs were started in each of the eleven centres by the Social Work Departments' Dietetic Advisor. All the trainees were weighed and measured, and their target weight determined from ideal weight charts. Each trainee was instructed on the dietary alterations necessary and the importance of exercise in the weight loss programme. A simplified diet sheet was designed to reinforce the message, and a copy given to each overweight trainee.

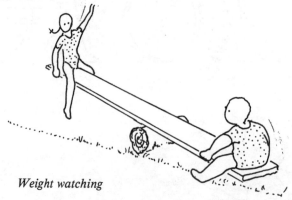

Weight watching

A talk was given to the parents at one of their meetings in each centre, and they were encouraged to participate in the programme themselves if they had a weight problem. They were all advised to check with their general practitioner before embarking on the diet.

As many fatty and starchy foods as possible were removed from the midday meal — potatoes were cut out and vegetables and salads increased. Puddings were replaced by fresh fruit, yoghourt, biscuits and cheese or jelly. During the winter, vegetable soups were allowed instead of sweet. That many of the staff in the centres participated in the weighing and dieting, greatly helped the trainees to both understand and comply with the restrictions. Extra physical activities were organised in the centres including keep fit, football and swimming.

110

The clubs have been operating for a year, with monthly weigh-ins to assess the progress. During the summer months results were very encouraging but losses during the winter slowed down. The difference in losses between different centres indicated the level of enthusiasm and interest of parents in helping the trainees to continue their diets at home. The response from parents has in general been good, but some parents refuse to deprive the trainee of anything. Individual consultations have been held with parents who refused to co-operate. 42% of the trainees were overweight to some extent and the average weight to be lost was 2½ stones. In the first year the average loss was ½ stone, but there were individual losses of 1½ to 2 stones in several cases. This average rate of loss is not as good as was hoped, but any loss is encouraging.

When weighing all the trainees and checking their weights against the Ideal Weight Chart, it was found that several trainees were underweight to a worrying degree. Advice has been given and a diet sheet provided, but the success rate has been disappointing. The biggest problem to be overcome if these trainees are to gain weight is the lack of feeding facilities in the Centres and also lack of finance. Regular high protein, high calorie snacks need to be provided in addition to the main lunchtime meal.

ASSESSMENT

There is no right or wrong way to teach movement and fitness training, as long as the teacher is always aware of the needs of the individuals in the group, and plans each lesson with these in mind — the teacher carefully assessing the progress of the group as a whole and of each individual. The method of recording the progress is the teacher's concern, but some record should be kept. Some centres record achievements on charts displayed on their notice boards — trainees and staff alike taking a great interest in the ticks or square-filling. One such chart of 'Physical Training Achievements' for the severely mentally handicapped is set out as follows:

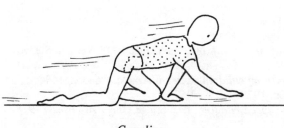

Crawling

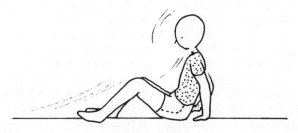

Moving backwards

Indoor activities

Phase 1

(i)   Crawl a distance of 9.5 m (30')
(ii)   Lying face down, using arms, travel forwards 6 m (20').
(iii)   Sitting, travel backwards 6 m (20').
(iv)   Lying, achieve 6 push ups.
(v)   Lying, roll sideways 3.6 m (12') to the right.
(vi)   Lying, roll sideways 3.6 m (12') to the left.

Phase 2

(i)   Slide under a partner who is kneeling on all fours.
(ii)   Slide through a tunnel made by 3 people kneeling on all fours and then help to make the tunnel.
(iii)   Roll a partner sideways like a log for 3.6 m (12').
(iv)   Sitting on seat only, spin right round using hands only to help.
(v)   Roll a large ball to the other end of the room and then collect it (any method accepted).
(vi)   Throw a large ball to a partner 3 m (10') away — sitting or standing.

Phase 3

(i)   Jump a distance of 1 m (3').
(ii)   Jump over an obstacle about 305 mm (1') high.
(iii)   Slide a partner along the floor for 6 m (20').
(iv)   Stand with arms extended to wall, lean against wall, achieve 6 push ups.
(v)   Bounce and catch a large ball 3 times.
(vi)   Dribble a large ball to the opposite end of the room.

Phase 4

(i)   In twos 3 m (10') apart. Throw and catch a large ball 3 times.
(ii)   Give a partner a ride round the room for about 6 m (20').
(iii)   Sitting back to back with partner, stand up and sit down twice.
(iv)   Keep moving round the hall, e.g. jogging for 30 seconds.
(v)   Keep moving round the hall, e.g. jogging for 1 minute.
(vi)   Create a mini circuit e.g. crawl under a table, over a low obstacle then run round a skittle at the opposite end of the room and return to the starting point — once, twice, three time without any pauses.

This method of encouraging movement is recommended for senior adolescents and adults. It can be used where there is no specialist help or where facilities are very limited. Tasks will constantly need to be revised to meet the particular disabilities of an individual or group. Distances mentioned are only intended to be guidance for the leader and should not be adhered to rigidly. There must always be the **potential for success.**

In this particular set of tasks Phases 1 and 2 provide scope for large body movements and can be attempted by the ambulant and non ambulant. They should often be repeated as warming up activities for those attempting the more difficult tasks in Phases 3 and 4. These demand increased concentration, co-operation, effort and motor skill. A playful presentation of these activities should always be encouraged.

FURTHER READING

ANDERSON, M. E. *Inventive movement.* Chambers, Edinburgh, 1970.

BUCKLAND, D.G. *Gymnastics.* Heinemann Educational, London, 1969.

CAMERON, W. M. and PLEASANCE, P. *Education in movement.* Blackwell, Oxford, 1963.

COLSON, J. *Getting into rhythm: music and movement and recreational activities for hospitals.* Yorkshire Regional Health Authority, 1974.

DIAGRAM GROUP. *Enjoying gymnastics.* Paddington Press, London.

GROVES, L. (ed.). *Physical education for children with special needs.* Cambridge University Press, 1979.

JENNINGS, S. *Creative therapy.* Pitman Publishing, London, 1975.

KNOW THE GAME SERIES. *Keeping fit, Gymnastics; Karate.* E.P. Publishing, Wakefield.

MEIER, W. and BARANEK, M. *Recreative movement in further education.* MacDonald & Evans, London, 1973.

MORGAN, R. E. and ADAMSON, G. T. *Circuit training.* Bell & Hyman, London, 1961.

MURDOCH, E. B. *Expressive movement.* Chambers, Edinburgh, 1973.

NORTH, M. *Composing movement sequence.* MacDonald & Evans, London.

ORAM, CHRIS. *Every woman her guide to fitness.* World's Work, Tadworth, 1978.

ROBINS, F. and ROBINS, J. *Educational rhythmics for mentally handicapped children.* Ra Verlag, 8713 Veriken Schwize, Switzerland, 1963.

ROBINSON, C. M. et al. *Physical activity in the education of slow-learning children.* Edward Arnold, London, 1970.

THOMAS, VAUGHAN. *Better physical fitness.* Kaye and Ward, London, 1979.

UPTON, G. (ed.). *Physical and creative activities for mentally handicapped children.* Cambridge University Press, 1978.

CHAPTER ELEVEN

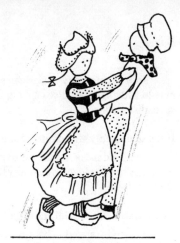

Dr Dance

Terminology – Teaching guidelines – Hints to teachers – Formations for simple dances – Simple steps for folk/country/national/social dancing – Composition of simple dance-like activities – Examples of adapted simple dances – American square dancing – Music – Scottish country dancing – Displays

Dance, however narrowly or widely interpreted, is a fundamental form of exercise, and the desire for rhythmic movement is inherent in most people.

Dance, which is both relaxing and exhilerating, is also one of the most popular of all social activities for fun and enjoyment. It can break down social barriers and provide excellent opportunities for all members of the community to share a common interest. Some mentally handicapped people have a well developed sense of rhythm and dancing can give them a feeling of normality not enjoyed to such an extent in other activities.

TERMINOLOGY

American square. A form of American folk dance originally developed in rural areas, in which a number of couples, usually in a square formation, perform changing figures with a caller.

Ballet. A classical form of theatrical dance which originally developed from Court dancing but took on its distinctive form during the 19th century. It presupposes a technique using an outward rotation of the legs which requires a lengthy training. An unusual feature is that women dance 'on the point'.

Ballroom. A social form of dance which has developed from the 19th century onwards. The English style of ballroom dancing developed during the nineteen-twenties and is famous throughout the world. Dances include the waltz, quickstep, slow fox trot and tango.

Clog. A form of tap dancing originating in Lancashire for which wooden shoes, i.e. clogs, are worn.

Disco dancing. A form of structured improvisation on and around the current pop music. The dancers usually dance independently and the finer details of content and style are dependent on the cultural origins of the music. Although a social dance, it has recently been used for display and competition among the dancers.

Folk/community dance. A simple form of dance developed by the people of a particular country and revealing specific characteristics determined by such factors as temperament of the people, historical and geographical background, costume, and musical instruments used.

Latin-American. The basic figures of the Rumba, Samba, Paso Doble, American Jive and Cha-Cha-Cha.

Modern educational dance. A method of teaching dance based on the set of principles devised by Rudolf Laban in the early years of the 20th century. This has been developed into a way of teaching creatively and is widely used in schools today.

National character dances. The steps are those used in the traditional dances. In both the music and dance arrangement, the characteristics of the country and of the particular type of dance are retained.

Both national and national character dances can be simplified to enable the non-dance specialist teacher to capture the style, quality, music and background of these countries.

National dances. Authentic traditional dances from Western and Eastern Europe, Russia and other parts of the world.

Natural movement. Natural movement is a free form of dance which trains an appreciation of beauty through the natural actions of human movement, and also lays emphasis on the importance of musical understanding. Its aesthetic appeal, and comparatively simple technique, allows pupils to respond eagerly to imaginative and creative opportunities, and develop a love of dance movement with a quality of expressiveness in interpretation which is of permanent value in their physical, musical and artistic education.

Old time. The sequence dances which were popular in the ballroom prior to the first world war. Such dances as Veleta, Boston Two Step, Military Two Step, Lancers and Quadrilles, come under this heading.

Sword and morris dancing. Sword and morris dances are danced by men only, often on village streets and greens or in the market place. They are suitable for displays and festivals.

Tap. A form of dance performed with metal plates on the shoes and characterised by the rhythmic tapping of the toes and heels on the floor.

Folk, community, American square, national and old time dances seem to be the most popular with mentally handicapped people, although they also enjoy and benefit from ballet, natural movement, ballroom and modern educational dance, taught by specialist teachers.

Introducing folk or country dancing

Simple dances indigenous to many regions and counties in England, Scotland, Ireland and Wales, danced by local groups and clubs can be taught to mentally handicapped people, as can the traditional national folk dances from Europe and other parts of the world.

Educational and social training

Dance is related to both educational and social training through its link with the country of origin, the music, art, history, geography, costume and customs of the people. It can also play a role in the drama production, pantomime, nativity play or musical show (maypole and country dances, national and tap dancing, for example).

TEACHING GUIDELINES

Enjoying working together and responding to the beat of the music should be established before teaching specific dances, e.g. sitting on chairs clapping or stamping with the leader, to the music. All can be helped to work together by following a leader in line formation with hands joined, leaders create floor patterns of their choice and finally individual groups join up in one large circle formation. Hand and eye contact help the group to gain confidence in working together, hence the value of a circle formation.

The organisation required for partner work is unnecessary at this stage. A variety of simple steps can be taught combined with easy floor patterns, e.g. moving towards the centre of the circle and back or travelling round the circle.

In contrast, dancers may then sit and experiment with clapping activities, at first following the leader and then creating their own clapping sequence to the music. They will now be ready to return to the simple circle movements as a climax to the session; this repetition will give the dancers confidence.

When the above dance activities can be performed with ease and enjoyment the dancers are ready to attempt simple partner dances. The teacher must assess how soon this stage is reached. Circumstances vary, the teacher with few helpers will take longer to reach this stage than one working in an integrated situation where there might be a one-to-one relationship.

When preparing a dance lesson, consider: the standard of movement and the sense of rhythm of the members of the group; the selection of dances and dance steps which can be easily learned by all; the need to repeat well known popular dances; the choice and availability of music and accompanists, e.g. pianists, accordionists, guitarists.

HINTS TO TEACHERS

1. Name the dance.
2. Listen to the music before dancing, talk about its characteristics.
3. Remember the gentleman **always** has his lady on his **right** unless otherwise indicated. Where there are more women than men in a class, the woman dancing 'man' should wear a band or some other identification.
4. Make sure the dancers know the formation and pattern of the dance.
5. Prompt well in advance when a change of formation or step occurs.
6. Link one phrase to the next by reminding the dancers of the steps at the end of one phrase and of those that are coming at the beginning of the next; practise these links to ensure continuity.
7. Coach good poise throughout.
8. Improve the standard of footwork even if it is a slow process.
9. Give as graphic a description as possible of the country of origin and its traditional costume.
10 **Repetition** is very important, especially when teaching links between two sequences or figures. The confidence gained by the success of learning two figures in the session far outweighs the value of attempting 3 or 4.

Adaptation and progress

Substitute easier steps for difficult ones.
Substitute or repeat a sequence of steps for ones that prove too difficult.
Delete a whole figure if necessary and repeat one of the other figures in its place, or omit it.
Simplify the formation and patterns.
Simplify the hold.
Use a longer phrase of music — 8 instead of 4, or 16 instead of 8 when teaching a step or pattern.

Although progress may be slow, improvement can be measured by:
quicker response to demonstration and verbal directions;
improved stadnard of performance;
improved continuity throughout the dance;
greater awareness of partner relationship and social responsibility;
ability to remember from one lesson to the next;
As dancers become more proficient, encourage those who are able, to create their own dance steps and patterns.

Steps, formations and holds

These examples of formations, steps and holds are based on traditional dances as recorded by the National Dance Branch of the Imperial Society of Teachers of Dancing, the English Folk Dance and Song Society and the Royal Scottish Country Dance Society, and have been kept deliberately simple to suit the needs of the adult mentally handicapped person whose movement, spatial awareness and feeling for direction is often limited.

Once a teacher has understood the basic formations, patterns and steps, and put them into short rhythmic phrases of 32, 16 or 8 counts it is possible without using complicated steps to choreograph a great number of dances designed to suit the abilities of any particular handicapped group. At a later stage a wider variety of steps and formations can be added.

Formations for simple dances

Processional
Longways set
Casting out and its variations
Turn your partner and its variations
Right and left hand star
Circles and variations, simple or more difficult
Arches and variations
Serpentine or snake
Back to back (Do-si-do)
Sets of 2 or 4 couples.

Steps for simple dances

Walking, forwards, backwards and turning
Running, forwards, backwards and turning
Skipping, forwards, backwards and turning
Skip change of step, leading to polka
Gallop or slip step sideways and variations
Side close and its variations (chassé)
Step and hop and its variations.

Steps for more advanced dances

French runs, forward and turning
Pas de basque 1 2 3 — 1 & 2
Waltz step
Pas Mazurka
Step and hops, with varying numbers of hops and change of direction
Balance step (setting)
Barn dance.

Although these more advanced steps are described in detail the most effective way for a teacher to acquire them is through practical experience with other dancers.

FORMATIONS FOR SIMPLE DANCES

Processional

Line up dancers to move in anti-clockwise direction around the edge of the room. The lady is on the gentleman's right side, i.e. ladies on outside, gentlemen on the inside.

Longways set (usually 4 couples)

Line up couples facing the teacher (thereafter referred to for this purpose as the top of the set). The lady is on the gentleman's right side, and inside hands, or right hands are joined.

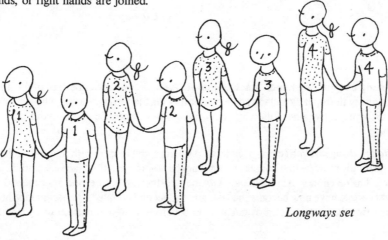

Longways set

In this formation the couples can move on behind each other, towards and away from the top of the set i.e. moving forwards and backwards.

Alternatively the couples can turn and face each other, and move forwards and backwards — towards and away from each other. Where a group has difficulty in doing this, the gentlemen's line link hands and the ladies do likewise.

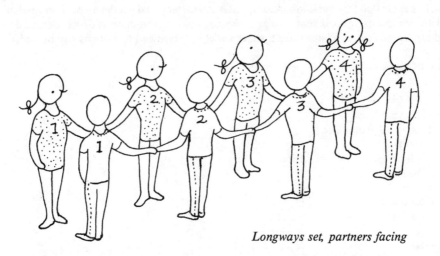

Longways set, partners facing

Casting out and variations

Casting out and back to place. Line up as in 2 without holding inside hands. Top lady and top gentleman cast outwards at the same time, the lady by turning to the right and the gentleman by turning to the left. They move to the bottom of the set, join hands, and walk to the top of the set, finishing when they reach their own places.

It might be helpful to chalk or mark the initials of the top couple on the floor in their own places, and also at the spot where they join together again.

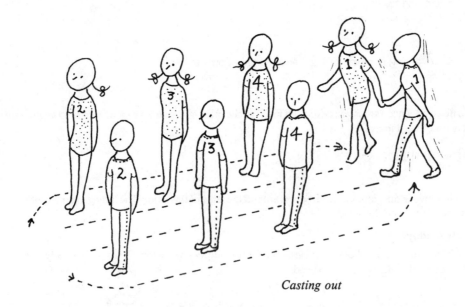

Casting out

Variations

1. Both lines casting out, joining hands, back to places. As in 3 casting can be repeated with both lines moving at the same time. The ladies following the top lady and the gentleman following the top gentleman. The leaders cast out and move to the bottom of the set, with their respective lines following them. Instruct each couple to 'find your partner, join hands and move forward to your own place'.

2. Casting out and making an arch (change leaders). As before, the leaders with their respective lines behind them, cast out and move to the bottom of the set. The first couple on reaching the 'joining position' face each other, join both hands, and raise them high to make an arch. The rest now join inside hands with their partners as before, and pass under the arch before returning to their own places. The first couple have now become the last, and the second couple have become the new leader at the top of the set. Each new couple practise the casting out movement as in 3 before using the pattern to change leaders.

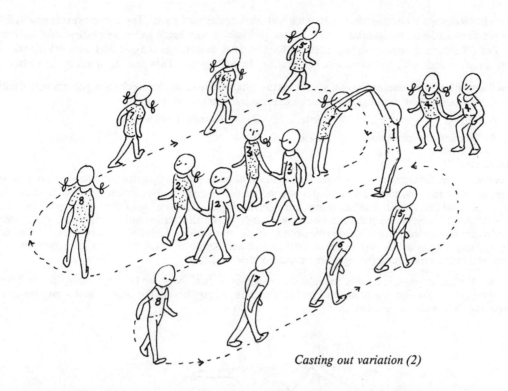

Casting out variation (2)

3. Casting out and all couples make an arch. As in 3, the top couple leaders with their respective lines behind them, cast out and move to the bottom of the set. This time the first couple join hands and walk forwards to their own starting positions, where they turn and join both hands and raise their arms to make an arch. Each couple in turn following their example, except the last couple who join hands and move forwards passing under the arches until they reach the top of the set. They have now changed places and become top couple, whilst the original top couple move into second place.

Turning your partners

This movement can be performed from a procession, longways set or circle formation.

Partners face each other, join right hands or both, turn clockwise, with either a walking, running, skip or slip step for an even number of counts, e.g. 16 or 8. The couples stop, and turn to go the other way, i.e. anti-clockwise. Where a one-hand grasp is used it is essential to change hands before setting off in the other direction, i.e. Right-hand grasp when turning clockwise; Left-hand grasp when turning anti-clockwise.

(1) Corner couples turning. In a longways set a turn can be made by: the top lady and bottom gentleman **or** the top gentleman and bottom lady (see diagram 11-5).

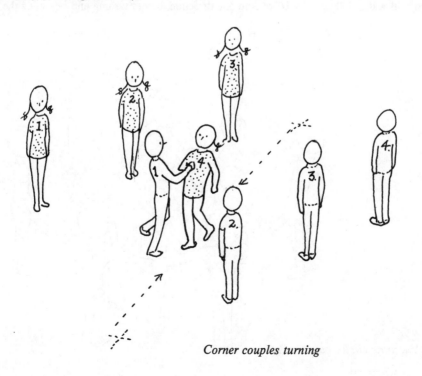

Corner couples turning

The couples in a longways set turn and face each other and take one step backwards. Top lady moves diagonally forward to the centre of the set, likewise the bottom gentleman. They meet, give right or both hands and move clockwise for an even number of counts e.g. 16 or 8. Walks, runs, skips or slipping steps can be used. They then change and give left hands, or keep a double hand hold and change direction and move anti-clockwise for a further 16 or 8 counts. They then fall back to their places.

Note: Practise with longer phrases of 32 counts if it helps to establish the pattern, before changing direction, and falling back to place. When this movement has been mastered, it can develop into the following turn:

| meet | 2 | 3 | 4 | | turn | 2 | 3 | 4 | (turning clockwise) |
| change | 2 | 3 | 4 | (turning anti-clockwise) | back | 2 | 3 | 4 | |

Right or left hand star

The last movement can develop into a right and left hand star, by 2 couples joining together. First couple extend and slightly raise their hands, at the same time turning towards the second couple. Second couple, extend and slightly raise their right hands, and turn towards the first couple. The ladies put their right hands palm down on top of their gentleman's right hand. The first gentleman puts his right hand on top of the second couple's hands. All finish standing with the right shoulders inwards, right arm extended and raised and the left arm stretched to the side to complete the star or wheel effect. The couples move in a clockwise direction, either walking, running or skipping forwards. Begin with a long phrase of 16 counts before going round the other way, with left hands joined in the centre, and the right arm stretched to the side.

Note: It is worthwhile stopping the music to make the change-over, until the group becomes competent to make a quick swing round to change arms. At first, the group will probably require talking through the change, and it may be necessary to physically correct and help with this movement.

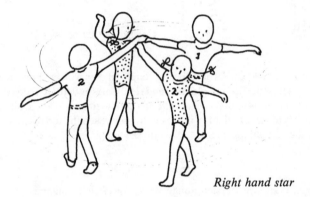

Right hand star

Circle formation (simple)

Make a circle with ladies on their partners' right. The group face inwards with hands joined. All move sideways to the right, with a slipping step i.e. side gallop. Keep to an even phrase before changing to move to the left, e.g. 32, 16 or 8.

Note: Where this proves to be difficult, make a circle and turn the left shoulder in towards the middle. 'Follow my leader'. Walk forwards in a clockwise direction for 16 counts. Any marching tune can be used for this and eventually the number of steps in any direction can be cut down, or the rhythm altered, to such as slow, slow, quick, quick, slow. Introduce short phrases of varying rhythm such as 8 walks, followed by 16 runs in one direction, before turning and repeating the other way.

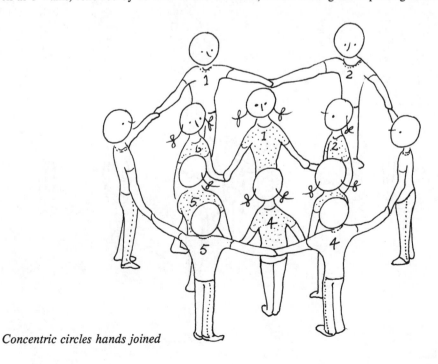

Concentric circles hands joined

Variations:

1.   Forwards and backwards to the centre. Join hands in a circle all facing the centre. 8 walks forwards to the centre and 8 walks backwards. Where the circle is too small, keep the same length of phrase but change the movements, e.g. 4 walks forward, 4 claps on the spot; 4 walks backward, 4 claps on the spot. With a more advanced group, a change of rhythm can be introduced, e.g. slow, slow, quick, quick, slow or variations introducing claps and stamps: clap, clap, clap, wait — stamp, stamp, stamp, wait. With a more advanced group the ladies move to the centre and back whilst the gentlemen remain in their places followed by the gentlemen moving whilst the ladies remain still.

2.   Concentric circles. Ladies join hands and make a circle on the inside. Gentlemen join hands and make a large circle round the ladies. The ladies turn left shoulder inwards and walk forwards in an anti-clockwise direction. The gentlemen turn right shoulder inwards and walk forwards in a clockwise direction. After 16 walks, both circles stop and change direction and repeat walks in the opposite direction. As the group becomes more confident, shorten the phrase to 8 counts. Running, skipping or stamps using various rhythms can be introduced.

Variation: Form two circles, one inside the other, facing the centre with hands joined. Slipping steps sideways, ladies moving to the right, and gentlemen to the left and vice versa. 16 or 8 steps.

Arches

The dancers make a circle or line, depending on the numbers with hands joined, arms raised to make arches. One dancer at a time weaves in and out of the arches, until either back in her place in the circle, or to the end of the line. As soon as the first dancer is back in place or at the end of the line, the second dancer then starts to weave in and out. The dance is repeated until all have had a turn. This sequence can be danced by a small group of dancers making a train-like formation, under the arches, as in 'Here comes a Bluebird through my Window' based on the Ladybird Series Singing Games.

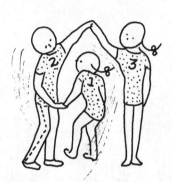
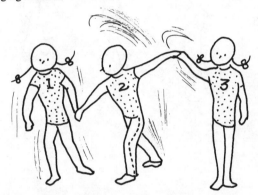

Arches

Variation: Three dancers, 1 gentleman and 2 ladies — gentleman in middle. The dancer on the right, No. 1, passes in front of the middle dancer, No. 2, and under the arch between dancers 2 and 3 and continues until back to place. The middle dancer, No. 2, turns under own left arm to complete the movement. Dancer No. 3 repeats the movement passing in front of dancer No. 2 and under the arch between dancers No. 2 and No. 1 continuing back to place. The middle dancer, No. 2, turns under own right arm.

Serpentine or snake

The dancers line up alternately, ladies and gentlemen one behind the other. The teacher is the leader to begin with. To any popular march or rag time tune, the leader weaves a snake-like pattern from one end of the hall to the other. Many dancers tend to 'overtake' the dancers in front, but must learn to keep their place in the line. This can be danced with hands joined.

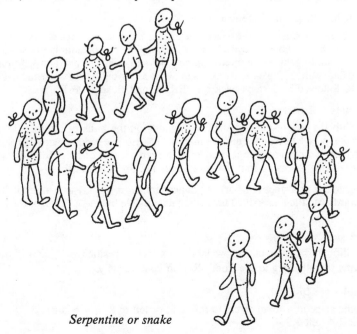

Serpentine or snake

Back to back (Do-si-do)

Start this movement in a longways set with the couples facing each other. Since each dancer walks in a square pattern, it is helpful to mark the pattern on the floor. To prevent confusion use two colours, one to show the lady's track, the other the gentlemen's. Give each couple the chance to work this out under supervision. The dancers pass right shoulders as they move forwards for 4 counts. They move sideways to the right with their backs to each other for 4 counts, backwards for 4 counts passing left shoulders and finally sideways to the left to face each other again.

Ladies and gentlemen can practise separately; this means they will actually move round their stationary partner, 4 forward, 4 to the right, 4 backwards, 4 to the left. If right and left is not understood, use terms such as 'sideways towards the music/door/window'.

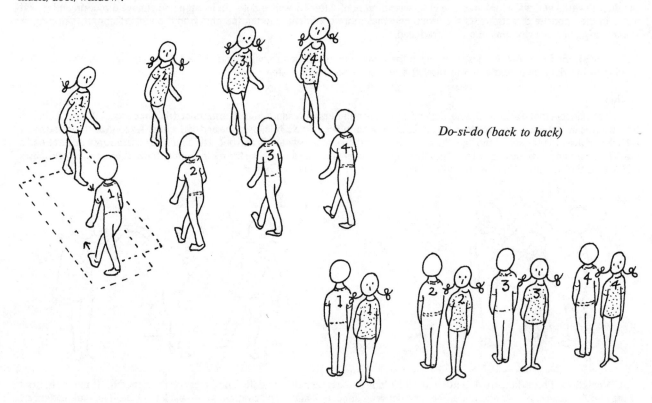

Do-si-do (back to back)

SIMPLE STEPS FOR FOLK/COUNTRY/NATIONAL/SOCIAL DANCING

R = Right foot

L = Left foot

The steps included in the first part of the glossary have been successfully used with older teenage and adult mentally handicapped groups. The steps described, although based on authentic footwork, have in some instances been adapted and simplified.

Walking Steps 4/4 time (a light, lilting tune 4 steps to 1 bar, 2 slow steps to 1 bar)

Encourage an easy lilting walk, in time with the beat of the music, and whenever necessary indicate which foot should start. Generally work on phrases of 16, 8 or 4, and be positive about counting the correct number of steps before changing direction. Walking backwards may take time to achieve, numerous dance-like activities in lines and with partners can be practised to improve moving forwards and backwards. The ultimate aim is to dance a step called 'forward and back a double' which is 3 steps forward R.L.R. close L. to R. followed by 3 steps backward R.L.R. and close L. to R.

Running steps 4/4 time (4 runs to 1 bar)

A light springing run with the weight pitched slightly forwards on the balls of the feet. Many older, heavy, mentally handicapped adults, hampered by a lack of balance and the inability to sustain a running activity for any length of time, find this movement difficult and awkward. If a running step is used keep to even phrases of 16 or 8, and combine it with a quieter less energetic movement such as walking to ensure that the group does not tire too quickly.

French runs 2/4 or 4/4 time (2 or 4 steps to 1 bar). A younger active group may well attempt these runs, with the weight of the body pitched slighly forwards and the toes kicked up as high as possible behind. (Think of the feet touching the seat whilst running).

Skipping 2/4 or 6/8 time (2 steps to 1 bar).

Many adults find this difficult, because of their weight and a lack of resilience. A skip is simple:
'Step forward, hop, bring the other leg to the front'. Repeat continuously.

Turn on the spot 4/4 time (4 steps to 1 bar)

Short walking or running steps in a small circle to the right or left to 8 or 4 counts.
Chant: Turn 2 3 4 or right 2 3 4, left 2 3 4.

Gallops forwards 2/4 or 6/8 time (2 steps to 1 bar)

A light springy step taken forwards, normally in phrases of 8 or 4 i.e. the right foot leads for 8, then change and bring the left foot through to lead for 8.

A gallop is a step forward on the right, followed by the left foot immediately closing with a spring so releasing the right foot forward again.

Simple version: Step R. forward, close L. to R., hop on the L. and lift R. foot up.

Chant: 'step, close, hop' 1 & 2.

Chant:	'step,	close,	hop'

Skip change of step 2/4 time (1 step to 1 bar)

This is a development of the forward gallop, and may well prove to be too difficult for some groups, because of its short phrasing (and 1 and 2). It is a lilting step that travels forwards, the leading foot changing at the beginning of every phrase. Start with the weight on the L. foot, and the R. foot free just off the floor. Hop L. and step forward R. quickly close L. foot to R. and step forward again R. Hop R. and bring L. foot through and step forward, close R. to L. and step forward again L.

	'Hop,	step,	close	step'
Chant:	and	1	and	2

Polka 2/4 time (1 step to 1 bar)

A springy step similar to the 'skip change of step' which has a rhythm of 'and 1 and 2' i.e. hop, step, close, step. Polka steps can be danced forwards, to one side or turning. Polka steps can be combined with skips, slips or runs, e.g. 2 polka steps followed by 4 skips.

Slip step or gallops sideways 2/4 or 6/8 (2 steps to 1 bar)

A bouncy step that travels sideways, normally in phrases of 16, 8 or 4. Encourage a good 'lift'. Step sideways with R. to the R. Quickly close the L. foot to the R. with a feeling of knocking the R. one out of the way. Immediately release the R. to the side and repeat the movement.

	1	and	2	and
Chant:	R.	close	R.	close
	1	and	2	and
or	step	close	step	close

This gallop step can be performed in circles, concentric circles, in lines or with partners, or by a solo dancer. It can be taken at a galloping tempo resembling the rhythm of horses hooves or more slowly and strongly, so that it is akin to the straddle step of men's morris dancing.

Many of the more advanced steps (9-13) may be unsuitable for some groups, but teachers can modify the steps and use the original folk tunes and rhythms to compose a variety of dances.

Step and close in different directions

If this can be mastered it provides a movement which is the basis of many central European dances, Afro/Carribbean and Disco dancing, as well as the beginnings of slow rhythm and social dancing.

(i)   Step right, close L. to R. and repeat travelling to the right with 4 or 8 steps. Repeat this step to the left i.e. step left, close R. to L. and repeat travelling to the left.
      The steps can be repeated 8, 4 or twice as required.

(ii) Step R., close L. to R. without weight, i.e. step right rest L., step left, rest R.
      Chant: step right, rest L., step left, rest R.
      This develops into a swaying movement alternately to the right and left and can be further developed into a forward and backward movement taken slowly or quickly.

(iii) Step R. forward, rest L. in behind, step back, L. and rest in front.
      Chant: forwards 2 3 4 back 2 3 4 **or** front 2, back 2.

Step and hop

A springy movement that can be performed in a variety of ways with or without a turn and or change of direction. Since it entails balance, co-ordination and control, it may take some time to achieve.

1.   Simple step and hop.
     Step R. to right. Swing L. up and across in front. Repeat to the L.
     Chant: Step, lift, step, lift.
     Later hop as the second leg swings up and across in front. Step, hop, step, hop (R. hop L. hop).

2.   More difficult version.
     If and when this is mastered a variety of rhythms can be introduced e.g.
     (i)   Step R. swing L. across and make 3 hops on the R. foot.
           Chant: 'step, hop, hop, hop.
           Repeat to the left.
           This movement and rhythm is to be found in the tarantella (6/8 rhythm) and other Italian dances.

(ii)   Glide, hop, hop (skating step) as in some Dutch, Danish and Swedish dances, 3/4 time (1 skating step to 1 bar). In couples, hands joined in front of the body right with right and left with left. Glide diagonally forward on R., 2 hops on R. repeat with L.

Chant: Glide, hop, hop. (Skate, hop, hop).

Pas mazurka 3/4 time (1 step to 1 bar)

This is a graceful step in 3/4 time, as in many Polish and Swedish dances.

Stamp, close, hop.

Teach it moving forward altogether.

Stamp, R. forward, close L. to R., hop L. raising the R. foot in front.

It repeats with the same foot leading and will combine well with runs or stamps e.g. Stamp R., close L., hop L. Stamp, close, hop

Stamp, step, hop. 3 runs R. L. R.

Repeat this starting on the L. foot.

Pas de basque 2/4 or 3/4 (1 step to 1 bar)

This step is taken from side to side, it is found in dances from Russia, Central Europe and in English and Scottish country dancing. One step has 3 beats and 3 changes of weight and is performed to a rhythm of 1 and 2.

Simplified version: Step R. to the right side. Quickly close L. into the R. and immediately stamp on the R. — in place. This whole movement repeats to the left. It is easier to chant: step, mark time, **or** R. mark time, L. mark time.

Note: This step requires a quick change of balance. It is, however, with a change of rhythm and tempo into a slow 3/4 (waltz), an effective simple way of teaching a step in waltz rhythm.

Waltz 3/4 time (1 step to 1 bar)

A gentle swaying movement in 3/4 time that can be danced with a partner. At a later stage, if this is mastered, it is possible to introduce a simplified close, change step, or 3 passing steps, long, short, short.

Basic waltz ryhthm step

(i)   Step R. to right

(ii)   Close L. to R.

(iii) Transfer weight back to R.

Holds. Holds can be varied to suit the ability of the class members. Here are some simple examples:

Partners stand side by side facing the same direction.

1.   Link inside hands
2.   Link inside elbows
3.   Cross arms in front, hold hands R. with R. and L. with L. (promenade hold).

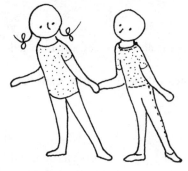 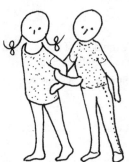 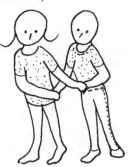

Holds (side by side)

Partners face each other

1.   Shake R. hands 'as if to say hello' and then turn side by side to move round the room (anti-clockwise).
2.   In coules, the gentleman puts his hands on the ladies' waist and the lady puts her hands on the gentleman's shoulders (lean away). They turn on the spot together. Gentlemen starting with the R. foot and lady with the L. foot.
3.   The gentleman puts his right arm round the lady's waist and grasps her R. hand with his L. hand. Keep arms at shoulder height. The lady places her L. hand on the gentleman's R. shoulder from behind (ballroom hold).

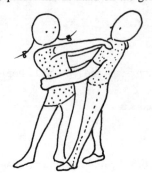 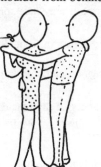 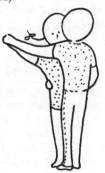

Holds (facing)

4. In a circle, the gentlemen put their arms round the ladies' waists and the ladies put their hands on the shoulders of the gentlemen on either side of them.

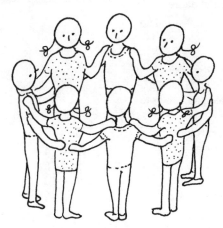

Holds (facing into circle)

COMPOSITION OF SIMPLE DANCE-LIKE ACTIVITIES

When practising the steps of a particular dance, it helps to compose a simple dance-like activity to an 8 or 16 bar phrase of 2/4, 4/4, 6/8 or 3/4 music according to the nature of the step(s). Keep the activities simple using one or two different steps only. Here are some examples.

Walking (promenade) 4/4 time (4 steps to 1 bar)

		Bars
Music	Any lively marching or walking tune (4 steps to 1 bar).	
Formation	In couples.	
Activity	Practise walking to the music (a light lilting step).	
	With inside hands joined partners walk anti-clockwise, round the room — 8 steps.	1 — 2
	With right hands joined (or right elbows linked) turn partner clockwise on the spot — 8 steps.	3 — 4
	Repeat (a).	5 — 6
	Repeat with left elbows linked turn anti-clockwise on the spot.	7 — 8
	Repeat all.	
Variation	Instead of bars 7 — 8, walk 8 steps to find a new partner: this makes the dance progressive and changes partners in a simple way.	

Slipping and skipping (in a circle).

		Bars
Music	Jig or reel. 2/4 or 6/8 time (2 steps to 1 bar).	
Formation	Couples in a circle hands joined.	
Activity	8 slipping steps (gallops) anti-clockwise.	1 — 4
	Repeat clockwise.	5 — 8
	4 skips into centre raising arms, 4 skips back to places lowering arms.	9 — 12
	4 stamps and 4 claps on the spot.	13 — 16
	Repeat all.	17 — 32
Variation	Instead of bars 13 — 16, drop hands, turn to face partner. 4 stamps, clap own hands, partner's hands twice.	

Gallops and Walks in longways set.

		Bars
Music	2/4 or 6/8 skipping tune (2 steps to 1 bar).	
Formation	Longway set of 4 couples, gentlemen facing ladies.	
Activity	Gentlemen and ladies walk forward towards each other and back — 8 steps.	1 — 4
	Gentlemen and ladies turn each other with right hand.	5 — 8
	Repeat from beginning.	9 — 12
	Repeat turn giving left hand.	13 — 16
	Top couple gallop down to the bottom of the set (both hands joined).	1 — 4
	Repeat back to place.	5 — 8

Dance

	Top couple cast right and left skip of walk to the bottom of the set.	9 — 16
	Repeat all with the new top couple leading the dance.	
Variation	The other dancers clap while the top couple slip down and up the set.	

Polka (Hop step close step = Hop 1 and 2).
Practise polka step round the room.

Music	Any lively polka tune 2/4 (1 polka step to a bar and 2 skips to a bar).	
Formation	In two's facing counter clockwise. Inside hands joined.	Bars
Activity	4 polka steps forward.	1 — 4
	8 skips forward finish facing partner	5 — 8
	Lady 4 polka steps round gentleman while he claps	9 — 12
	4 polka steps round the lady while she claps	13 — 16
	Finish side by side ready to start again.	

Waltz or triple run

Music	Any waltz 3/4 time (1 waltz step to a bar).	
Formation	Sets of 6. Two lines of 3 facing each other. 1 gentleman and 2 ladies in each line	
	L G L	
	L G L	
Activity	Lines waltz towards each other 2 steps. Lines waltz away from each other 2 steps.	Bars 1 — 4
	No. 1 lady cross diagonally 4 steps	5 — 8
	No. 2 lady cross diagonally 4 steps	9 — 12
	The gentlemen change places — 4 steps	13 — 16
	Repeat all back to places	17 — 32

A musical medley

Use tunes suitable for different steps, skipping, polka, slipping, waltz, walking etc. The dancers listen to the music, identify the step (s) verbally and then dance them.

EXAMPLES OF ADAPTED SIMPLE DANCES

Shepherd's hey

Music	*Shepherd's hey 4/4 time (4 runs to 1 bar).*	
Formation	All dancers stand facing the teacher with hands by sides.	Bars
Dance	4 runs forward, 4 runs backwards	1 — 2
	Jump feet apart rebound, jump together	3
	Repeat jump	4
	Chant: Out – wait – in – wait – out – wait – in – wait	
	Repeat Bars 1 — 4	5 — 8
	Clapping pattern	
	Clap, clap, 'slap' slightly raised right knee	
	Chant 1 2 3, wait	9
	Chant 1 2 3 wait	10
	3 claps under right knee 1 2 3 wait	11
	Repeat claps under left knee 1 2 3 wait	12
	Repeat the clapping pattern	13 — 16

Country gardens

Music	Country gardens 4/4 time (4 steps to 1 bar).	
Formation	The couples line up one behind the other in longways set formation with the lady on the gentleman's right.	
Dance	The ladies following the top lady, cast out to the left and walk round the gentlemen's line and back to their places.	Bars 1 — 4
	The gentlemen following the top gentleman cast out to the right and walk round the ladies' line and back to their places	5 — 8
	Casting out	
	Both leaders cast out simultaneously, the ladies to the right and the gentlemen to the left	9 — 12

The first couple meet join hands and walk forward to their starting positions. They face each other. They raise their arms to make an arch. 1st and 2nd couples follow and do likewise	13 — 16
4th couple meet and join inside hands and pass under all the arches until they reach the top of the set	17 — 20
They have now become the top couple, and the former top couple become the 2nd couple	
The new top couple turn on the spot 8 steps clockwise — 8 steps anti-clockwise	21 — 24
Repeat the dance sufficient times until all the couples have led the dance.	

Here comes a bluebird (Based on the song in the Ladybird Series Dancing Rhymes 1976).

Music	Here comes a bluebird — 3/4 time (1 waltz step to 1 bar)	
Formation	All the dancers form a circle or line with hands joined and arms raised to make arches. A dancer at the end of the line dances with the teacher with the waist hold.	
Dance	The teacher and dancer weave in and out through the arches	Bars 1 — 8
	They separate and join hands with the nearest dancer to them, and each couple turns his new partner on the spot	9 — 16
	At the end of this phrase, the dancers left in the line make their arches, and the 2 couples now make a line one behind the other and weave in and out of the arches	17 — 24
	Each time the dance is repeated the number of couples dancing doubles and the number in the line decreases	25 — 32
	This is a simple dance in which everybody can join. It can also be danced in a circle formation.	

A-hunting we will go

Music	A-hunting we will go. 2/4 time (2 gallops to one bar)	
Formation	Longways set (4 couples)	Bars
Dance	1st couple gallop down the set	1 — 4
	Repeat back to places	5 — 8
	First gentleman and lady cast out right and left to the bottom of the set followed by the rest (skipping or walking step)	9 — 12
	1st couple make an arch — all dancers pass through ready for 2nd couple to become the new 1st couple and lead the dance	13 — 16
	Repeat until each couple has led the dance	
	It may be necessary to lengthen the phrases to 8 bars = 16 gallops or skips at first.	

Handkerchief dance

Music	6/8 time (2 steps to 1 bar)	
Formation	Couples linked by large handkerchief or scarf held in right hands throughout.	
	Do not break the hold	
	1st lady stands between and below the second couple.	Bars
Dance (skips or lilting walk)	Star clockwise (right hands raised)	1 — 4
	Star anti-clockwise (right hands raised)	5 — 8
	1st man under 2nd couple's arch	9 — 10
	2nd couple under 1st couple's arch	11 — 12
	1st couple under 2nd couple's arch	13 — 14
	End couple under 1st couple's arch	15 — 16
	Swing and change 1st lady under 2nd couple's arch	1 — 16

Pop goes the weasel

Music	Pop goes the weasel — 2/4 time (2 skips to a bar)
Formation	Circles of 3 dancers with hands joined. 1 dancer in the centre of each circle (the weasel). 1 free dancer.

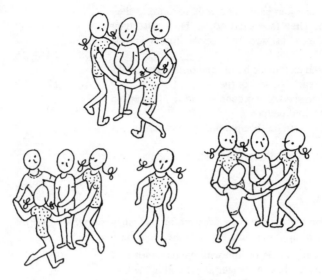

'Pop goes the weasel'

Dance	Skip round clockwise singing	Bars

Dance — Skip round clockwise singing
Half a pound of tuppenny rice
Half a pound of treacle
That's the way the money goes   1 — 6
'Pop' goes the weasel   (12 skips)
On **'Pop'** the dancers lift their arms high and the 'weasels'
'pop' out and run into another circle   7 — 8
The free weasel runs into a circle leaving another weasel free.
Repeat skipping anti-clockwise.
Walking steps or slip steps can be substituted for skips.

Two circles

Music — Barn dance — 4/4 time (1 barn dance step to 1 bar, 4 walks to 1 bar)

Formation — Two circles — gentlemen outside, with hands joined, ladies indise facing the gentlemen with hands joined.   Bars

Dance — 8 barn dance steps to left (1 – 2 – 3 hop)   1 — 8
Gentlemen grab a partner from the other circle and promenade
her towards the teacher (8 walking steps)   9 — 10
Promenade away into a space   11 — 12
All swing partners   13 — 15
Reform 2 cirles and start again   16

Promenade dance

Music — Waltzing Matilda — 4/4 time (4 steps to 1 bar)

Formation — In two lines facing each other, hands joined down the line partners side by side (not opposite).

Dance — Top and bottom gentlemen lead their lines up or down the
room with 8 walks, turn, ladies lead lines back to places, 8   Bars
walks   1 — 4
Each gentleman stamps to the lady opposite to him to attract
her attention, then turns and walks away from her across the
room while she follows — 8 steps: turn, and the lady leads
back to places, 8 steps   5 — 8
Partners link right arms and turn with 8 walks: link left arms
and turn with 8 walks   9 — 12
'Thread the needle'. Top gentleman and lady lead the others
with 8 polka steps or 16 walking steps down the inside of the
set under an arch made by bottom couple, and divide back to
places.   13 — 16

Teddy bear's picnic (walking step)

Music — Teddy bear's picnic. 2/4 time (2 steps to 1 bar).

Formation	In three with elbows linked, or hands joined, facing counter-clockwise. One gentleman between two ladies.	Bars
Dance	Eight walks forward	1 — 4
	Eight walks backward	5 — 8
	Eight walks forward	9 — 12
	Gentleman turns the lady on his left under his left arm, then the lady on his right under his right arm	13 — 14
	All clap hands 4 times	15 — 16
	Ladies four walks forward to the gentleman in front to make the dance progressive.	

Skipping dance based on a French folk dance.

Music	Any 6/8 skipping tune e.g. Girls and Boys come out to Play, Sur le pont d'Avignon.	
Formation	6 or 8 dancers — the couples stand facing each other holding right hands.	
Dance	Fig 1. The outside dancers skip back leading their partners away from the centre.	Bars 1 — 4
	Repeat skipping back to original places. Repeat all.	5 — 8
	Fig 2. All join hands in one circle, skip round to the right — 16 skips.	9 — 16
	Fig 3. The two dancers at the front of the circle break hands while the two at the back of the circle make an arch. The front two turn inwards and lead through the arch turning to left and right respectively, skipping round to the front to reform the circle the rest all following, hands joined. The two forming the arch turn under their own arms.	1 — 8
	Fig 4. Repeat Fig 2, end divided into 2 lines facing each other	9 — 16
	Fig 5. 4 skips forward, 4 skips backward, 8 skips forward across to opposite side passing right shoulders	1 — 8
	Fig 6. Repeat Fig 2.	9 — 16
	Fig 7. Repeat Fig 3.	1 — 8
	Fig 8. Dance in one long chain in any direction and back to original places to start the dance again.	9 — 16
Adaptations	Use a lilting walking step at first until the formations are known. Use longer phrases of music e.g. 16 bars for Fig 3. Slipping step sideways can be substituted for skipping in Fig 1. Dancers would stand sideways to the centre to do this. Slipping step sideways can be substituted for skipping in Fig 2.	

Polka

Music	Any polka tune ('See me dance the polka'). 2/4 time (1 polka step to 1 bar or 2 skips to 1 bar of music).	
Formation	In couples with inner hands joined, facing anti-clockwise.	
Dance	Starting with foot away from partner 4 polka steps forward, finish facing partner	Bars 1 — 4
	With both hands joined, 8 skips round clockwise	5 — 8
	Repeat 1 — 4	9 — 12
	Repeat 5 — 8 skipping round anti-clockwise	13 — 16
	Repeat all	
Variation	Instead of 13 — 16, spin partner on the spot arms straight, pulling away from partner (very small steps).	

Circle walk

Music	4/4 gay walking tune (4 steps to 1 bar).	
Formation	In threes with elbows linked, facing counter-clockwise. One gentleman between two ladies.	Bars
Dance	16 walks forward, i.e. counter-clockwise	1 — 4
	4 step-hops, stepping on left foot and swinging right leg across	5 — 6
	Gentleman joins hands (cross grasp) with outer lady and they spin round on the spot, leaning away from each other and taking very small steps	7 — 8

Dance

Repeat 5 — 6 and 7 — 8 starting the step-hops on the right foot, and gentleman spinning with inner lady	9 — 12
Join hands in circle of three 8 skips to left and finish in a line	13 — 14
Gentlemen, 8 walks forward to the next two ladies, join elbows ready to repeat dance	15 — 16

Four meet

Music	Walking tune. 4/4 time (4 steps to 1 bar).	
Formation	In twos, side by side. An even number of couples, in circle formation, alternate couples facing counter-clockwise. One longways set is a better formation for an uneven number of couples.	
Dance	4 walks forward to meet the opposite couple, 4 walks backward to places	Bars 1 — 2
	Join right hands in a star and walk halfway round with 6 steps, falling back to the other couple's places on 7 and 8	3 — 4
	Giving left hands, ladies change places; gentlemen do likewise giving right hands	5 — 6
	Join in circles of four. 6 slips clockwise (one and a half times round), drop hands with opposite couple (partners keep hold) and move on to meet new couple	7 — 8

Circle waltz

Music	Valeta or any quick waltz. 3/4 time (1 waltz step to 1 bar) (3 running steps to 1 bar).	
Formation	One circle, hands joined, gentlemen and ladies alternatively, four couples.	Bars
Dance	All 'balance' toward and away from centre	1 — 2
	Gentleman hands the lady on his left across to his right side. Lady moves counter-clockwise in front of gentleman with 6 small runs or 2 waltz steps	3 — 4
	Repeat 1 — 2 and 3 — 4 three times, finish holding both hands with a partner, gentleman back to centre, lady facing him (on the last handing the lady is handed from left to right and further to form an outer circle — she faces the gentleman)	5 — 16
	'Chassé' anti-clockwise step close, step close	17 — 18
	Repeat clockwise	19 — 20
	Repeat 17 — 18 and 19 — 20	21 — 24
	Waltz in two's counter-clockwise; all finish in a circle with hands joined.	25 — 32
	Repeat all.	

If the above dance is performed with five or more couples in a larger circle, different partners will be secured each time. This is useful as a 'mixer'.

American Square dancing

With a basis of folk dancing steps, formations and holds, mentally handicapped people will develop confidence to respond to American square dancing where there has to be a quick response to a caller.

People from all parts of the British Isles who settled in America not only kept alive traditional dance music (jigs, reels and hornpipes), but also developed a modern form of community dancing in true country style.

Cecil Sharp discovered this American dance from collecting folk songs of English origin in America. At a 'Frolic' in the Southern Appalachian Mountains our own songs like 'Billy Boy' and 'On Top of Old Smokey' and others were being sung by the mountain fok and they were dancing 'sets' similar to those still danced in English country villages. Square dancing, with other forms of community dancing, should be included in the physical activity programme. It is fun, social and useful as a display item. It can fit into a composite lesson as a final dance or form part of a social evening of dancing and games. In some places square dance groups met frequently. These groups often welcome new members and might, if asked, give a demonstration of simple dances with a 'join in session' to follow.

Square dancing is particularly suitable for mentally handicapped because the steps are simple and because of the way it is presented; the calling (promoting) is a continuous reminder of what comes next and the repetition in the various figures and choruses provides opportunity for practice.

Presentation

Steps and style. The steps and style of square dancing are adapted to suit the local people, local music and conditions. In some areas it is danced more vigorously using the country polka step. When introducing these dances to beginners, start with the single 'dancy-walk' step (when covering the ground): an occasional shuffle or double step can be used to cover less ground or the balance or setting step on the spot.

Dance – walk step. Although this is simply a movement from foot to foot like a walk, it is very different from the everyday street walk. There is a lilt in the movement and the steps are shorter. The heel is not dropped. Swings can be modified at first by using a flat walk step from foot to foot and the propelled pivot introduced at a later stage.

Traditionally the dancers carry themselves upright with arms relaxed at the sides.

Gentlemen always look after their partners and often dance more vigorously than the ladies. Good dancers appear to be on skates as they move smoothly round. Skipping and the pedestrian walk or march should not be used.

Calling. The caller is the person who directs the dance either by warning, 'prompt calls' or singing calls. The dancers should always know beforehand what figures they are going to perform.

'Warning or prompt calls' are used to prepare the dancers and action calls give them the actual moment of starting. The singing calls fit in with the rhythm of the music and the word synchronise with the movements as they are being danced. Singing calls should only be used when the dancers are more experienced.

Music. Square dance music is usually jigs, reels, hornpipes or waltzes. 2/4, 4/4, 6/8, 3/4 time. Piano and square dance band records are obtainable. (See Further Reading p. 136).

Square sets. The set is made up of four couples numbered counter-clockwise from couple No. 1.

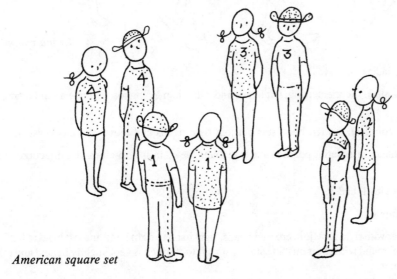

American square set

Remember: the gentleman always has his partner on his right; the gentleman has his **corner partner** on his left; the lady facing him is his **opposite**; the lady has her own **partner** on her left; the lady has her **corner partner** on her right; the gentleman facing her is her **opposite**.

Big set. Some simple figures can be practised in a circle of more than four couples e.g.

Circle right	Break the chicken's neck
Circle left	London Bridge
Forward and back	Single file Indian style
Promenade	Swing

Glossary of simple square dance terms and figures

Allemande left. Corner partners join left hands and walk round each other in an anti-clockwise direction. One complete turn and back to own places.

Allemande right. Partners join right hands and walk round each other in a clockwise direction, one complete turn and back to own places.

Circle left. All join hands in a ring and walk round in a clockwise direction.

Circle right. All join hands in a ring and walk round in an anti-clockwise direction.

Do-si-do corners. Corner partners walk forward passing right shoulders, step sideways back to back. Walk backwards to places passing left shoulders.

Do-si-do partners. See do-si-do corners.

Grand chain. Partners face each other and join right hands. They move forwards round the set giving left and right hands alternately to the oncoming dancer. Gentlemen move anti-clockwise and ladies clockwise.

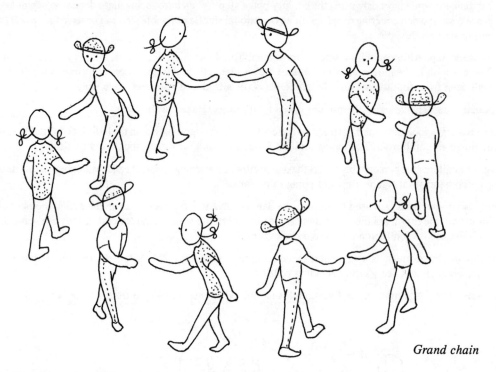

Grand chain

Honour. Gentlemen bow, ladies curtsey.

Left hand star (for two couples). Gentlemen join left hands and ladies join left hands, forming a star and move round in an anti-clockwise direction.

Right hand star (for two couples). As left hand star but join right hands and move in a clockwise direction.

Promenade. Partners join hands in a skating position and lead round the set in an anti-clockwise direction (unless otherwise directed by the caller).

Top or head couples. Couples 1 and 3.

Side couples. Couples 2 and 4.

Swing. Step towards partner with right foot, join crossed hands, right hand to right hand and left hand to left hand. Keep the weight on the right foot and propel round with short pushing steps with left foot which is kept slightly behind and to the side of the right foot. Lean away from partner.

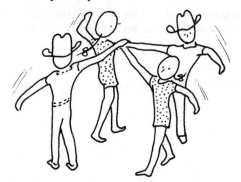

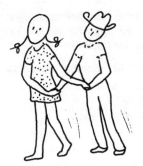

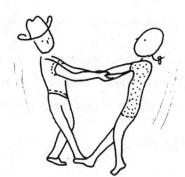

American Square – star-promenade-swing

Examples of big set figures (any number of couples in a circle).

Music   Yankee Doodle — 4/4 — 4 steps to 1 bar
                John Brown's Body — 6/8 — 2 steps to 1 bar
                White Cockade — 2/4 — 2 steps to 1 bar

Linking figures

	Bars
All join hands and circle right 8 steps	1 — 4
Turn round and come back left 8 steps	5 — 8

Call: 'Back track, back track, circle back on the same old track'

All to the centre and fall back twice	
4 steps into the centre	1 — 2
4 steps back to places	3 — 4
Repeat	5 — 8

Call: 'Advance and retire, forward and back,
Make those feet go whichetty whack'

'Everybody Swing'. Swing your partner	1 — 8

Call: 'Swing your partner round and round
till the hollow of her foot makes a hole in the ground'

Promenade your partner round the set	1 — 8

Call: 'All promenade your honeys, take them around the green,
Be sure you take them home again,
no matter where you've been'.

Examples of figures and calls

Break the chicken's neck

While hands are joined in a ring, the leading couple moves under an arch made by the opposite couple, they break hands, separate left and right taking the two ends of the ring round until it joins again. The couple who made the arch finish by turning under their own arms. 16 steps — 1 — 8

Call: John and Joan break the chicken's neck
Break to the right and break to the left.
Repeat until all dancers have led the dance.

London Bridge

This is called when all couples are promenading in a circle. The first couple make an arch and turn back on their tracks, and each couple makes an arch in turn and follows the first couple. These figures and calls can be put together in any order as the caller directs, but each couple should lead the figure in turn.

Bars
1 — 16

e.g. 1 Hold your partner.	Chord
Honour your opposite.	Chord
Circle right and left	1 — 8
1st couple Break the Chicken's Neck	9 — 16
All to centre and fall back twice	17 — 24
2nd couple Break the Chicken's Neck	25 — 32
3rd couple Break the Chicken's Neck	1 — 8
Promenade your partner	9 — 16
4th couple Break the Chicken's Neck	17 — 24
Everybody swing	25 — 32

If there are more than 4 couples, repeat until all have had a turn to lead the dance.

2 Honour your partner.	Chord
Honour your opposite.	Chord
Circle left	1 — 4
Circle right	5 — 8
All promenade	9 — 16
1st couple London Bridge	17 — 24
Promenade	25 — 32

Dance

2nd couple London Bridge	1 — 8
Promenade	9 — 16
3rd couple London Bridge	17 — 24
Promenade	25 — 32
4th couple London Bridge	1 — 8
Promenade	9 — 16
Swing your corner	17 — 24
Swing your partner	25 — 32

These figures can be danced in square sets of 8.

Displays. Simple American square set dances can be used for display purposes.

Suggested costume* for a display team. *Ladies:* Three-quarter length brightly coloured cotton skirts, plain or patterned gathered into a waistband and pretty white cotton blouses with short puff sleeves and round drawstring neckline. Low heeled shoes and stockings. *Gentlemen:* Slacks all the same colour — navy. Brightly coloured shirts to tone with the girls' skirts. Red, green, yellow or blue. Low heeled shoes and socks.

*(See also **Costume** on p. 135).

Set figures

Suitable set figures are:

		Music
1.	Hinky Dinky Parlez Vous	Mademoiselle from Armentiers
2.	Solomon Levi	Solomon Levi
3.	Circles All	Oh dem Golden Slippers
4.	Texas Star	Camptown Races

Once the lilting walking step is mastered and the group understand the square set, many simple patterns can be made up by the teacher and class members from the Glossary of square dance terms (see p. 129).

Phrases of music can be lengthened to give more time. The call 'promenade your partner' can overcome problems such as couples losing their places or dancing out of time with the music, by bringing the phrase or dance to an end or continuing until dancers are back in their own places.

Hinky Dinky Parlez Vous

Music: Mademoiselle from Armentiers or other 6/8 tune.

Introduction	Bars
Honour partners	chord
Honour corners	chord
Circle left	4
Circle right	4
All promenade	8

Dance

	Call	Instructions	Bars
1.	Two head ladies forward and back parlez vous	1st and 3rd ladies advance to the centre and back 4 steps in, 4 steps out	4
	Repeat	Repeat	4
2.	Two head ladies turn around parlez vous	1st and 3rd ladies advance join hands, turn once round and back to places	4
3.	Swing your partner round and round parlez vous	All swing partners	4
4.	Promenade her up and down — promenade her round the town	All promenade partners anti-clockwise	8

Chorus

As introduction without honours	16

Repeat the dance 3 times starting with side ladies (2nd and 4th) followed by head gentlemen (1st and 3rd) then side gentlemen (2nd and 4th) in turn.

The Chorus can be used after each pair has danced as indicated by the caller.

Solomon Levi

Music: Solomon Levi or any 6/8 tune.

Introduction	**Bars**
Honour partners	chord
Honour corners	chord
Do-si-do corners	4

Do-si-do partners	4	
Promenade round the set back to places	8	

Dance

	Call	Instructions	Bars
1.	First couple separate out around the ring, pass your partner going out, meet her coming in.	1st couple divides and walks round outside the set passing each other behind 3rd couple back to place.	8
2.	Pass right by your partner salute (honour) your corner girl	When they reach their own place they pass and honour the corner girl	4
3.	Turn your partner round and round and promenade the set	Turn and swing partners	4
		Promenade round anti-clockwise	8

Repeat the dance 3 times, 2nd, 3rd and 4th couples starting in turn.

After the 4th couple have led the dance the call can be 'promenade the hall' — the gentlemen lead the ladies off to a chair.

Circles All (pick up two, four and six)

Music: The Irish Washerwoman or any 6/8 tune.

Introduction	Bars
Honour partners	chord
Honour corners	chord

Dance

	Call	Instructions	Bars
1.	Ist couple to the 2nd couple, circle four circle four around the floor.	Ist couple walks to 2nd couple, joins hands in a circle and circles once round left (clockwise)	8
2.	Pick up next couple and cirle six circle six around the floor.	1st gentleman breaks hands and leads the line of 4 to 3rd couple, all join hands and circle once round to the left.	8
3.	Pick up the last couple, circle left	1st gentleman breaks hands and leads line of six to 4th couple and circle round to left.	8
4.	All do-si-do with your corner girl, back to back	Back to back with corner girl.	4
5.	Do-sildo with your own back to back till you reach home.	Back to back with partner	4
6.	Turn and swing your corner girl	Swing with corner girl	4
7.	Promenade your partner Promenade your own Promenade around the track Promenade till you get home	All promenade with partners	12

Repeat the dance 3 times with 2nd, 3rd and 4th couples leading in turn.

Texas Star

Music: Camptown Races

Introduction	Bars
Honour your partners	chord
Honour your corners	chord
All forward to the centre and back	4
All swing partners	4

Dance

	Call	Instructions	Bars
1.	Ladies to the centre and back to the bar	Ladies advance to the centre and back to place.	4
	Gents to the centre with a right hand star	Gentlemen to the centre join right hands in star.	4
2.	Right hands round don't be slow Now with the left and home you go	Gentlemen walk round in star formation clockwise; on the last beat they turn about and form a left hand star	4

Dance

3.	Pass your partner give her a whirl Now link up with the next wee girl	Gentlemen walk round in star formation anti-clockwise, ladies turn with left shoulder to centre; as the gentlemen pass they give their partners a little push on the shoulder causing them to spin once round on the spot. Gentlemen then link arms with the next lady (new partner).	4
4.	Ladies swing in and gents swing out Turn the Texas Star about	Gentlemen walk on with a new partner, then drop left hands and move back, with arms still linked, they swing the ladies into the centre. The ladies join right hands and form a star.	4
5.	Keep the new one and cirle back	Ladies move round the set clockwise back to the gentlemen's home.	4
6.	Swing your little girl round and round, Swing her up and swing her down	All swing partners	4
7.	Then promenade away you go, Chicken in the bread pan Kickin' up the dough Promenade with a whickety-whack All around till you get back	All promenade partners	4

Repeat the dance 3 times until gentlemen get their own partners back.

The Texas Star can be danced with your own partner throughout. In 3. the gentlemen return from the star with their **own partners.**

MUSIC

Selection

Music needs to be carefully selected. Most traditional folk dance records and tapes are recorded at the proper tempo for folk dance groups. As these records appear to be the only ones available, many of the steps and sequences will require twice as much music as normal when taught to mentally handicapped people, e.g. if a step takes 2 beats normally, allow 4 beats at first to complete it. If a sequence of steps takes 4 bars, allow 8 bars, or 8 bars allow 16 bars.

Live music

The ideal situation is to have a musician, a pianist, violinist, accordionist or guitarist either paid or voluntary. The accompanist can contribute so much to a dance lesson not only musically but as a person and friend to both class members and teacher.

A musician can help in the selection of tunes, quicken or slow down a phrase as necessary, repeat a phrase over and over again for practising steps or sequences, and slow down the end of one phrase and the beginning of the next phrase to enable the linking of one sequence of steps with the next.

Cassette tapes

If live music is not available, try to find a musician who can make a cassette tape with tunes for walking, skipping, running, clapping, side slipping 16 or 32 bars of 4/4, 2/4, 6/8 time followed by a short sequence of steps based on these steps e.g.
In couples — round the room
8 walks forward — 8 walks backward
8 claps — 8 walks round partner clockwise
Progress by substituting skips or runs for the walking steps
Clap own hands, different parts of the body or partner's hands. The turn can be made by crossing one or both hands with a partner and either walking, running or skipping.

Count a steady beat, which one of the group can maintain, and ask the accompanist to play a tune suitable for the steps chosen and record it at the right tempo. A slow version should be made for practice and a further one for the better performers.

It is advisable to leave **spaces** on the tape between the practices to give time for the teacher to prompt and coach without having to switch the tape on and off.

Tapes can be made of all the other steps and dances recorded in the same way.

Note: Although there is some repetition in the Dance and Movement Training music sections, it is necessary to emphasise the special use of music in both.

SCOTTISH COUNTRY DANCING

Scottish Country Dancing is another popular form of dance. A Scottish Country Dance teacher, has taken classes in Hansel Village, Ayrshire — a happy well balanced community for mentally handicapped people where young people are trained to reach their full potential in living and working.

Development

Since starting in 1969 as a one night per week recreational evening of country and pop dancing, the class has flourished. In 1973 a mixed team of dancers entered the Ayrshire and Edinburgh Music Festivals winning certificates (with merit) on both occasions. The team danced against Branch teams but as no other mentally handicapped teams entered, the judges judged them for their overall ability. In 1978 there were three teams, mixed, ladies and a demonstration team all correctly dressed. These teams compete in festivals, give displays and help the less able dancers in the classes.

Once a year other groups come to a dance in the village. The less able dancers look forward to this occasion as they never dance outside the village. The guests are happy to dance simple dances with them.

Presentation

9 years of interest and patient teaching has produced this development and the standard is still improving. The teacher has built a team of helpers round her — an assistant teacher, a pianist and an accordianist. The age range of her class members is 16 – 55 years.

She starts her beginners by getting them moving. She says, 'Moving around is more important initially than actual step learning — let them "skip" round to the music'.

Gradually skip steps, skip change of step and pas de bas are introduced — some take a very long time to perform them and others never seem to quite manage it. Nevertheless many do reach a reasonable standard. Only team members dance Strathspeys.

Once the simple steps are known, the teacher makes up her own very simple dances before using those from Scottish Country Dance books, often adapting the formations to suit the ability of the dancers.

During the class, some 'pop' music is played by the accordianist — they sing and dance to this which adds variety. The more severely handicapped people who cannot country dance can join in the pop.

The teacher finds it is necessary to be firm and make them change partners from time to time or they will always dance with their 'best friend'. She also dances with them herself. Having an assistant and live music makes this possible. Dancing with the class members is specially important when training the teams.

Simple dances

The following dances have been taught successfully, all are from the Scottish country dance book series.

Book 1. Petronella
 1 Rory O'More
 1 Cumberland reel
 2 Soldiers joy
 3 Blue bonnets
 5 Linton ploughman
 9 More Lady Catherine Bruce
 21 My only Jo and Dorrie O.

The team's dances in 1978 were:
 Montgomeries fant (mixed)
 Strathglass house (mixed)
 Durham ranger (ladies team)
 The Earl of Home (ladies team)
 Bonnie Ann (demonstration team)

The teacher and her helpers hold the opinion that if anyone contemplates teaching mentally handicapped people to dance, it is worth 'having a go', 'little by little you will see your efforts bearing fruit and the pleasure and enjoyment it brings to the handicapped is ample reward at the end of the day'.

DISPLAYS

Simple folk, national and national character dancing can be used effectively for display purposes.

COSTUME*

As many characteristics of the dance are related to the costume and because it helps to create an atmosphere it is important that the costume is as authentic as possible. It would be unrealistic to provide a costume for each nationality but the following simple basic costume can be made — authentic headdresses, waistcoats, aprons and footwear can then be added, appropriate to the country.

----

*For illustrations and descriptions of costume see Mann, Further Reading, p. 136.

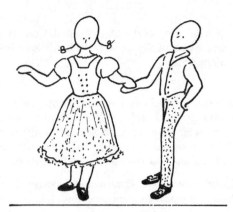

Basic costume

Ladies' basic costume. *Skirt* Three-quarter length brightly coloured skirts, plain or patterned, gathered or pleated into a waistband. *Blouse* White blouse, with short or long puff sleeves and a round drawstring neckline. *Bodice (waistcoat)* This can be made with a side opening made with an open-ended zip. 6 small brass or silver buttons sewn in a double row down the front will give the effect of a double-breasted fastening. *Petticoat* Stiff taffeta or paper nylon — frilled to suggest petticoats.

Gentlemen's basic costume. *Trousers* Slacks or jeans all the same colour. *Shirts* White or brighly coloured shirts. If coloured, to tone with or contrast with the ladies' skirts. *Waistcoat* As for the ladies but with a high neckline. *Collar and cravat* White plastic collar. Large soft bow with ends like a cravat to be worn outside waistcoat.

Footwear *Stockings* White stockings or socks. *Shoes* Black leather low-heeled shoes. The same for lady and gentleman. The gentleman should wear a wide elastic garter round the foot and the shoe with a large buckle attached to the top. *Boots* These can be improvised by making a black gaiter in felt or canvas with a zip side fastening and elastic straps worn under the shoes.

FURTHER READING

CARROLL, J. and LOFTHOUSE, P. *Creative dance for boys.* MacDonald & Evans, London, 1969.

HAYLOR, P., SPENCER, P., and WALSHE, G. *Teach yourself dancing – ballroom, Latin-American, social.* Imperial Society of Teachers of Dancing, London, 1977.

KNOW THE GAME SERIES. *Dancing; English folk dancing; Scottish country dancing; Sequence dancing.* E.P. Publishing, Wakefield.

LADYBIRD SERIES. *Dancing rhymes; Action songs; Singing rhymes.* Ladybird Books, Loughborough.

LAVELLE, DORIS. *Discotheque dancing.* Imperial Society of Teachers of Dancing, London, 1970.

LAVELLE, DORIS. *Latin and American dances.* Pitman, London, 1969.

LINGARDE, ANNE (ed.). *Party dances and games.* Imperial Society of Teachers of Dancing, London, 1972.

LOFTHOUSE, P. *Dance: activity in the primary school.* Heinemann Educational, London, 1970.

MANN, CATHLEEN. *European peasant costume.* A. & C. Black, London, 1968.

SLATER, WENDY. *Teaching modern educational dance.* Macdonald & Evans, London, 1974.

SMEDLEY, R. and TETHER, J. *Let's dance: country style.* Elek, London, 1972.

EMI RECORD RLS 720. 20 European dances mostly from Scandinavia — *'Dances and folk dances from many lands'.* English Folk Dance and Song Society publishes catalogues of dances and records (see Appendix 3), also 'Folk Mail', a bulletin of folk song, dance and music.

Information on dances, records and music can be obtained from the following:
Royal Scottish Country Dance Society, The Secretary, 12 Coates Crescent, Edinburgh, EH3 7AF;
Society for International Folk Dancing, The Secretary, 33 Orchard Avenue, Southgate, London, N14 4NB.
Welsh Folk Dance Society, The Secretary, Dolawenydd, Betws Ammanford, Dyfed SA18 2HE.

CHAPTER TWELVE

Outdoor Pursuits

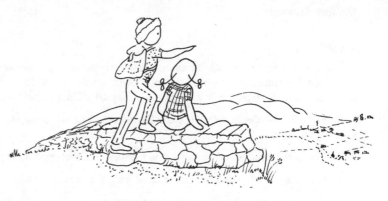

Facilities – Types of Activities – 1. Individual outdoor activites and water sports – camping – canoeing – rambling – riding – route-learning – sailing – walking – 2. Schemes of training in outdoor pursuits combining several activities – Sheffield training centres – Pinewood Adventure Training Centre – Churchtown Farm Field Studies Centre – Outward Bound – Calvert Trust Adventure Centre – Katherine Elliot Cottage Project – Gildersleets Yorkshire Dales Adventure Centre – 3. Holidays providing an introduction to outdoor pursuits.

Outdoor pursuits make a valuable contribution to the social and educational training and to the health of mentally handicapped people. Fresh air alone is health-giving and outdoor activities place the individual in situations which can never be simulated in the hospital, classroom or workshop.

FACILITIES

Many hospitals have extensive grounds — some have natural sites for camping within easy reach of the buildings yet out of sight; most have wooded areas, paths and playing fields where simple orienteering games, route-finding and nature trails can be organised. Few adult training centres, on the other hand, have suitable on-the-spot facilities but the staff of some centres have investigated their immediate surroundings, and found fields, woods, country walks, hills, mountains, the sea, inland lakes, lochs or canals and rivers, and also co-operative farmers and qualified coaches expert in a variety of outdoor pursuits and water sports. Further afield, they have found outdoor pursuit or adventure training centres which have been used successfully for adventure training and holidays. These centres are usually run by national and local voluntary organisations or local authorities.

TYPES OF ACTIVITIES

The following activites are being practised in one or more areas in England, Northern Ireland, Scotland and Wales:

angling (see Appendix 3, NAC book, p. 57)
camping (see p. 138)
canoeing (see p. 139)
caving (see p. 148)
expeditions (see p. 147)
map reading and compass work (see p. 154)
mountaineering (see p. 146)
orienteering (see p. 147)

potholing (see p. 157)
rambling (see p. 139)
riding (see pp. 140-142)
rock climbing (see pp. 147-148, 152)
route learning (see p. 142)
sailing (see p. 144)
youth hostelling (see p. 191)

There is no reason why other activites such as go-karting, ski-ing and tobogganing should not be included in the outdoor programme when facilities are suitable and equipment available for the few who show an interest and have the capacity.

This chapter gives details of the ways in which local authorities, managers, instructors, recreation officers and nurses have pioneered their schemes. It is hoped that many others will feel inspired to examine the possibilities of encouraging mentally handicapped people to take part in outdoor pursuits and to make use of existing facilities and expertise. It is also hoped that parents and other members of the family will find ways of participating in some form of outdoor activity in which the handicapped person can be involved and be more ready to consent to their son or daughter joining in planned outdoor pursuits be it in hopsital, centre or Gateway Club.

Although at first sight some of these activities might appear dangerous, with expert knowledge, co-operation and total attention to the details of safety and prior preparation, they are being enjoyed by and are challenging to some mentally handicapped people.

This chapter has been divided into three sections — listed at the beginning.

1. INDIVIDUAL OUTDOOR ACTIVITIES AND WATER SPORTS

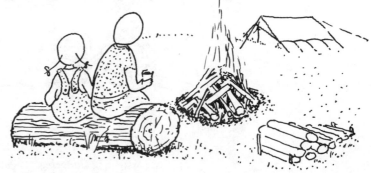

Camping

CAMPING

Several hospital and adult training centres are becoming interested in camping under canvas (see the Sheffield scheme, Pinewood Adventure Centre and Outward Bound, pp. 146, 148, 154). Scouts, guides and the Camping Club of Great Britain have considerable expertise in camping, and may be willing to help train nurses and instructors in camp-craft.

For a few residents, camping could be arranged within the hospital grounds if a suitable site could be found out of sight of hospital buildings.

Those responsible for camping with mentally handicapped adults and children should consider the following points.

Camp sites. Make sure: it is sheltered from the prevailing wind — that it is level — never pitch a tent on a slope!

Water — water should be within easy access.

Toilets — whatever type of toilet is used it must be stable — some have found the commode chair most suitable for severely handicapped people provided it is on a firm base.

Tents — advice should be taken on the type of tents used: don's overcrowd them — it is necessary for each individual to be able to get out during the night without falling over and waking the rest.

Guy lines — mark the guy lines with flags or pieces of cloth. It is all too easy to trip over them.

Camp beds/Sleeping bags — both need ground sheets underneath and make sure there is plenty of warm material underneath — a lilo air bed, old eiderdown or blankets; closed foam insulating mats are now in common use. Roll up sleeping bags and bedding during the day.

Wellingtons and plimsolls — use wellingtons and plimsolls first thing in the morning because of wet grass.

Battery night-lights — battery night-lights will help the strange night environment.

Those leading the camp should be qualified to do so. Alternative indoor accommodation should be available in case of bad weather.

All equipment should be in first class order and regularly inspected and repaired.

Safety regulations applying to all camping should also apply to camps for the handicapped.

A group from Aston Hall Hospital in the Trent Region camp every year, sometimes as far afield as Devon and the Lake District. Several mentally and physically handicapped residents, both children and adults, some in wheelchairs, enjoy the freedom of open air life — perhaps exploring the dried-up river bed or helping to feed the donkeys and chickens on a farm. Some help fetch water while others help with preparing food and washing up, and some make their own beds. Others may only be able to lie on the grass contentedly listening to their radio or picking the long grass.

What do they get out of living under canvas? The following are comments by the camp staff and campers:

'See their faces and listen to the things they have done — probably for the first time ever'.

'I saw a cow putting its milk in a pipe'.

'I saw a doggy collecting sheep'.

'We saw a man on a rope up a mountain'.

'We went through a dark cave',
and many more.

Some venture to the local pub, pushing wheelchairs and helping those who are unsteady on their feet.

Last year Aston Hall played host to the Orpington Gateway Club who camped in the hospital grounds and used the hospital equipment. This proved to be a very successful venture.

CANOEING

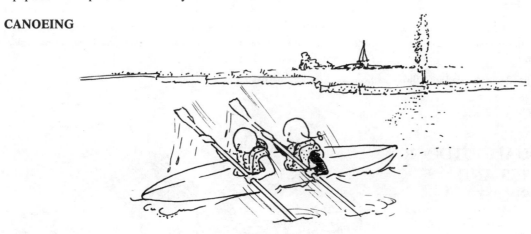

Canoeing

Canoeing can be taight to mentally handicapped people if qualified instruction is available, usually at outdoor pursuit centres where a member of the staff has the British Canoe Union instructors award.

One successful method of teaching mentally handicapped adults to canoe is described by an instructor at an adventure training centre.

'The water is 'still water' — a lake 76 m by 50 m, the depth in the centre is 1.75 m (5'6"). An adequate water depth is required to allow escape from a capsized canoe.

Who should canoe?

'All taking part in water-born activities should be able to swim or at least able to cope in cold water.

Staff

'The ideal staffing level is one-to-one. The ability of the members of the group must be considered when deciding staff ratio.

Equipment

'A two-man rubber dinghy — fibre glass canoes and paddles. Trainees wear a swimming costume with a warm sweater, plimsolls and a life jacket — any jacket with a BSI Kite Mark and designed to keep the face up and clear of the water is suitable.

Teaching method

Stage 1.   An instructor takes a trainee out in a two-man rubber dinghy at first; this allows the trainee to get the feel of sitting in the water.

Stage 2.   The trainee is taught to paddle or row this craft.

Stage 3.   The instructor and trainee then transfer to a double seater canoe, the instructor in the rear teaching the actual paddling stroke and steering techniques.

Stage 4.   Transfering to a single canoe is the most critical time in the teaching of canoeing. 'The first time the trainee is in complete command of his or her own destiny'. At this stage the trainee canoeist will feel just how light a fibre glass canoe is — how easy it is to rock and how the wind can spin it around.

Each stage must be practised over and over again until the trainee canoeist is confident and can move to the next stage.

Safety

Before going on the lake trainees are taught:

1.   how to put on a life jacket;

2.   how to fasten it correctly and securely;

3.   that the life jacket must be worn at all times. It is useful to let them wear a life jacket in a swimming pool to get the feel of it and so boost their confidence;

4.   how to get afloat when capsized;

5.   'Eskimo roll' for the more able people — in a swimming pool.

Note: One of the problems with capsizing is that most people lean back when they feel they are falling overboard — this has the effect of stiffening the body so that the canoeist gets jammed in the canoe. It is imperative to teach people to lean forward and so roll out of the canoe once it is upside down.

Epileptics

Recommendations on water sports and epilepsy, compiled after consultation between the Advisory Panel on Water Sports for the Disabled, the British Epilepsy Association, and the Disabled Living Foundation, and a number of doctors, will be published in the revised edition of *Outdoor pursuits for disabled people* by Norman Croucher and in a Sports Council leaflet *Water sports and epilepsy*.

Canoe building

There are opportunities for mentally handicapped people to build canoes under expert guidance (see p. 154).

RAMBLING

Rambling is a simple and informal activity which can be enjoyed by all except the most severely handicapped people.

The equipment needed obviously depends on the type of walk planned. The main items are a rucksack, a pair of stout boots and some waterproof clothing, none of which need be very expensive.

Mentally handicapped people are invariably welcome to take part in walks organised by the many local clubs and groups, as long as it is appreciated that the people leading the walks will not necessarily have any special expertise in looking after mentally handicapped people. People living in London, for example, can take advantage of the public rambles

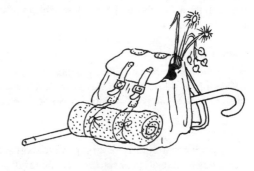

Rambling

organised by the Ramblers' Association. Low-priced transport by coach and train is provided to different parts of the attractive countryside around London, the walks being conducted by experienced leaders. Information about these excursions can also be obtained from the Association, which provides fact sheets giving basic information about walking in the country and equipment for ramblers.

Many groups of the Ramblers' Association have prepared slide talks which can be adapted, if necessary, for presentation to groups of mentally handicapped people. There is usually no charge for this service.

RIDING

Riding is exceptionally popular with mentally handicapped people, but because of the limited facilities and the lack of transport and finance, relatively few have the opportunity to ride. The Riding for the Disabled Association (RDA) is always willing to give help and advice to any establishment or club thinking of encouraging its members to ride.

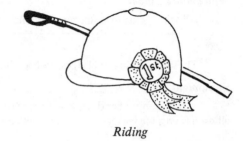

A few hospitals and adult training centres situated near a riding school with riding instructors and voluntary helpers can offer riding, and one or two hospitals have ponies or donkeys on site.

Riding

The Diamond Riding Centre

The Diamond Riding Centre in Surrey was first opened in 1968. The idea was to give handicapped children the opportunity to experience the joy of riding a real pony. Since then the group has expanded. Today it has eighteen ponies with their own stables and a large indoor riding school where four hundred people come riding every week. Many of these young riders are now adults because no one had the heart to say they could not come any more as they grew older. The following account is based on the experience of Helen Henn, a physiotherapist, who has worked at the Centre since it began.

Riders

Many of those who come for lessons at the Diamond Riding Centre are mentally handicapped. They come from adult training centres, special schools and hospitals around South London. Pupils from the schools go on to the adult training centre and, having ridden while at school, are proud to show their colleagues at the centre what they have achieved, be it the rising trot or just mounting successfully from the floor. Sometimes they have a sympathy and rapport with the pony which makes their hour at the centre the only time in the whole week when they can demonstrate to themselves and others their skill in managing to make a pony go where they want.

Rides usually end with a game of some kind: this is the moment when the rider becomes sufficiently excited to use his legs strongly enough on the pony's side to win. If the same rider is likely to be the champion every time, the helper leading the pony can hobble the best and let the slowest have a chance of the accolade.

Organisation

A full ride consists of eight people. Some adult training centres have so many who wish to ride that they take sixteen people each week, eight watching for half an hour while the first eight ride. However, this half hour can be instructive and fun. The waiting trainees can go down to the stables and see the ponies in their boxes and perhaps help to tack up or watch the ponies being groomed. After the ride is over the riders learn to run up the stirrup irons and, if the ponies are not wanted again immediately, they assist their leaders to put them away in the stables.

Helen Henn says: 'Perhaps one of the many good things that develop from riding is when a clumsy hyper-active person slows down and is gentle and kind to that warm soft creature waiting so patiently to allow them to mount. Often the pony is a better teacher than we are'.

Preparation

Before any group starts riding, those in charge, be it head teacher or manager, should visit the centre to see for themselves what riding involves. There is more to riding than sitting up and staying on, and a careful assessment must be made of which trainees gain most from it. To help them appreciate this to the full, the instructors/teachers are asked to ride if they have never done so before; often they are surprised to find it is not as easy as it looks. Riding requires balance, co-ordination and concentration, and those who are slow to begin with and need a lesson to be repeated many times often become better riders in the end.

Ponies and weight limit

The ponies at the Centre are mostly native breeds — small and stocky — but even these ponies will suffer back trouble before long if ridden by someone over eleven stone sitting like a sack of potatoes. The fact that riders cannot weigh more than twelve stone is often an incentive to some who are overweight to slim.

Cost

Unfortunately riding is an expensive sport and always will be. Ponies must be fed and buildings maintained, so it is essential that every minute of riding time is used to the full and to the maximum benefit of the rider. Riders pay something towards the cost of their ride but the charity supports about two-thirds of the actual cost.

Anyone who has balance problems in learning to walk or run will find riding a great stimulant and an incentive to hold himself upright and maintain a better posture. Trotting, cantering or going over small jumps are some of the goals, but everything achieved can be a real morale booster, especially to those who score very few goals during their lives. Meeting their voluntary helpers is a two-way event rewarding for both helpers and riders who are so often isolated in their institution or home. Relaising how much they rely on their helpers as well as the pony for an enjoyable ride can make them less self-centred, and remembering to thank both helper and pony at the end of the session with a handshake or a pat can mean a great deal.

Physiotherapists and instructors

Considerable responsibility is put on the shoulders of the riding instructor and this is shared by the honorary physiotherapists who provide the necessary link between the medical and horse riding worlds. Physiotherapists often attend during rides and will advise on the best ways of helping the people with different disabilities. The riding instructor is not only responsible for the safety of the ride but needs to have eyes at the back of her head to keep eight ponies and riders working hard, but not on top of each other, also to see that those who are impatient to learn wait their turn. Everyone is encouraged to have a kind feeling for the pony they are riding.

A good instructor will incorporate many things into the lesson which will not only teach the trainee to ride but help him in his day-to-day living. Trotting over poles can be exciting, a lesson in good rhythm, and the rider can count out loud — an exercise which can help those with communication problems. 'At the Diamond Riding Centre a non-communicating person has been heard to shout out a whole sentence in the excitement of a game'. Those who succeed in mastering the rising trot have achieved a real feeling for the movement of the pony and have learnt to move in rhythm with him. All **good** movement is rhythmic. Learning which is 'left' and 'right' can be a problem, but anyone whose pony goes the opposite way from everyone else's when the instructor asks for a right turn, soon understands the difference between the right and left rein.

Liaison

Good liaison is essential between the adult training centre, school or hospital and the Riding Centre. Also, before riding lessons commence the instructor must be told as much as possible about the trainees, in particular about any aspect of their condition which might affect their attitude to riding, especially if any of them have a fear of animals or of heights.

Helpers

Good leaders should build up personal relationships with the riders so that they know them as individuals and anticipate the moments when they are most likely to need help during the lesson: Johnny may ride quite safely on the straight, but a sharp turn during a game may unseat him; Jane can reach and take a hat off the pole quite easily, but Mary requires her pony to stand quite still before she will stretch out for the hat, and even then the helper may have to offer a little assistance.

Clothing and equipment

Riders must have a good riding hat, lace-up shoes with a heel or boots, and trousers; these things are necessary for safety and comfort. Shoes that are likely to catch in the stirrup must not be worn. The bridle and girth must be checked for each rider if he is unable to do so himself; the bridle and saddle and the health of the pony are the responsibility of the riding school.

Insurance

A riding centre which is a Member Group of the Riding for the Disabled Association is fully insured for public liability. The Diamond Riding Centre is a Member Group of the RDA and is also approved by the British Horse Society.

Safety

Mounting must be taught carefully and those who have no spring will need some assistance, either a helper's strong arm, a stool or a mounting block, so that the saddle is not damaged or the pony's back hurt.

Riding holidays and other events

Sometimes 'hacks out' are arranged from the Centre during the summer months. The RDA organise very successful riding holidays. Sponsored rides, horse shows and gymkhanas all add interest to the sport; even the slowest poney and rider can win a rosette in the fancy dress parade.

The NSMHCA Riding Fund

An anonymous gift of £3,500 enabled the NSMHCA (National Society of Mentally Handicapped children and Adults) to set up, in 1977, a riding fund so that the society could offer free riding sessions to special schools, hospitals, Gateway Clubs and other organisations. The society hoped that, as a result of these lessons, the beneficial effect of riding on even severely handicapped people would be realised and that such lessons would continue to be made available.

For the majority of mentally handicapped people the degree of competence needed to be successful in the RDA's tests is beyond their ability, but the few minutes they spend on horseback every week can represent an achievement and be of a therapeutic value quite disproportionate to the time involved. It is with this kind of 'riding' that the Society's fund is especially concerned.

Evidence suggests that a handicapped child can gain in confidence from the knowledge that even he, for a change, is in control of, and responsible for, a creature who is dependent on his whims and wishes — he who is usually so heavily dependent on the support of parents and friends. Difficult children learn to relax, non-communicating children to adopt a more responsive attitude.

In addition, some mentally handicapped people, for example those at Lufton Manor, NSMHC's rural training unit for horticulture and farming, have the opportunity to learn stable maintenance.

Riding with a difference

To overcome the difficulty that very severely handicapped people cannot sit astride or even side saddle on a horse, on riding school found a trap, refurbished it and trained a pony a draw it. It was then possible to lift people into the trap so that they too could experience 'riding'. It is worth inquiring locally to see whether a local farmer has a forgotten pony trap hidden in the corner of a barn.

Donkey riding

At a donkey sanctuary at Slade House Farm, Salcombe Regis, Devon, the first indoor donkey riding centre for disabled people is nearly complete. Donkeys are placid and very suitable for the young to ride.

The founder of the Slade Centre, a qualified teacher, assesses the value of donkeys on trial visits — 'The results are shattering: autistic children begin to relate, the hyperactive quieten while riding, and even spastic and severely handicapped children make movements previously thought impossible by doctors, therapists and teachers'.*

The intention is that the Slade Centre will be used by schools during the week and that on Saturdays the Centre will welcome parents with disabled children.

ROUTE LEARNING

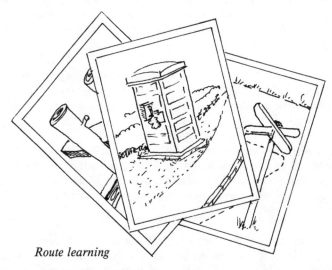

Route learning

Route finding is necessary for some types of physical recreation, such as rambling, orienteering or even finding the way to a sports centre field or park. The following account of a study carried out by the Deputy Manager of Redditch Adult Training Centre, Worcestershire, may help some trainees and hospital residents to use photographs as clues to finding their way about.

Anyone using a route which he has used before looks for certain 'cues' along that route. The object of the Redditch study was to see whether mentally handicapped people could be taught to find their own way over a set route by looking at photographs of cue points.

The route

The chosen route — a mixture of roads, lanes and field footpaths — had a number of junctions giving a choice of direction and suitable cue points at each junction.

A number of factors had to be taken into consideration in choosing the route:

1. it had to be sufficiently far away from the trainees' home for them not to be already familiar with it;

2. although the ultimate aim was for the trainees to be able to traverse the route alone, the leader was still responsible for their safety and well-being while the study was in progress so that the route had to be in a fairly traffic-free area;

3. mentally handicapped people in general do not have the same chance to get out into the wider environment as the non-handicapped, so any opportunity to get away from built-up areas should be taken.

Photographs

The route was photographed, suitable cues at every corner, and when the road was too long between these corners to see the next junction, or there was a bend in between, reinforcers such as a 'no waiting' sign, a 30 mph sign, a lamp post within a garden, or some distinctive railings or piece of brick wall were photographed.

Prints were developed and printed, and extraneous areas of sky and foreground trimmed off. They were then mounted on uniform size cards in a ring folder.

---

*Therapy, Dec. 7, 1978.

Selection of trainees

Three trainees, of varying degrees of intelligence, were selected. An elementary form of assessment was necessary to attempt to get an idea of the functional level of the trainees involved. In selecting the three people for the experiment two factors were taken into account:

1. that the trainees must be able to walk at a reasonable pace for a distance of 1½ to 2 miles, some of it over rough paths;

2. that, because of the mileage involved in travelling between the centre and the route, all three had to be taken together, two being left in the car while the other one was taken round the route.

Alan, the brightest of the three trainees selected, could read fairly well by ATC standards, and would probably have been working had he not had other problems. Brian suffered from Down's Syndrome and Charles also, but he was less able than Brian. He was only able to do simple repetition work at the centre and could seldom repeat three digits accurately.

The first trip

On the first trip round the circuit the three trainees were driven to the car park at the beginning of the course and, after ascertaining that the other two would be all right sitting in the car together, the manager got out with Alan, showed him the first photograph, and asked him what it was.
'A telephone box', he replied.
'Can you see one anywhere round here?'
'Yes over there', said Alan, pointing to 'phone box about a hundred yards away.
'let's go down to it then'.
The box stood at a junction, with the main road bearing slightly to the right and a narrow lane branching off to the left. When they arrived at it the manager showed him the second photograph, taken from the telephone box, which depicted the main road going straight ahead and also the broken white lines across the junction with the minor road, as well as some cars on a car park further down. Alan quickly got hold of the idea and had no difficulty in finding his way round the course, taking forty-one minutes.

Brian had more difficulty than Alan and needed a few prompts. His biggest fault was his tendency to make up his mind before reaching the next cue point and before seeing the photograph relating to the following cue point.

Charles, the least able of the three, was a rather slow walker, and sometimes had difficulty balancing on uneven ground, though he negotiated the stiles without any help. The sixty minutes he took for his first trip — half as much again as each of the other two — was, however, due more to the time he spent at all the major cue points than to his slow physical progress. At a cross roads, where the correct route to the right was denoted by a fence of white palings, Charles could not make up his mind which way to go, so the manager pointed to each road in turn and asked him if he could see any white railings as in the photograph. In each case he answered 'yes' and when asked which way he thought he ought to go, he indicated the road straight ahead.

Cueing points

It soon became obvious that what the manager had considered good cueing points were not necessarily so to the trainees. At one stage he had taken a photograph to include a 'slow' sign for traffic, but when asked what they could see, both on the photograph and along the route, each of the trainees remarked on a brick wall, some tall trees and a house, but none noticed the 'slow' sign until it was pointed out to them. It had not occurred to the manager that, being unable to read and not being drivers, the sign would have no meaning for them.

Second and third trips

The manager went round with the trainees three times altogether, on the second and third journeys letting them carry the book of photographs while he walked a yard or two behind.

Alan amanaged very well, not having to refer to the book at all. Brian thought he could do without it on the second journey, but had to be helped occasionally. Charles got in a complete muddle, not because he did not know the route, but because he could never find the photograph relating to the point he was already at.

Solo trips

Finally, each boy did a solo run. Thjey all made it successfully, and then another boy, Dennis, who had walked twice with the manager round the course without seeing the photographs 'had a go'. He almost confounded the manager's theories and nearly ruined his study by going round without any help and with no mistakes!

Conclusions

As the manager commented, this was a preliminary study and by no means a scientific investigation. A lot more needs to be done before any decisions can be made as to whether photography can play a useful part in teaching social competence to mentally handicapped people.

Because Alan, Brian and Charles used photographs on their initial journeys this is not to say that they would have found it any harder to have learnt the route without them. Dennis appears to have managed just as well with the photographs, memorising the course without being expected to.

If this method of teaching route learning was continued with a particular group of people, would they eventually build up a strategy of movement whereby they look for cues on all journeys?

The four trainees dreived a great deal of pleasure from taking part in the experiment. Most mentally handicapped people seem to enjoy open-air activities, and these four were no exception. They would have liked the experiment to have continued for a much longer period. The satisfaction which they obviously obtained would of itself have made the whole project worthwhile.

SAILING

Sailing is considered by some to be dangerous and outside the capabilities of mentally handicapped people. However, a few adult training centres include sailing in their programme, one of the more successful being the Blantyre Adult Training Centre, St. Austell, Cornwall.

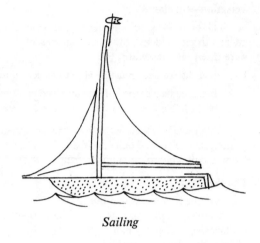

One of the centre's instructors has been sailing with groups of mentally handicapped people for five years. The progress made has proved to be intellectually stimulating, socially valuable and emotionally satisfying, and has proved an enjoyable way for the participants to exceed society's expectations and to formulate ideas and beliefs of their own.

Experience of Blantye suggests that anyone planning a sailing programme for mentally handicapped people should bear in mind the following guidelines.

Sailing

Precautions and safety

1. Prepare yourself, your craft and your crew, and get to know local conditions.
2. Wear correct clothing and footwear.
3. Practise survival techniques in water.
4. Take life jackets to the local swimming pool and use them in shallow, warm water. Instruct the correct method of wearing and fastening them and how to remove them.
5. Discuss capsize and man overboard drills and, when the trainees are confident, practise these skills.
6. Read and use the Department of Trade and Industry Seaway Code and/or use the various British Waterways pamphlets.
7. Acquire a good stable tender, and never overload. It is better to make three safe journeys than one fatal one.
8. Check weather conditions.
9. Carry safety equipment — flares, fire extinguisher, life jackets, anchor — and know how to use them.
10. Understand the use and storage of toxic materials, and carry emergency spares for boat and marine engine(s).
11. Leave details of where you are going and how long you expect to be away with a responsible person.

Suggested plan

1. Carry out a feasibility study.,
2. Discuss it with those in authority.
3. Look at what resources are available; create resources where none exist.
4. Look at the area of risk (see Chapter 16 'Insurance').
5. Acquire the necessary skills and expertise before attempting to instruct.
6. Discuss the programme fully with all interested parties — management, parents, guardians, colleagues.
7. Acquire necessary safety equipment before acquiring the necessary craft. It is all too tempting to use a boat without the necessary safety equipment and an initial programme can be made using safety equipment only.
8. When all equipment has been secured, choose a pilot group of people to work with, set short term goals for long term plans. Consider the ethos 'do your homework if you don's know where you are going any road will take you there'.

Resources

Allied forces establishments	Royal National Lifeboat Institution
Outward Bound centres	Sea scouts
Sailing clubs	Sea cadets
Boatyards	Youth service
Chandlers	Technical colleges
Ocean Youth Club	British Waterways Board
Royal Yachting Association	(also many local charities and organisations)
HM Coastguard Department of Trade	

WALKING

A well planned purposeful walk whether taken in a large city, town, country area or by the sea provides many opportunities for learning.

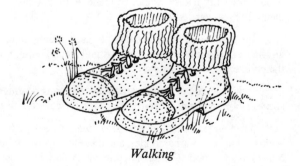

Here are some ideas for walks and ways in which they can be planned: a nature walk; a farm visit; a route finding walk leading to orienteering; a shopping expedition; a discovery walk; a hide-and-seek walk.

Walking

A nature walk

1. Draw attention to some natural objects — a catkin, a stone, a flower, leaf. See how many of these things can be brought back.

2. Find a dark green leaf, a light green leaf and a yellow leaf. Gradually learn the tree names — later those of the different flowers and fruits.

3. Birds. Identify some of the common birds. Show pictures first, e.g. robin, magpie, chicken, tit, thrush, blackbird, duck, swan.

4. Collect coloured pebbles from the beach.

5. Collect anything of interest in the neighbourhood.

A farm visit

Many farmers are willing for small groups to visit their farms — to see the animals, a tractor, a plough, farm buildings, dogs and cats, chickens.

A route finding walk (see p. 142)

This method has many possibilities.

A shopping expedition

This expedition needs careful planning and can only be undertaken with those who are learning about money.

A discovery walk

1. Plan a walk to find out the different types of buildings existing in the immediate environment, e.g. church, hotel, pub, post office, ambulance and fire stations, swimming baths, sports centres, adventure playground.

2. Take walks with different themes: how many different kinds of transport were seen on the walk?
   'Uniform' walks — how many different uniforms were seen, e.g. police, nurses, firemen, soldiers, bus drivers and conductors etc.
   'Work' walks — visits to factories, building sites, stores, to see people and their different kinds of work.

Hide and seek walk

This type of walk is particularly appropriate in places where there are low bushes or shrubs, logs, benches — instruct the walkers that, at the whistle signal, they should all try to get off the ground or get out of sight — when two whistles are given, all should get to base.

Note: Suitable for hospital grounds. It is necessary to fix the route precisely and know the members of the group well.

Picnic walks

Walk to a picnic area with a good view, perhaps a lake or the beach. Take a picnic with you and sometimes cook outside.

Quiet walks

1. Sounds — how many sounds can you hear? What makes the sound? — a bird, an animal, a bus or a train?

2. Smell — what do you smell? Is it the exhaust from a car, a flower, a factory?

3. Look — take a magnifying glass with you, study leaves, flowers and trees — what can you see?

4. Feel — what does the bark of a tree, pine needles, a stone, the water in a stream, feel like—

Note: To speed up walking, follow 12 to 20 walks by 12 to 20 runs (this also helps counting). Gradually lengthen the period of time allocated and encourage long strides.

2. SCHEMES OF TRAINING IN OUTDOOR PURSUITS COMBINING SEVERAL ACTIVITIES

Two well established schemes are described in detail, the Sheffield Adult Training Centres' Outdoor Pursuits Scheme, and the Pinewood Adventure Training Centre in Croydon. Both of these, the first based on weekends and single days, the latter on residence for a longer period, show what enterprise can ultimately achieve.

Two other schemes – one involving the use of the Church-town Farm Field Studies Centre in Cornwall by a Surrey adult training centre, and the other of Outward Bound Wales by groups from a Birmingham Hospital and an adult training centre from Bournemouth — are described in some detail. Other groups attend the centres at the same time, so that the trainees have the opportunity not only to participate in the outdoor activites, but also to meet other students, to work together and learn to understand each other.

Some details are also included of three other well known training centres for outdoor pursuits for mentally handicapped people — the Calvert Trust Adventure Centre in the Lake District, the Katharine Elliot Cottage Project in Scotland and the Gildersleets Yorkshire Dales Adventure Centre.

SHEFFIELD TRAINING CENTRES — OUTDOOR PURSUITS SCHEME

Ways and means

The adult trining centres in Sheffield are successfully answering the question as to how the natural desire of mentally handicapped people for adventure can be directed into exciting yet safe channels and at the same time arouse a worthwhile interst that will survive in later years and be of use in their future training, giving them new motivation and means of communication.

About ten years ago a few of the more able mentally handicapped trainees were taken on country rambles and fishing trips. One of the instructors was a leader with the Edale Mountain Rescue team and, with the help of other team members, was eventually able to introduce rock climbing, fell walking, bivouacing, caving and mountain hut weekends.

Field studies are a part of all expeditions: the trainees observe local flora and fauna and items of geological interest. Collections can be made and mounted during the 'back at Centre' study sessions, but only of items which do not deplete the natural resources of the area. Other means such as sketches, plaster casts and rubbings are used for these. In some areas there are museum services which loan out collections and specimens.

Drawing and painting are often used as means of recording experiences and discoveries. This is helpful to those who cannot read or write, and can take the place of a log book. A group mural can also record the activities. The instructor comments, 'From experience over the years, the young men and women trainees so far involved have, without doubt, benefitted physically, socially and as individuals'.

Co-operation

What is it that makes a specialised team of instructors' objectives work? The co-operation of not only a few but of all the centres involved, and the parents of the trainees taking part; the staff who are not outdoor pursuit minded but willing to have extra class numbers in order to benefit the few; the kitchen staff who not only provide food for expeditions but also help to supervise the trainees in such tasks as sandwich making; also the other specialists such as the senior instructor engineer who has spent many hours canabalising obsolete wheelchairs in order to make one to our specifications, based on the principles of mountain rescue equipment. Sheffield now has a prototype chair with not only wheels but also sledge runners and anchorage points for stabilising ropes to be tied. This project is now in the hands of Sheffield University who hope to produce a new chair of maximum strength for maximum lightness, incorporating modifications found necessary on test runs.

Many of the Edale team members became interested in this rewarding work; they could see, from weekend to weekend, an improvement in the trainees' self-confidence and self-reliance and, in some cases, a marked improvement in gross motor co-ordination and balance. These outings also helped the trainees to become aware of the needs of others, and to be less self-centred. These activities were considered voluntary and because they took place at weekends, the adult training centres were not officially involved. The work continued and a few far-sighted managers began to accept the importance of the venture. After a successful managers' meeting the activities were incorporated into the Centre's timetable, i.e. one day per month and the Friday afternoon prior to a weekend expedition. The use of the Centre's transport was granted and some time was allocated to the administration and paperwork involved.

The Outdoor Pursuits scheme is now accepted as part of the day-to-day training and assessment programme. Independence in curriculum and organisation is maintained and use is still made of voluntary help at weekends as well as centre staff. In this way contact is kept with other interested agencies, the Special Schools and the Society for Mentally Handicapped Children and Adults for instance, as well as the many individual experts who sometimes offer assistance.

Leaders' training

Before the more adventurous outdoor activities can be envisaged, the problem of training staff must be realised. Their extra voluntary training should be of a standard acceptable not only to the parents of trainees, but also to the authority. In Sheffield, staff are selected and trained not necessarily for their academic qualifications but, in the first instance, for their experience and suitability as mountaineers, cavers and rock climbers. Not only do they have to possess expert knowledge in any one subject, they must have an active interest in many others. They should also be able to work individually and yet be self-disciplined and able to work as a team. The staff as a whole must be prepared to work with enthusiasm. A harmoniuos staff relationship is 'Utopia' in any situation but this must be achieved if the aims of adventure training are to succeed.

A field team

A field team consists of an adviser — who takes full responsibility for safety and staff training — an organiser — who is responsible for equipment, bookings of huts and hostels and also acts as treasurer — four senior staff — all experts in their own field — and ten instructors who have completed an annual in-service training course. The organisation of the team mentioned above now includes four women which makes possible such events as female bivouacs.

Outdoor Pursuits development in the Sheffield training centres is not a full-time occupation for the staff, but one to which they give their time voluntarily, and with the exception of a few mid-week outings, carry on their normal teaching duties within the centres. The instructor training programme is a yearly event designed to include a great deal of navigation both night and day. Mountain safety and rescue techniques are covered with emphasis on First Aid and medical knowledge. Any medical condition, heart disease or tendency to chest infections more serious than is accepted as normal with trainees suffering from Downs Syndrome, must be known to the instructors, so that the programme can be modified to suit each group. In most Outdoor Pursuits centres the courses are aimed at the limits of strength and endurance of the individual, but a different approach must be adopted with handicapped people to allow a good margin of reserve strength and energy. Experience is vital; the instructor must know when to get off the hill or, more importantly, when not to be on the hill in the first place. Potential instructors are also given the opportunity to visit unfamiliar mountain countryside and to spend a night out in bivouac conditions, usually in winter.

A year's programme

A programme in booklet form is published each year and given to any interested trainee. The 1978 programme included about 72 different expeditions. The 1979 programme had 92. The activities undertaken are fairly comprehensive and are aimed at all levels of intelligence: they vary from simple nature trails, including those for wheelchair cases, to mountain expeditions to over 3000'. Some are mid-week day expeditions, others take place at weekends.

Selection of those to take part

Individuals from adult training centres, Gateway Clubs and hospitals are selected and invited to join whichever expeditions coincide with their own particular level of training and ability and to join those which may expand their potential.

Planning the expedition

The types of expeditions, walks or scrambles undertaken and the length and strenuousness of the routes will depend on the individual trainee. However, walks of all grades can be found in any mountainous area and each course starts with the less strenuous and builds up to an expedition of suitable length and duration, including a camp under canvas, or, if the weather is poor, in a youth hostel. If the physical prowess of those taking part is such that they are not capable of carrying the tents, sleeping bags, and cooking equipment, the route can be so planned that equipment for camping is taken by transport and dropped off at a pre-arranged camp site, and collected later. If by using a shorter route the trainees could be self-supporting, however, they would benefit from the feeling of being self-dependent.

Obviously each walk or expedition requires a great deal of thought and planning, taking into consideration such factors as the medical condition of each individual, the time of year and, above all, the weather. Although orienteering is perhaps beyond the capabilities of most trainees, simple map reading can be interesting; for instance, north, south, east and west without the complication of degrees, and map references up to four figures can be within their scope. The use of simple conventional signs can help to teach observation, while looking for churches, woods and streams marked on the map can add interest.

Rock climbing

Rock climbing, an exciting activity, well within the powers of most trainees, undoubtedly helps to build self-confidence, and provides the novice with a great sense of personal achievement.

Climbs of many hundreds of feet can be tackled with selected trainees if the safety rules are strictly observed, but the outcrop type of climbing reaching a height of not more than about 24m (80′) provides trainees with sufficient scope and a spice of danger, while making an accident almost impossible.

The Peak District National Park is by far the best area for outcrop climbing. Gritstone Edges now boast many hundreds of climbs all named and graded according to severity. For instance 'easy': with large footholds suitable for beginners; 'moderate': not much more difficult, but having one or two places that are a bit 'sticky'; 'difficult': usually steeper and more exposed than the first two grades, but with adequate footholds and handholds, which there may not be in a climb that is rated 'very difficult' or 'severe'. The climbs get progressively harder and are graded 'very severe', 'extremely severe' and so on. Mentally handicapped people should not undertake climbs any harder than 'difficult', as the harder climbs (although no more dangerous on a top rope) do demand an extremely good sense of balance and co-ordination. To tackle climbs graded higher than 'difficult' a much higher intellectual ability is required than can generally be found among mentally handicapped people. No doubt a trainee could be 'dragged' up harder climbs, but not only would this have no practical value, it would kill his enthusiasm.

Rock climbing would probably be number one on any list of dangerous pastimes. In fact this is not true; if certain rules are obeyed (i.e. if there is a ratio of two expert climbing instructors to one trainee actually climbing, and if equipment such as harnesses and crash helmets is used) the likelihood of a trainee falling more than a few inches would be slight, especially if the climbers were using an outcrop where the total height is not more than a rope's length. Rock climbing is also a suitable activity for the less robust; it is a test of balance and co-ordination rather than of pure strength.

Caving

Caving is an activity which can be graded in severity from the easy, open-to-the-public commercial caves, to the complex systems of the famous and often notorious potholers' caves. It rarely depends on the weather except after very heavy rain. Caving can usually be undertaken when rock climbing cannot. A wet day on the rocks can be a chilling experience and far less agreeable than a day spent in the constant temperature of the caves. This too is a sport involving little danger if treated with respect.

A pot-hole is a cave that has been formed or eroded so that it is vertical, or nearly so. Exploring a horizontal cave is usually quite exciting and quite difficult. A pot-hole can only be safely negotiated by a team of experienced people with ropes, ladders, wet suits and inflatable dinghies as well as many other items of equipment. This would be quite beyond the resources of even selected trainees. The commercial caves open to the public and several other famous caves can be used by small parties of trainees, but even then only after individual trials, since psychological factors could well be involved, i.e. some trainees may suffer from claustrophobia or be afraid of the dark.

Water sports

Activities such as swimming, canoeing, and fishing can all be practised with success. Both swimming and fishing have been carried out in the Sheffield area for many years.

Pony trekking and horse riding are other possible activities — in Sheffield they are organised on a contract basis with a local riding stable.

PINEWOOD ADVENTURE TRAINING CENTRE, CROYDON *

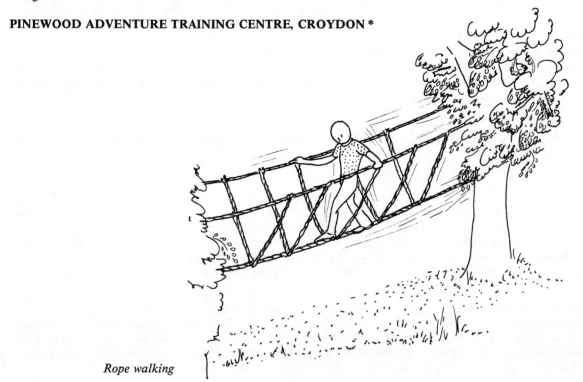

Rope walking

---

*The material for this section was extracted from James Ross' Pinewood Adventure Training Courses 1972.

The experiment

In 1972 the Assistand Director of Social Services, London Borough of Croydon, set up the first long term adventure training centre for mentally handicapped people in the country at 'Pinewood', the Scout training centre in Croydon, leased from Monday to Friday for six months of the year. It was felt there was a need to offer opportunities to the trainees beyond the scope of day centres, in particular opportunities for social and personality development as well as for independence.

The Centre

The Centre is situated in about seven acres of very rough woodland with a small lake, surrounded by rhododendrons and blackberry bushes. The centre building on a hill consists of a large brick built hall, with two small rooms leading off to one side, male and female toilets, kitchen, office and a store room. Around the outside are a number of clearings where the trainees sleep in tents.

The trainees

Because of the rough ground the first course was made up of reasonably physically capable, mentally handicapped trainees from day centres and ESN schools in Croydon. Each course lasted two weeks, with the trainees returning home at weekends. During the first year an average of nine trainees attended Pinewood on each course, making a total of ninety for the six-month period.

Staffing

The staff in the first experimental year consisted of a leader and a deputy leader, both active Scout leaders employed by the social services as instructors in day centres, and two male and two female staff recruited from international voluntary services. These four volunteers lived and worked from Monday to Friday with the trainees for free board and accommodation, plus a small pocket money allowance.

Selling Pinewood to parents

Details of the proposed scheme were sent to all the parents who were asked to attend a meeting at one of the day centres. Understandably, a lot of parents had reservations about their sons and daughters sleeping in tents and canoeing or taking part in other physical activities; very few, however, withdrew from the scheme.

Questionnaires

Next, as much information as possible was obtained from a questionnaire answered by the trainees' own families, hospital or hostel. It soon became apparent that most parents underestimate the potential of their sons and daughters.

Consent forms

Parents were requested to complete a consent form, with details of pocket money for the period of the course and a medical free-from-infection certificate, together with details of medication and/or drugs and an address where they could be contacted should any emergency arise.

Adventure training programme

The programme was designed to develop social and self-help skills, communication and confidence. Because of the opportunities the Centre provided, trainees could be placed in a variety of unfamiliar situations, conditions and experiences which were both an adventure and a challenge.

Although mainly an outdoor, open-air programme, it nevertheless provided ample exercise in normal, everyday life skills and was designed to increase each member's sense of responsibility for himself for his friends, for his team and the group as a whole.

In most instances it was felt that by taking members away from their families, familiar surroundings, regular routine and parental supervision, they were stimulated, challenged and extended, in fact the results surpassed the highest expectations. Most members demonstrated that they were able to cope with situations and activities which they had not previously encountered and acquired simple skills which they had never been allowed to perform previously — washing and dressing was a typical example. Few of the members had cooked a meal at home, but after patient instruction encouragement and supervision, more than 80% were able to cook their own breakfasts without supervision before the end of the course.

Some trainees were apprehensive about the adventure sections of the programme and were afraid of going into the canoes until they were assured and coaxed. These initial fears were quickly overcome and the most timid were able to complete all the activities in the programme.

Ten days of adventure: the programme

Activities during the day were divided into three main observation categories:

Individual activities. Each day commenced at 07.30 hours and the first hour was occupied with dressing, washing, making the camp bed, tidying personal belongings.

Team activities e.g. tidying the tent; preparing breakfast and setting tables etc.

Group activities e.g. all the members on the course working together. Breakfast was at 08.30 hours and each member was expected to prepare and cook his or her own breakfast. Preparing meals and eating properly took longer than was intended but the extra time spent in this aspect of the training proved enormously valuable and influenced the pattern of behaviour in all the other activities.

Before members and staff left the breakfast table, a short time was spent discussing the day's plans; what they were to do and how? This encouraged considerable enthusiasm and the leadership gained excellent response from even the most slow and disinterested. The intensive part of the programme began at 10.00 and continued until 12.00 noon. The programme included:

Danger training (safety) — striking matches; lighting kitchen stove; lighting picnic type stove; lighting open type camp fire; using sharp knife or tool; first aid for cuts and bruises; emergencies – what to do; danger – care and thought.

Adventure training — erecting tent; building camp fire; cooking on camp fire; making simple camp gear; building rope bridges, ladders and swings; climbing; tracking; exploring site; nature treks; boating – canoes, pontoon.

Social training — consideration for others – relationships; manners and behaviour; washing and dressing, personal hygiene; laundry – personal clothes; money; letters – writing; telephone; shopping; what to buy; what to eat; police; fire station; bank; post office; singing; dancing; music; drama, games.

The pre-noon period was planned to be intensive, stimulating and full of variety and challenge. The activities were changed frequently and only the more absorbing adventurous type of activity was allowed to continue longer than thirty minutes. Boating and nature trails were some of the exceptions. This meant that members usually practised four or five different activities each morning.

At noon the group divided into teams (there were two teams to each course), for camp duties, which were arranged to give each team an alternate days responsibility for preparing lunch and evening meal. That most members became efficient at this in a remarkably short time was ascribed to the team-task-pattern which allowed the lower grade members to have a very clear lead from the more able. The high staff ratio afforded the all-important praise-reward-encouragement combined with the assurance of support if it was necessary. After lunch the team who prepared the meal was responsible for clearing tables and washing up. On alternate days the team cleared the main hall, prepared the gear (e.g. the canoes), cleaned wash-rooms, etc., while the other team prepared the meal.

In the afternoon team activities included sports, swimming, canoeing, adventure trails and initiative team projects, which included nature trails and a special adventure trail. The adventure trail led the team to the lake which they had to cross on their own initiative, either by canoe or pontoon.

One day each week they went to another scout adventure training centre in Sussex, with an open-air swimming pool. This was one of the much enjoyed special excursions which included a long drive in the mini-bus, a picnic lunch, and extremely attractive change of scenery and, for most members, the enjoyment of swimming. Again, the more timid were encouraged by the confidence they had gained living in the 'adventurous life'.

At the end of the afternoon activities, the members were expected to wash themselves, tidy or change their clothes, before preparing the evening meal for the benefit of the group.

Each evening there was a social hour which included games, dancing and singing, this was a preparation for the end of course camp fire and barbecue, to which all parents and many friends were invited. New songs and games were learnt to demonstrate on the final evening. Most were ready for bed after a supper drink and biscuits at 22.00 hours. Sleeping in a tent was a new experience for most and sleeping without a light on all night for an even larger number.

In the first few days the members showed obvious signs of being tired after the evening meal, but, towards the end of the course, most trainees adjusted to the new open-air life and change of routine. Most appetites increased as expected.

Consultation with parents

Two follow-up parents meetings were held and the enthusiasm shown was extremely gratifying. The most significant opinion expressed by parents was the increased insight they had gained by visiting Pinewood and seeing their son or daughter doing a variety of activities they themselves would never have thought possible. Secondly, the parents said they felt that their son or daughter had gained the confidence to do many more things because of the nature of the adventure training course.

One boy's parents expressed delight that their son, who had previously been afraid to go up or down stairs on his own, now objected to any form of help or supervision. The same parents could not believe their eyes when they visited Pinewood and saw him walking across a rope bridge slung between two trees. Another mother said she had seen a 'marvellous change in her daughter . . . it's almost a miracle. She now wants a flat of her own'. J's mother said her daughter had to be persuaded to go on the course but there was no hesitation to return for the second week. The parents were unanimous in their wish that this type of project be continued.

Since 1972 Pinewood has gone from strength to strength, the number of trainees attending courses has increased steadily every year — over a five-month period 150 trainees took part in 1975; for some it was their fourth session. For the more able trainees more ambitious programmes are devised, in order to meet the challenge and the demands that they themselves make — rope bridges have to be higher, aerial runways need to be longer and faster, and 'death' slides steeper. In 1978 two groups were taken away from Pinewood for a week and spent the whole time living under canvas in small two and three man tents.

Cooking was done entirely over four calor gas stoves and took quite a time, especially breakfast, when everyone cooked their own. Toilet facilities consisted of one male and one female toilet with small wash-hand basin. Washing in cold water in the middle of a field caused some concern at first, but everyone soon got used to it. During the day time was spent on rock climbing at Harrisons Rock, near Groombridge, Kent, which again proved that mentally handicapped people are capable of a lot more than they are sometimes given credit for.

In the evening four trainees and two members of staff went with tents and food to another scout camp site, where they spent the night camping in a very large wood. The intention was to try some deer stalking in the early morning. Bedding down for the night followed a midnight swim in the out-door swimming pool, which proved to be a new experience as did cooking breakfast and supper over a wood fire.

CHURCHTOWN FARM FIELD STUDIES CENTRE

Churchtown Farm Field Studies Centre, which operates under the auspices of the Spastics Society, provides field studies and linked educational and adventure holiday courses for all types of handicapped children and adults. It has well equipped laboratories, classrooms with a range of audio-visual aids, a library and a photographic dark room. The dining hall and common room are in an old converted and modernised barn and an exciting feature of the development is an indoor pool. The Centre can accommodate 24 to 30 students plus the necessary visiting staff. Accommodation has been specifically designed for the handicapped with particular emphasis on the toilet/shower areas.

Selection

In 1977 the Colebrook Day Centre in Redhill decided to investigate the possibility of offering holidays involving more active pursuits than those provided by the usual seaside holiday. The Centre contacted numerous organisations including the Ramblers Association, Holiday Fellowship, Youth Hostel Association and National Students Travel, all of whom were willing to consider mentally handicapped people with certain reservations regarding their handicap. Finally, the Churchtown Farm Field Studies Centre, Bodmin, Cornwall, was selected because of the varied facilities it offered and the Centre's willingness to accept mentally handicapped people.

Staff

The Centre has its own team of fully qualified, experienced instructors and is admirably situated close to the coast, rivers and Bodmin Moor. It has its own nature reserve and trails. It was believed that clients would derive considerable benefit from physical pursuits and the staff of Churchtown Farm submitted the following programme:

1. coastal footpath walks;
2. rambles on the moor;
3. horse riding;
4. sailing;
5. rock climbing.

Preparation

With this range of activities in mind, plans were made to formulate a preparation programme, having first invited applications from clients. It was decided that a group of between 9 and 12 should be chosen at random, since the Centre did not know what response to expect and because it was difficult to select clients. A group of 10 women and 4 men with varying mental and physical abilities was chosen, in addition to 2 staff from Colebrook and a voluntary worker.

As walking would be the main activity on the holiday, part of the preparation consisted of a series of hikes which not only prepared the group physically but also gave them the opportunity of participating together as a team. Details about Bodmin and its environs given in the classroom proved valuable as some of the clients had little experience outside their own locality or had never been away from home or the family before.

The justification for preparation soon became apparent as many of the clients had little walking experience and some had never even encountered a stile. The group were taken out on three separate day hikes over different terrains, each hike being longer and more difficult than the previous one. It was evident after the first that adequate footwear and waterproof clothing were essential. This preparatory programme enabled clients to adjust far more readily to new situations and experiences during the holiday itself.

Aims and objectives

While primarily a holiday, this venture was also intended to provide the participants and those with whom they come into daily contact, considerable additional benefits. A major aim was to instil confidence through experiencing many new and challenging situations; to achieve this, each individual was extended to his maximum potential so that he should understand his capabilities. It was hoped that the holiday would also help to develop:

understanding and mastery of fear;
awareness of safety factors;
language;
acceptance of criticism;
ability to listen and comply with simple unaccustomed instructions;
stamina;
body awareness;
confidence and trust in others;
ability to make choices and make decisions;
self-help and hygiene;
understanding that different activities require different skills, perseverence, speed, patience etc., with changing emphasis;
anticipation and recollection.

In addition, it was hoped to:

    integrate academic education with constant reference to basic concepts;

    Enhance the client's standing in the family, as their experience on the holiday may well have exceeded those of their brothers and sisters;

    reinforce socially acceptable standards in a different environment;

    improve staff's understanding of individual members of the group;

    provide parents with opportunities during the absence of their son or daughter to have a vacation themselves without the normal pressures inherent within a family with a handicapped member;

    make it clear to various authorities and fund-raising organisations that, given the opportunity, handicapped people can participate in a wide variety of pursuits and that learning through participating in outdoor activities can very often prove to be more profitable than learning in the classroom setting.

Activities undertaken on the holidays

Walking. These walks, which included walks along coastal footpaths and over rough moorland, were graded — the most difficult, moorland walk, being undertaken towards the end of the holiday.

During the initial walk when obstacles were encountered, some people needed help and encouragement to overcome the awkward section. As their confidence increased they became more self-reliant and encouraged each other rather than awaiting staff assistance. The slower walkers raised their speed and on occasions a handicapped client, rather than a member of staff, led the party. The group also became more aware of their surroundings through looking for flora and fauna, some of which they collected for later use in the production of log books. The need to observe the environment was made apparent because of the different types of conditions underfoot. For example, anyone who did not walk carefully over rocks and boulders was liable to bruise and graze his hands, knees and shins, while the unobservant got wet when walking through marshland.

Stepping stones provided an excellent opportunity to improve confidence and co-ordination — at first several members negotiating them were unable to balance on the stones and received a bootful of water. This did not seem to upset them unduly, but on the second attempt fewer feet became wet.

Horse riding. This took the form of a one-hour ride, the horses being led by experienced riders on foot. At first clients were anxious at the prospect of mounting such large animals but, eventually, all but two did so and one of those was too large for the horses available. One girl remarked that 'she felt like a queen as she looked on everything'. By the end of the ride all the riders were far more relaxed, they conversed not only with the helpers but also with the horses, and were sufficiently confident to stroke the horses' manes.

Swimming and sailing. The Centre has its own fine swimming pool available each evening. During swimming sessions it was found that none of the clients were unduly frightened of the water even though a number were non-swimmers. This was important when considering sailing, as the boats were taken not only up river but also out to sea. Boating was an exciting exercise as the water was not calm and all learnt a certain amount about the sea and wind. Furthermore, a number of clients were given the opportunity to take the tiller for a short time.

Rock climbing. Individual clients climbed a small rock face and, on hearing that they were to climb and seeing the equipment, one comment was 'people like us aren't supposed to do things like this', and the general feeling was one of considerable apprehension. This was no doubt due to the fact that no preparation had been given for rock climbing due to lack of facilities and lack of experience on the part of the organisers. To help them overcome their fears, the most able and active client was selected to make the first ascent. Having seen that one of their peers was able to negotiate the climb, most of the other members were prepared to attempt the face. They all appreciated the importance of listening to the instructions carefully and of complying with them. During the second holiday, all clients were prepared to climb the face and showed far less apprehension.

The climb had been extremely well prepared by the staff from Churchtown Farm who had anticipated that some would find the climb very difficult, they were, however, not prepared to let any member of the group fail, although this meant that several clients needed a great deal of encouragement and some assistance. Each client experienced the exhileration of having achieved what seemed to him at the outset an impossibility. The thrill was further enhanced by the knowledge that he had possibly achieved something which was unique within his own family. How many brothers or sisters had climbed a rock face?

Waterfall — climbing the rapids (second holiday only). This unexpected and therefore unprepared venture was more readily accepted than on the first holiday — no doubt prior experience helped many of the clients. The group were taken to the rapids of a fast running river — first three clients, and later the others, slid into the water fully clothed and were immediatelyu engulfed in extremely cold, foaming, white water, varying in depth from 1' to about 4½'. all were afraid but were able to control their fear and negotiated the river, crossing with some difficulty because they were unable to find secure footing since the numerous rocks beneath the surface were of different sizes. In addition, the strong current retarded their progress and the noise of the rushing water made the instructions of the staff virtually inaudible. although staff were in the river and in close attendance, the clients were very much on their own, in that they had to rely on their own initiative to make headway across the river, where they then had to climb up through the rapids. All the group were exhilerated by this adventure and proof of its popularity was the request of some clients that they be allowed to make a second crossing, which they did if time allowed. (Only one client did not take part in this activity because it was felt that the unpredictability of the individual might endanger her safety and that of others). This physical and tactile experience obviously fired the clients' imagination and it proved to be the outstanding feature of a very successful second holiday.

Safety

The Churchtown Farm staff, who stressed the need for safety throughout the holiday, provided all the necessary specialised equipment and explained the various safety procedures to the Centre staff accompanying the group. All activities were undertaken by clients voluntarily, persuasion rather than compulsion being employed. In fact, little persuasion was needed as the excitement generated by the activities themselves created sufficient stimuli.

Follow-up activities. Memories are precious to everyone, and since mentally handicapped people have great difficulty in recalling events, it was decided to follow up the holiday with a series of sessions designed to help them remember and retain as much about their holiday as possible. Clients were encouraged to express their thoughts and feelings on the events of the day into a cassette recorder and this was used later at Colebrook to aid memory. Sessions were devoted to compiling individual log books, dictating a transcript, painting pictures and discussing photographs and films taken during the holiday.

Colebrook have since approached organisations in the hope that some of their clients can continue the activities in which they expressed most interest. Last year the Centre was able to arrange horse riding lessons not only for the group who had been to Churchtown Farm but also for other clients and, after the second holiday, the staff contacted sailing organisations in the hope that this could be included in the facilities offered at Colebrook.

Films were made of both holidays to create and foster interest among parents and other people who may have little knowledge of the capabilities of handicapped people. In this way the Centre is able to provide visual proof of the ability of the participants.

OUTWARD BOUND

Outward Bound Wales has two centres, Aberdovey and Rhowniar. Courses of a week's duration for mentally handicapped people from a hospital and an adult training centre have been held at Rhowniar. This Centre is situated mid-way between Tywyn and Aberdovey and is a large private house surrounded by woods, meadows and large gardens, which has been extended and modernised. It is situated half a mile from the sea wall above sea level. Cadir Idris can be seen in the distance and other peaks of 700 and 900 m.

The Centre has comfortable dormitories, living and dining room, a large assembly hall for drama, music and movement, and good facilities for laundering and drying clothes.

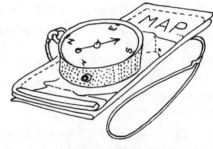

Outward Bound

Courses

'Each course strikes a balance between physical and mental challenges. The adventures and risks are real, so is the satisfaction of achievement. The classrooms of Outward Bound are the mountains, the sea and the storms; the elements become the examiners of young people brought up in the urban industrial environment created by man'. (Duke of Edinburgh, Patron of Outward Bound).

The first course for mentally handicapped residents

Six 'higher' grade residents (3 men and 3 women) with 3 members of the nursing staff from Chelmsley Hospital, Birmingham, were the first mentally handicapped people to attend a course at Outward Bound Wales. This venture happened as a result of one member of staff hearing a BBC programme featuring Outward Bound Courses.

Preparation

To prepare for the course the residents and hospital staff walked and pursued other activities at weekends.

The first course for adult training centre trainees

The first adult training centre to take trainees on an Outward Bound course was the Bournemouth Adult Training Centre. A group of 12 men and 2 training centre staff arrived in the second week of a standard/Junior course, age range 14 to 20 years.

The concurrent Outward Bound courses

The mentally handicapped groups arrived in the second week of a three week course. Each group of Outward Bound students worked with the mentally handicapped group for 1 day in a one-to-one ratio. The handicapped group seemed to adapt very easily to the different faces and were not confused by having different students with them each day. They also enjoyed relating the day's events to students they had worked with earlier in the week.

Course aims

1.   to give the mentally handicapped students a challenging and enjoyable 'holiday';
2.   to give the students on the Outward Bound course the opportunity to mix with handicapped people and vice versa.

Programmes

Since the Outward Bound staff had little previous knowledge of the mentally handicapped individual's abilities, the programme had to be somewhat flexible — but all took part in the following activities:

camping	disco	rope course
canoeing	exploring the shore	shopping
canoe building	games	swimming
cleaning camping gear	life line	trampoline
climbing practice and rock climbing	picnics on beach	walking
compass course (competition in pairs with one student)		watching badgers

Meals

Both mentally handicapped groups shared tables in the dining room with the students on the Outward Bound course who were working with them on that day. This arrangement seemed to help the students to mix and communicate with one another.

Comments — from staff of hospital, adult training centre and Outward Bound

From the Voluntary Service Department — 'The first year, "higher" grade patients took part in the second week of a normal three week course so that usual course members, especially those working for their Duke of Edinburgh's Gold Award, became involved with our patients and their activities. During the first venture the patients were able to make their own small canoe, which was brought back to the hospital, where it is used quite often in our hospital swimming pool.

'The following year six of the more dependent patients, were selected to attend a one week course. Unfortunately, there was no involvement with other course members, as there were no three week courses on at that time. However, this venture was still very successful and our patients very obviously benefitted from the experience.

'It was generally agreed that in future we would endeavour to take part in the usual three week course, as experiencing these activities with other young people was beneficial to everyone'.

From the Senior Nursing Officer's report — 'The instructor had obviously given a great deal of thought to our activities programme. In fact, all the instructors had prepared the ground with each group of students who assimilated our group into their group activities. They all showed a great deal of interest, kindness and understanding for our residents.

'I am sure that many people would be surprised to know that those suffering from Down's Syndrome and epileptics can climb and swim in the sea quite safely provided due precautions are taken. Swimming in the pool and surf were greatly enjoyed. All residents wore life jackets'.

Canoe building — 'I never thought that building our own canoe would stimulate so much interest, but thanks to the instructor who organised this activity it turned out to be a very interesting venture. He gave us all a task to do, some had to polish the mould, some had to cut the fibre glass mat, some had to stir the resin and we all had a hand in stapling and rolling on the resin. The canoe was taken back to the hospital'.

From Outward Bound instructors — 'For Outward Bound students and staff it was interesting to work with six such different people and to learn to adapt to each. Judy was always happy, whereas Elaine lacked confidence and needed a lot of encouragement. Martin would remain interested in what he was doing until the task was completed whereas Kevin wandered from one thing to another. Michael had a good sense of humour, always wanted to know "why", and could reason things out for himself. Barbara loved to use the tambourine to the record player and had a marvellous sense of rhythm. She seemed to live in a world of her own but would give a big affectionate hug when something pleased her . . .

'Our two walks were quite short but we found that they got pleasure from simple things like shouting to get an echo. They each managed a roped scramble during the rock climbing day, and the boys and Barbara went on to do a second route'.

From the Bournemouth Adult Training Centre report — 'The week which trainees from Dorset spent at the Outward Bound school was a time they will never forget. Ten out of the group of twelve men have already asked "when can we go again"?

'A sense of achievement and most important of all, an increase in their own self respect may be brought about by attempting activities which some of their families and friends had not tried'.

(Another mixed group from this centre went to Rhowniar in September 1978).

From parents 'We feel that, in the final analysis, all must be on the credit side. I was certainly prepared for our son to find things too much for him, but, to your credit, he didn't, and we knew that the basic idea and aim of your course was a good one.

'Christopher particularly liked the rock climbing, rope swinging, trampolining and his first experience of sleeping under canvas. This has been a big step forward . . . I am sure this venture has helped him to gain more confidence in doing things for himself and another big factor is the chance for him to mix and converse with complete strangers. It has also given me a "break" from normal routine'.

'Although Stephen has always enjoyed outside activities and has usually been ready to have a go at any new challenge, as parents we were a little apprehensive about this venture, not knowing to what extent Stephen would be able to participate. At the same time having a chance to be able to get involved with so many different activities where normally because of the handicap he might not have ever had such an opportunity, was a challenge not to miss . . . Also, mixing with a group of girls (other than those he meets every day at the Centre) would possibly help to develop a more social understanding between the normal and handicapped person'.

From one of the Outward Bound Students who worked with the Bournemouth ATC — 'On Wednesday while I was helping to make breakfast in the barn, Stephen came over to me and said that this holiday was the best he had ever had and he would like the staff and girls to know how grateful he was. Nobody had told him to say this . . .

'I must admit that as time went on I found it a lot easier to talk to them and the atmosphere became more relaxed. They told me about their lives, and what they do at the Centre where they work. I think it was of great value for these young men and an experience they will enjoy for the rest of their lives'.

A social worker who spent the entire week with the second group of trainees from the Bournemouth ATC sums up his experience of the course as follows: 'This week had proved to be one of the most wonderful I have spent in my career in social work. I saw these twelve people become caring, capable individuals whose ability to make their mark on all they came into contact with will never be forgotten. The probably touched some hundred people during their week at Rhowniar and the impression they made would make anyone proud to have known them. The development in self esteem and physical and co-ordinating skills was truly remarkable. They became sharing and caring people both as individuals and as a group. I could never express my gratitude to them for allowing me to have been associated with them and I shall never forget our week at Rhowniar. I don't believe that any other type of experience could have made the impact that this did, and it must be the beginning of a continuing process of providing opportunities for mentally handicapped people to show what they are capable of'.

THE CALVERT TRUST ADVENTURE CENTRE, KESWICK

The aims of this Centre are to provide the facilities for disabled people to enjoy the Lake District National Park as far as possible in the same way as able-bodied people.

The Centre is built in traditional Cumbrian style, and is set in two acres of grounds overlooking Bassenthwaite Lake, below is the mountain range of Skiddaw, 931m. It commands a beautiful panoramic view of the nearby fells.

The Centre is open from mid-January to mid-November for archery, angling, birdwatching, riding, hill-walking and nature trails, whilst between April and September, sailing and canoeing are added to the programme, thus offering facilities for purposeful and enjoyable community life throughout the year. The accommodation is suitable for both sexes, in mixed groups, and is specially designed for wheelchair usage. Twenty-seven people can be accommodated in pleasant 2-bedded rooms, with adequate bathrooms, showers, toilets and drying rooms; two dining rooms, a lounge (with TV), a games room and a shop complete the accommodation. A key purpose of the Centre is self-sufficiency. The course members will cook and cater for themselves in the fully-equipped kitchen. Food stores may be purchased from the Warden.

KATHARINE ELLIOT COTTAGE PROJECT, HAWICK

The Katharine Elliot Centre, having decided to develop an outdoor pursuits programme, discovered a likely base for their project in a cottage on an estate in the Border country; they contacted the Factor and the Hawick Rover Scouts, and the Scouts, the owners, decided to give the Centre the use of the cottage and donated a gas cooker and light fittings.

The cottage roof was repaired and a new window added; the guttering was renewed and the walls repaired for decorating. A fireplace with surround was built and flooring apoxy resin was laid. A local Women's Guild donated two calor gas fires and several pieces of furniture were forthcoming from other sources. A path was laid and rock and stone embedded in the cart track to 'firm up' the ground. All this was accomplished through the hard work of staff and trainees. Curtains and bed covers were made from offcuts of material donated by local mills.

Angling and canoeing in Williestruther Loch

The Centre investigated the possibility of using a local loch for angling and canoeing. This was not possible, but did lead to discussion with the Border's Education Outdoor Activities Staff and the Roxburgh District Council, who offered 'Williestruther Loch', providing certain guarantees were given to angling clubs, shooting clubs and other bodies.

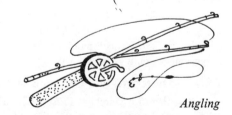

Angling

A suitable seasonal timetable was evolved. A shingle beach is ideal for canoeing and dam stonework offers a suitable dinghy wharf. The 'Spetch', part of the River Teviot, running through the Hawick Park, also offers ideal canoeing on grade 1 water for training canoeists.

The Hawick Angling Club allows members from the Centre complimentary passes to use any of their waters.

Equipment

A two-seat kayak was built from a Moonraker kit and has proved an ideal trainer stability craft on loch and river.

The three/four seat dinghy was built from plans and base materials and given rubber section safety grabs by the Centre; over 50% of the Centre members use this. It can be, and is, used:

1. as a basic paddle craft — Canadian paddles;
2. as a basic rowing boat;
3. with an outboard motor as a recovery and motor vessel.

A Water Bat KW7 and KW4 are the property of the Katharine Elliot Centre and small Water Bats — Panthers and Snipes are available via Selkirk High School Canoe Club.

Integration (Border's 'Snap In' Club)

The Manager of the Katharine Elliot Centre joined the Teacher's Train In's organised by the Education Outdoor Activities. As a result of this the following year Selkirk High School staff and Canoe Club members, with Selkirk baths staff, developed facilities for evening 'integration sessions' with Selkirk High School Canoe Club, Friday evening 'Snap-In' Club, Joint Weekend Slaloms (river races, camps and youth hostel tours), Thursday lunch time Katherine Elliot Centre swim/canoe preparatory sessions in which the Selkirk High School teachers and baths staff work together with Centre staff.

GILDERSLEETS YORKSHIRE DALES ADVENTURE CENTRE, GIGGLESWICK

In 1967 a group of Yorkshire Dales enthusiasts, who became Trustees, converted a farmhouse and equipped it to provide regular courses to foster a love of the countryside and face the challenge of wild and difficult country.

Francis Johnson, one of the founders, says: 'Our progress can be attributed to the work of many instructors who enjoy encouraging youth to try something new and difficult, to build upon their own success no matter how small this may be. My mind goes back to a meeting with some doctors in 1966 when it was agreed that there was scope for a place like this giving short courses, with moderate discipline, to selected patients and individuals who need this sort of natural medicine. Some of our hopes then have been fulfilled'.

For most of the year children, young men and women, enjoy the facilities of the Centre, enthusiastically sharing potholing, rock climbing, mountaineering, camping expeditions, forest orienteering and exploring lakes and rivers of the north.

The Project Training Officer of the Trent Regional Health Authority, which has sponsored staff and patients from hospitals for mentally handicapped people for the last seven years describes the work of the Centre: 'The patients and staff are selected by the individual hospitals and a meeting is held prior to their going on the course, with Mr. Johnson and myself and the staff who are to attend. A detailed programme is worked out and contingencies are made so that the programme can be altered very quickly according to the weather. Since we started this scheme a number of hospitals have sent staff and patients independently to the Yorkshire Dales Adventure Centre, one started up its own Adventure Centre in Derbyshire, a number of outdoor pursuits have been undertaken and as a direct result of the success of this experiment, the Regional Health Authority has purchased a quantity of camping equipment which is available on free loan to hospitals throughout the region'.

3. HOLIDAYS PROVIDING AN INTRODUCTION TO OUTDOOR PURSUITS

The holiday schemes described serve primarily as an introduction to one or more of the foregoing activites or just to 'the out-of-doors'. Such is the popularity of some of these schemes that facilities, clubs, qualified instruction and help are searched for locally, so that some of these pursuits become a part of the hospital's or ATC's general programme.

More and more hospitals and ATCs are looking for holidays for residents and trainees where new activities can be tried and new ideas born. An activity enjoyed on holiday can easily become a part of the everyday programme.

Some examples of such holidays are given in this chapter. Many more exist, organised either by local authorities or voluntary organisations. It is a case of 'shopping around' to find the best package, not only from the financial aspect but from also the standpoint of instruction and safety.

Brighouse ATC

Brighouse Adult Training Centre in West Yorkshire took nineteen adults to Low Mill Askrigg (a centre set up by the village trust). From this village in the dales the trainees took part in a wide range of activities which included, for the more active — climbing, walking, canoeing and potholing — and for the less active — country walks with visits to a cheese factory, a 96-year-old fairground organ, a farm and a pottery.

Peter Le Marchant Trust, Colston Bassett

The Peter Le Marchant Trust, based in Nottinghamshire, arranges day and weekend boat trips for handicapped people of all ages and with all types of disability. Those with severe mental or physical handicaps can and do enjoy the exhilerating experience of travelling through some of Britain's loveliest countryside. 'A day of brightness' was the way one visitor summed up his experience.

In 1976, only one 40' narrow boat was in use, now there are more, including a 70-footer.

The Trust will accept bookings from all sources, voluntary organisations, social services departments and families with a handicapped child.

Avon ATC

An Avon Adult Training Centre staged a pilot scheme in 1977 which has now been extended.

The Manager of the Blackhorse Adult Training Centre suggested that, rather than take a large group of trainees to a holiday camp, it would be far better to take small groups throughout the summer, on a variety of holidays according to the apparent individual need. It seemed likely that many trainees would benefit from living in small groups rather than in the more overpowering environment of a large holiday camp. It was therefore agreed that, as a pilot scheme, two separate groups of twelve trainees would spend five days in an area of wild country to assess the suitability of some adventure activities for mentally handicapped adults.

It was found that the Fedw Adventure Centre owned by the Methodist Asssociation of Youth Clubs would be a suitable place for the initial trials. The hostel, high on Llangattock Hillside above Crickhowel in the Brecon Beacons National Park, is an old converted farmhouse.

During the first week the most exacting activity was the climb by three trainees from Llangenny to the summit of the Sugar Loaf (1950'). However, during the second week six trainees from a similar group to the first, climbed the Sugar Loaf and three later in the week climbed Pen-y-Fan (2907').

From two groups of 12 in 1977, four ATCs visited the Fedw Centre in 1978 with 90 trainees. The choice of activities has widened to include pony trekking, boating on a nearby canal and visits to caves and castles in the district. Fedw is not staffed by qualified outdoor pursuits instructors, but the Avon Authority feels that this is no deterrent. 'For the present, an unstaffed Centre such as Fedw would appear to offer the greatest potential. It allows our staff to structure their programme to suit their group, without the constraint of fitting it to a standard day common to most staffed centres.

'If it is found that there are small groups with a particular interest, such as pony trekking, climbing, canoeing etc., consideration might be given, in the future, to mixing trainees from more than one centre for a specialised week, with an accent on that activity.

Should specialised groups be formed, then the use of a staffed centre with expertise in that activity should be considered. Numerous centres of this kind would tailor a course to cater for groups of disabled people'.

FURTHER READING

GENERAL

CROUCHER, NORMAN. *Outdoor pursuits for disabled people.* Disabled Living Foundation, London, 1974; (revised edition) *Adventures of their own.* Woodhead Faulkner, Cambridge (in press).
DEPARTMENT OF EDUCATION AND SCIENCE. *Safety in outdoor pursuits.* HMSO, London, 1972.
GIRL GUIDES ASSOCIATION. *Guiding for the handicapped.* Girl Guides Association, London, 1972.
SCOUT ASSOCIATION. *Extension activities handbook: guide to scouting activities with the handicapped.* Scout Association, London, 1972.
SMITH, ROGER. *Outdoor directory.* Holmes McDougall, Edinburgh, 1979.
SPORTS COUNCIL, ADVISORY PANEL ON WATER SORTS FOR THE DISABLED. *Water sports for the disabled.* Royal Yachting Association Seamanship Foundation, Woking, 1978.

ANGLING

KNOW THE GAME SERIES. *Course fishing; Game fishing; Float fishing; Sea Angling.* E.P. Publishing, Wakefield.
NATIONAL ANGLERS' COUNCIL. *Guide to fishing facilities for disabled anglers.* National Anglers' Council, 1977 (see Appendix 3).
WRANGLES, ALAN. *A line on sea fishing techniques.* Kenneth Mason, Havant, 1979.
WRANGLES, ALAN. *A line on sea fishing tackle, rigs and bait.* Kenneth Mason, Havant, 1979.
WRANGLES, ALAN. 2 books on coarse fishing. Kenneth Mason, Havant (in press).

CAMPING

KNOW THE GAME SERIES. *Know the game camping.* E.P. Publishing, Wakefield.
SCOUT ASSOCIATION. *Enjoy camping.* Scout Association, London, 1973.

CANOEING

BRITISH CANOE UNION. *No. 1 Choosing a canoe and its equipment; No. 2 Canoe handling and management; No. 7a Canoe building (soft skin moulded veneer); No. 7b Canoe building (glass fibre).* British Canoe Union (see Appendix 3).
KNOW THE GAME SERIES. *Kayak canoeing.* E.P. Publishing, Wakefield.

CAVING AND POTHOLING

KNOW THE GAME SERIES. *Potholing and caving.* E.P. Publishing, Wakefield.

MOUNTAINEERING

BLACKSHAW, ALAN. *Mountaineering.* British Mountaineering Council, Manchester, 1970.
BRITISH MOUNTAINEERING COUNCIL. *Booklet on safety on mountains; leaflets on helmets, ropes and hypothermia.* British Mountaineering Council, Manchester (see Appendix 3).
LANGMUIR, ERIC. *Mountain leadership handbook.* Scottish Sports Council, Edinburgh, 1973.

ORIENTEERING

DISLEY, JOHN. *Orienteering.* Faber, London, 1978.
HARRIS, NORMAN. *Orienteering.* World's Work, Tadworth, 1978.
KNOW THE GAME SERIES. *Orienteering.* E.P. Publishing, Wakefield.

RAMBLING

Mann, John. *Walk.* Paddington Press, London, 1979.

Sharp, David. *Walking in the countryside.* David and Charles, Newton Abbott, 1978.

Spurbook of map and compass (2nd ed.). Spur Books, Bourne End, 1980.

RIDING

Peacock, G. and Saywell, S. *Introduction to riding for the disabled.* Riding for the Disabled Association (see Appendix 3).

Riding for the Disabled Association. *RDA handbook (articles on riding for mentally handicapped people).* Riding for the Disabled Association (see Appendix 3), 1978.

Sayer, D. K. *'Look at this!' Signs for deaf and non-communicating riders.* The Diamond Riding Centre for the Handicapped, Carshalton, Surrey, 1979.

SAILING

Bond, Bob. *Sailing manual.* Pelham Books, London, 1973.

Know the Game Series. *Sailing.* E.P. Publishing, Wakefield.

Royal Yachting Association. *Learn to sail (a guide to RYA recognised teaching establishments).* Royal Yachting Association, Woking.

WATER SAFETY

RoSPA. *(Several publications on specific sports including water safety).* RoSPA (see Appendix 4).

CHAPTER THIRTEEN

Adventure Playgrounds

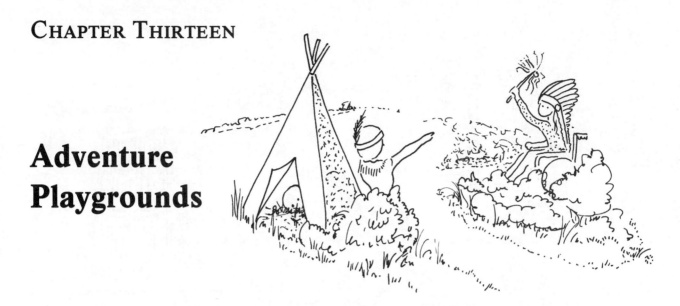

The object of an adventure playground is to stimulate the mental and physical development of a child or adult by the use of imaginative, adventurous play.

A number of hospitals have built an adventure playground within their grounds. Without doubt, these playgrounds afford excellent apportunities for residents to explore, to be 'active in' or to be quiet.

Drummond Abernethy, Consultant to the NPFA (National Playing Fields Association) says:
'In this country we are belatedly beginning to realise the urgent and imperative necessity for children and young people to be able to play in the manner which nature predestined. In other words. the process is so diverse that it includes physical and mental growth, learning, fun, experiment, social conduct and many other skills. Because of the extraordinary conditions in which we live in this (so-called civilised) modern society, this whole growing up process is now quite impossible in its original and natural form. Twenty years' experience of ordinary adventure playgrounds has taught us this: as soon as children identify with the scheme and with the adult and teenage workers and helpers one is constantly staggered by the initiatives and liveliness which stem from what at first sight had seemed the most unpromising child and teenage material. The same goes for the parents and adults who begin to move into these schemes. Over and above all this, one also releases a torrent of help from able-bodied young and old'.

The handicapped Adventure Playground Association and the National Playing Fields Association are working together to find ways and means of establishing more adventure playgrounds for handicapped children, and will advise anyone considering setting up any facilities for mentally and/or physically handicapped children, young people or adults on lay-out, equipment, building, organisation and leadership, and can arrange for them to visit a handicapped adventure playground scheme in progress. Owing to the complexity of an adventure playground and the wildly varying ideas as to what constitutes such a playground, it is essential to discuss all plans for development with one or other of the two organisations mentioned.

PLANNING AN ADVENTURE PLAYGROUND

The success of an adventure playground depends on the initial planning and the skill and imagination of the play leader and many experienced leaders feel that the following ideas should be taken into account when planning a playground.

Layout

See the section on informal play areas in Chapter 5 (see p. 13) and consult the National Playing Fields Association and/or the Handicapped Adventure Playground Association (see p. 182).

Equipment

Everyday removeable equipment, which can be replaced or interchanged, should be the basis for a good adventure playground and trainees should be taught to handle and care for these items. Equipment which can provide the concepts of 'up', 'down', 'height' and 'through' 'round', etc., to provide stimulation should be emphasised. Natural mounds or cuttings help to provide such stimulation.

Swings, see-saws, slides and roundabouts are expensive pieces of equipment both to buy and to maintain but could become a more economic proposition if a group of parents, ATCs and hospitals co-operated in purchasing and using the equipment.

Types of playground

For those who are only slightly handicapped the playgrounds outlined in *Adventure playgrounds for handicapped children* (see Further Reading, p. 162) can be suitably adapted, although some of the equipment could be expensive. For the more severely handicapped the playground need not be sophisticated. Simple equipment, such as wooden boxes, wooden planks on bricks (so that the height can be adjusted quite easily), old car tyres and everyday functional items not normally seen in the hospital (such as suitably placed old tree trunks, immobilised old cars from which all projections and wheels have been removed, old road rollers etc.) can be easily used to provide obstacle courses. It is a good idea to keep a store of such objects for creative play.

Climbing ropes should be trailed down natural or artificially made banks rather than, or in addition to, being hung from trees. People can pull themselves up such banks and are not likely to injure themselves should they fall.

Artificial sand dunes rather than sand pits, or sand in small holes to allow people to dig easily, should be provided. Trees and shrubs and the whole of the natural terrain of the area can

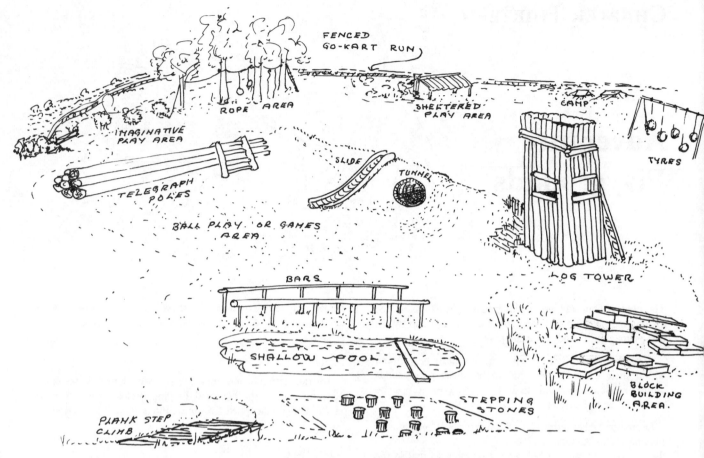

Examples of adventure playground equipment

be utilised for exploration leading to adventure play. It is, however, essential that the equipment provided for this group is readily adjustable to meet their needs.

Profoundly physically and mentally handicapped people can also benefit from the use of adventure playgrounds — their handicaps are no bar to some form of physical play. Water pools at ground level fro water play and gardens with sand dunes in which to dig can be particularly enjoyed by this group.

The various types of adventure playgrounds suggested for different types of patients are not separated functionally. In many hospitals with large numbers of people with various handicaps it may be necessary to provide a full range of adventure play. In smaller hospitals with perhaps only a small number of children, most with profound mental handicap, the type of playground required will have to be adjusted in relation to the abilities of the users.

Adventure playgrounds need not be limited to outside areas: the use of wards as indoor play areas should be considered. Everyday, cheap equipment coming into the hospital and used on the ward, such as cardboard boxes, packing cases, tins, string, can be adapted for play in these areas. Ropes, hoops, coloured ribbons, large blocks of wood, can all be used in imaginative play on the wards.

Storage of equipment

It is desirable, whatever the type of adventure playground, that suitable storage space for material and equipment is provided adjacent to the playground itself.

Staffing

To get the best out of either outdoor or indoor adventure play areas, trained play leaders should be employed. These play leaders, together with help from volunteers, staff and interested parents and friends, can make an adventure playground work.

A description of the planning, building, development and running of the adventure playground at St. Lawrence's Hospital, Caterham, Surrey, illustrates the variety of resources that can be utilised, and how a playground can be equipped and managed.

PLAYGROUND AT ST. LAWRENCE'S HOSPITAL

At the beginning of 1974 the League of Friends considered whether some of the old farm buildings in the hospital grounds could be used as a centre for the League's first major project — a new adventure playground. The Regional Board's Surveyor reported that the old buildings could be repaired.

An ambitious fund raising campaign was launched and contact made with various local youth organisations. The National Playing Fields Association immediately gave encouraging advice and a promise of financial help; local volunteers also offered to help.

Boys from a local school started to clear the site after which a mechanical digger excavated a huge sandpit, the earth being used to form a landscaped range of hills. The pit was lined with concrete and surrounded with an 8' wide patio.

Materials — including wide concrete pipes, railway sleepers, telegraph poles, timber and polystyrene cylinders — were very generously provided by a local firm. The band of the First Battalion the Irish Guards worked for a week moving a line of fencing to extend the area of the playground, levelling and grassing part of the site, building a drainage sump, two concrete jumping pits, an area of stepping stones and constructing a balance walk and a barbecue.

The derelict old three bedroomed farmhouse was repaired with the first instalment of the NPFA grant and voluntary labour. The outside was painted by a group of International Volunteers and the interior reconstructed and decorated to professional standards over a period of a year by members of a local organisation — the materials used being supplied by the organisation.

In October 1974, the first play leader was appointed and, although much of the playground and buildings was still under construction, she withstood cold, wind and rain and organised order from chaos. At this stage, the support of the NPFA was invaluable and in May 1975 they organised a Study Day on 'Play in Sub-normality Hospitals' at St. Lawrence's. Speakers included Mr. Alfred Morris, MP, then Parliamentary Under-Secretary of State for the Disabled, and Lady Allen of Hurtwood, Chairman of the handicapped Adventure Playground Association.

By this time a new toilet block and washroom had been built, 50 yds of Go-Kart track constructed and also a fountain, waterfall, stream, paddling pool and a castle moat. Local school children gave great support.

In the summer of 1975 regular users of the playground included the children of St. Lawrence's, many adult residents (who particularly enjoyed paddling during the hot weather), members of the hospital staff children's club and several groups of handicapped children. With the help of donations and grants from trusts, charities, business interests, private individuals and groups of children as well as the Croydon Area Health Committee, two old barns have been re-roofed, re-floored, made stormproof, decorated and equipped with gas-fired warm air central heating and fluorescent lighting. Additional play features provided in 1975 included a fibre-glass 'igloo', an aviary with budgerigars and a look-out tower, built as a leaver's project by pupils from a local school.

On the first Open Day held in October 1975 the playground's specially designed flag — made and given by a local firm — was hoisted. It depicts a bluebird of happiness and a yellow background symbolising the role of the playground as a place where the handicapped children and adults can emerge from the hospital ward and spread their wings in the sunshine.

The playground was well used during the winter by residents and staff, children and parties of handicapped children from the community. By the beginning of 1976 the project was so well established and successful that Croydon Area Health Authority sanctioned the appointment of an Assistant Playleader. The large barn was used as a Play Hall for games and play, singsongs and concerts and the occasional film show, and the small barn was ready for fitting out as a 'Soft Play' Gymnasium with specially designed equipment for blind and severely handicapped children and adults. Extra features added included a rabiit hutch (with rabbits), a guinea pig hutch, an embankment slide, swings, a climbing-tower and a cyclodrome.

The hours of opening have gradually been extended to enable more of the older residents to use the facilities. Time is divided between play sessions on the wards and others on the playground. Many more departments are now using the facilities and the older residents enjoy erecting tents, building Go-Karts and mask making.

The headquarters now consists of eight rooms — playrooms, storerooms, office, kitchen, washroom and toilets, connected to the barns and soft play area. Outside the adventure playground has a great variety of unconventional and challenging equipment. Adjoining is a camping ground of one acre.

Extensive and increasing use is being made of the playground by handicapped children from the community. The reputation of the playground has spread and several teams of medical and administrative staff from other hospitals, anxious to provide similar facilities, have visited St. Lawrence's.

The Playleader

The author talked to many playleaders and feels that the points made by the St. Lawrence's Hospital Playleader are generally applicable.

Seeking co-operation

Armed with little but enthusiasm the playleader at the hospital began to develop the playground. During the mornings, when she visited every ward and department in the hospital she found out the Sisters' problems and observed those under their care who would eventually use the playground. The afternoons were devoted to building equipment, cleaning the paddling pool and painting floors, and in the evenings many of the adults who worked during the day helped to build pedal go-carts or helped the local kids and volunteers doing their Duke of Edinburgh Award paint pictures on all the walls. The art therapy department provided paints, paper and sticky paper, and the two small rooms in the house were used for general crafts. After a Baby Belling cooker was installed, cookery was included.

Equipment

Rather than expensive equipment, most playleaders favour sturdily made improvised equipment which can be easily replaced when worn out, hence the need for skilled volunteers. Equipment in the large barn includes an eight-seater rocker-box, made out of two table tops and two bed frames; a circular bicycle on a track with two wheelchairs, two seats and four seats with pedals; a trampoline (1' high) made out of a bed frame covered with a plaited and woven nylon wool, and a boat to climb in and out of, given to the hospital. Some of the most used objects are balls made out of foam bits stuffed into a nylon stocking, and plastic hoops. A milkfloat, virtually given by a dairy for transport was adapted by volunteers.

Using the playground

The playground was eventually used by patients from most of the departments and from as many of the wards as the playleader and her two assistants could collect. Most of the groups begin by pushing, rolling and swinging in the soft play room which not only gave the adults more freedom of movement but made them more independent. After this they began to explore and make up their own activities, and could soon get themselves on to the swings, down the slides and up rough grass.

Camping

During the summer the residents with behaviour problems were taken camping. At the end of their camping holiday, the young men looked content, well fed, and had developed the initiative to take themselves to bed at night. A similar scheme was successfully tried with female residents.

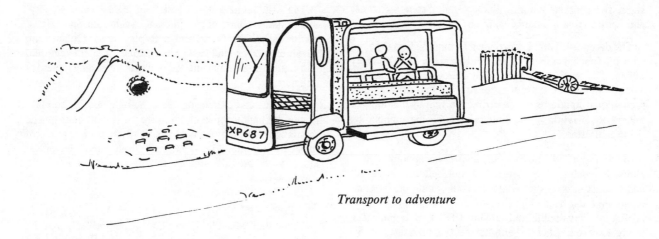

Transport to adventure

Voluntary help and integration

The playground has grown from empty buildings to a community centre. As the playleader says: 'Local mums with their own handicapped children come. Adult training centres trainees 'drop in' for an afternoon. Help is given by six local schools doing term time community service. It is nice having one to one ratio for our severely disabled groups, and cups of tea at four sort out any problems. These young adults often lend a hand on Saturdays and during school holidays as well. Adult residents now help with the children in a very understanding and caring way. Sunny days can be used spontaneously by four or five wards as well as organised groups. Nurses from different wards then find time to chat when everyone is occupied. Sometimes even the hospital workmen drop in for a chat and a repair. One could say that the playground now belongs both to the hospital and the local community. It is easy meeting a stranger when both are involved in an activity, the job now is facilitating the right activity'.

Safety

Playleaders find that if heavy equipment is placed where it is not easily moved, and light equipment put where it will not injure anyone if it is thrown, there is little chance of accident. Broken toys are always repaired quickly or thrown out if they are irreparable. Every new piece of equipment is tested by the playleader and by volunteers.

FURTHER READING

HANDICAPPED ADVENTURE PLAYGROUNDS ASSOCIATION. *Adventure playgrounds for handicapped children.* H.A.P.A., Fulham Palace, Bishops Avenue, London SW6 6EA.

CHAPTER FOURTEEN

Gateway Clubs

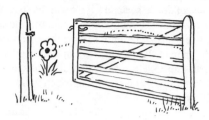

In 1966 the National Society for Mentally Handicapped Children and Adults, recognising the need to co-ordinate and develop the many clubs for handicapped children which were springing up as a result of the initiative of parents, promoted the National Federation of Gateway Clubs as a national voluntary youth organisation with the needs of mentally handicapped people particularly in mind. Since that time the Federation has been particularly concerned to secure the recognition of these needs in the field of leisure and recreation by both central government and local authorities with the result that Gateway Clubs are now recognised throughout England, Wales and Northern Ireland as an integral part of the Youth and Community Service, many of them receiving assistance from their local authorities in a variety of ways, including payment of leaders, provision of premises, assistance with transport and equipment and allocation of teaching resources. In these activities sport and physical recreation have played a prominent part, stimulated by the organisation of competition at regional and national levels and, as yet to a lesser degree, by the physical activities sections within the Gateway Award Scheme.

Gateway clubs exist to privide for mentally handicapped people in the community what the rest of the community enjoys as of right in a mixture of youth clubs, community centres, sports centres and evening institutes. The integration of mentally handicapped people into existing organisations is not necessarily in their best interests. Needs, pace and performance are too disparate to enable them to obtain full value from services shared with the rest of the community. Gateway Clubs attempt to achieve a degree of integration through the services of helpers and friends and through access to the resources at the disposal of the local authorities, though at present only a few clubs make use of facilities for informal further education in the form of teachers taking responsibility for games coaching or special activities such as dance, drama and cookery.

THE MEMBERS

In broad terms the mebership of Gateway Clubs is drawn from two categories: the severely mentally handicapped of whom there are some 124,000 in England. Wales and Northern Ireland, with about 77,000 in the age-group 15-64, and those who, while less severely mentally handicapped, are nevertheless at a considerable social and cultural dis-advantage to the extent that they are unlikely to integrate

successfully in normal youth clubs and organisations of a similar nature. So far as the latter category is concerned it is possible only to guess at a figure, but it is unlikely to be less than 100,000 and could be considerably greater.[1] With nearly 500 clubs and a membership of about 25,000 and with a potential membership in excess of 200,000, the National Federation can be said to be only touching the fringe of the problem.

It should not be concluded that Gateway Clubs are intended more particularly for, and are largely the preserve of, the less severely handicapped members of the community, through which they can enjoy participating in sporting activities. Gateway Clubs, quite rightly, are seen as places in which their members can enjoy their leisure time in relaxation. It is, however, not always fully appreciated that relaxation may take an active form and call for more stimulating interests and experiences than being entertained or 'occupied'. This applies particularly to the more severely handicapped members of the community, especially those with multiple handicaps, for whom simple movement exercises, with or without music, and even simpler dance-drama can provide new and pleasurable experiences.

THE CLUBS

As part of the preparation for this publication information was obtained from nearly 300 clubs representing approximately 80% of the total number of clubs affiliated to the National Federation at that time. Of particular interest were the type and size of clubs, the nature and quality of the accommodation in use and the sporting and physical activities engaged in.

Type and size

Over 70% were 'open' clubs of which two-thirds were for members over the age of 16, one quarter catered for members of all ages and the remainder were junior clubs. Of all the clubs included in the survey 13% were based on schools, 8% on training centres and 8% on hospitals.

The majority of Gateway Clubs, nearly 60%, had a membership of between 20 and 50, with a further 30% in the bracket 50 to 100. School clubs tended to follow this pattern whereas, perhaps understandably, hospital clubs tended to be larger.

1. Stuart, Francis. *Leisure services for the mentally handicapped. The role of Gateway Clubs.* NSMHC, 1976.

Accommodation

The most popular meeting places appeared to be schools, the premises of local societies for mentally handicapped children, local authority youth centres, church halls and adult training centres. However, only 15% of the accommodation in use at the time of the survey was considered adequate for club purposes and 25% was classified as unsatisfactory. The clubs were fairly evenly distributed between those having the use of only one space, those having two spaces, and those having three or more spaces within which to operate. In most clubs indoor facilities for sport and physical activities other than dancing were limited. Nor was there any indication that this deficiency was compensated for by access to outdoor facilities, other than grassed areas and public parks.

Sports and physical activities

The range of interests and the range of abilities require that Gateway Clubs should offer a wide programme of activities covering the whole spectrum of interests associated with youth clubs, community centres and adult education of an informal nature. So far as sport and physical recreation is concerned almost any activity, with appropriate modifications to the rules, is likely to be found in a Gateway Club. However, closer examination of the actual number of clubs engaging in the more imaginative and adventurous pursuits reveals how comparatively few of the members have the opportunity of participating in them. For this, a major share of responsibility must fall upon the shortcomings of the accommodation available and the absence of qualified instructors and helpers. Few Gateway Clubs have access on a regular basis to such specialist facilities as gymnasia, sports halls and swimming pools, even in urban areas. Even the use of playgrounds and all-weather surfaces does not feature prominently in reports of activities undertaken by clubs.

The results are predictable: the activities receiving the most frequent mention are dancing, especially jiving, darts and table-tennis. The various forms of football, five-a-side, six-a-side and eleven-a-side, came well down the list after swimming, rounders and country dancing. Gymnastics, movement and music, netball, keep fit classes and athletics come even lower, emphasising the deficiencies noted above. Yet the members of some clubs can enjoy riding, camping, relaxation classes, tennis, cricket, and trampolining and individual clubs have experimented with roller skating, squash, ten-pin bowling, volley ball, canoeing and sailing. Gateway and similar clubs need greater resources to develop interest in activities which promote self-confidence as well as pleasure, such as sailing, canoeing, trampolining, riding, climbing and especially swimming. One of the conclusions of an International Symposia on the Leisure Time Needs of the Retarded[2] was that: 'The forms of leisure activities for the retarded need to be even more varied than those for the rest of the community'.

Competitions

Two or the features of the Gateway year are the national competitions for five- and six-a-side football and rounders. Darts and table-tennis competitions at a similar level are under consideration. Behind these events are the regional competitions which attract wide-spread support and which in turn are based upon inter-club competitions at a local level. Several regions also organise athletics meetings which arouse considerable enthusiasm among the comparatively few clubs which participate and which effectively demonstrate the value of athletics as a Gateway activity. Both track and field events produce good standards of performance and the rules and track disciplines are well understood by the majority of competitors.

Junior Gateway Clubs

The demand for and the provision of leisure-time interests and activities for children of school age has been a feature of youth work for as long as voluntary organisations have been active in this field. Mentally handicapped young people are no exception; indeed it can be argued with some justification that their need for participation in stimulating activities and experiences outside the home is greater than that of normal children. From the point of view of parents and siblings the opportunity for a handicapped child to belong to a club, if only for one evening a week, comes as a welcome break from the tasks of constant attention and constant amusing out of school hours. Junior Gateway Clubs have therefore featured in the work of the National Federation of Gateway Clubs from the earliest days of its existence and there is now a growing number of such clubs operating either in their own right or as a special evening (or Saturday) of Gateway Clubs which cover the full age-range.

Activities centre around games, music and movement, simple crafts and art. A high ratio of helpers to members is required, with leaders who have at their command special knowledge and experience of handling children whose need of physical expression is quite inconsistent with their comparatively low mental ages. Collaboration between club and school and the incentives offered by the Gateway Award Schemes at the upper end of the age-range can do much to supplement the work of the schools and the resources of the home.

Gateway Clubs in hospitals

As a result of past policies many severely multiply handicapped people can still be found in sub-normality hospitals, together with a still large population of active mentally handicapped people who by now are so thoroughly 'institutionalised' that life outside the walls can offer little prospect of security and happiness.

For the residents of the hospitals themselves the organisations of Friends and Visitors almost invariably offer a lively programme of activities and entertainments covering most evenings of the week. A growing number of hospitals, however, are beginning to appreciate the value of Gateway Clubs as being something in which the residents cannot only be actively involved as members of their own right but also where they can share the activities with helpers from outside. In this respect a Gateway Club can be a valuable adjunct to a programme of preparation for transfer from hospital to living in the community, while encouraging discharged residents to retain their contacts with Gateway Clubs in the area.

---

2. National Development Group for the Mentally Handicapped. *Day services for mentally handicapped adults.* Pamphlet No. 5 HMSO, London, 1977.

One hospital club has found that, because of a lack of helpers, the members have had to learn for themselves how to be self-sufficient and to be concerned for their less able fellow members. Not only has there been a noticeable improvement in social behaviour but members have also learned to participate in club policy-making in entertainments, in running a tea-bar and in the collection of subscriptions.

The same hospital encountered a problem of how to provide physical recreation for a group of high-spirited adolescent girls. The boys, with football and cricket on a competitive basis, were already catered for. The result was the formation of a keep-fit class team which, with coaching and practice, became so successful that it now gives public displays. Special features of the displays are rhythmic exercises to music, sword and country dancing, mat-work, Indian club swinging and solo gymnastics.

Gateway Clubs in schools and training centres

Comparatively few Gateway Clubs are based on a school or adult training centre although there are signs of growing interest, especially arising from a desire to participate in the Gateway Award Scheme. There are two inhibiting factors: in the first place there is a feeling that leisure time is more profitably spent in an atmosphere and surroundings which are quite distinct from those associated with the daily routine of school and work; secondly, the need for leisure to be seen as distinct from work programmes in terms of time as well as of place. Also, it must be accepted that however generous the response to transport needs, it is often impracticable for children to go home after school and return for club activities in the evening, especially when they are likely to be drawn from a very wide area. The same can be said of the adult training centres which serve mainly rural areas, with the added disadvantage that there are often few opportunities for activities outside the centre and the home in these circumstances.

Staffs in both establishments might examine ways in which either the daily programme can be extended into the 'twilight' hours to enable the people or trainees to enjoy leisure activities, especially those of an informal nature, or ways in which links can be established with existing Gateway Clubs or new clubs formed as the need requires. 'For many mentally handicapped people their visit to, for example, the Gateway Club is the high spot of the week. SEC (Social Education Centre) staff should maintain contact with their local Gateway organisers to explore areas in which they might usefully co-operate[2]'.

THE GATEWAY AWARD SCHEME[3]

The main objectives of the Gateway Award Scheme, which is open to all members of Gateway Clubs who are over the age of 14, are to encourage participation in new activities and interests, to develop self-confidence and to increase powers of concentration and perseverance. There are no pre-determined standards and there is no element of competition; the determining factors are the degree of handicap and the initial level of ability of the entrant, however minimal, and the extent of the improvement achieved during the course of participation in the Scheme.

At present the Award comprises two stages, entry to the second of which is possible only after the completion of stage one. Thus, each stage represents an objective in its own right, Stage One being regarded as within the reach of most members of Gateway Clubs whereas Stage Two may not be practicable or even desirable for a more severely handicapped member. Both sections include athletics, swimming, walking, team games and trampolining.

EXAMPLES OF GATEWAY CLUB PROGRAMMES

Sport schemes — Halesowen and Stourbridge Gateway Club

1.   Monday — Swimming class — held at local swimming pool (reserved for Gateway Club)
7.30 p.m. — 8.00 p.m.   Main pool (swimmers only)
7.30 p.m. — 8.30 p.m.   Learner pool.

2.   Wednesday — Football practice (Autumn/Spring term) — held at the local High School gymnasium.

3.   Friday — Keep Fit and Sports Club (Spring and Summer term). A large number of mentally handicapped people are overweight, and do very little exercise. The club's aims are therefore:
     (i)   to help those who are overweight to do exercises to help lose excess weight as well as using dormant muscles;
     (ii)   to teach new skills from darts to rounders.

The club divides into: (i) the less able and fairly old and even severely handicapped; (ii) the more able and younger and so more active members. The first group is divided into three sections: 1/3 time exercises – teaching; 1/3 time equipment – bikes, sculling machines, weights, chest expanders, hoops; 1/3 time games – darts, quoits, skittles, etc.

Every three weeks the above members attend the local school and use the hall, equipment and benches, and are taught how to lift and carry them.

The second, more able members, use the local school gym: 1/3 time jogging; 1/3 time exercises; 1/3 time ball skills, etc.

In good weather all groups are taken out into the school fields and divided into three groups for the teaching of skills:
(i)   the severely handicapped people: skittles, medicine ball, etc.
(ii)   the more able boys and men: jogging, football, athletics, shot, relays, sack races, cricket.
(iii) the more able girls and women: jogging, rounders, ball skills, athletics.

Each year a team is selected for the West Midlands Gateway Regional Sports and, although these tend to be the best athletes, the other are not neglected, and on the club's own sports day the members are again divided into two sections: advanced and novice.

---

3.   Full details of the Gateway Award Scheme can be obtained from the National Federation of Gateway Clubs, NSMHCA Centre, 117-123 Golden Lane, London EC1Y 0RT.

Members of the advanced group take part against each other in the usual sports events and in 1980 will compete for a cup based on a point system.

The novice group containing the less able club members are dividied into two groups:

(i)   those who can take part in track events but are not very fast, and those who can just compete in field events.

(ii)   the more severely and older handicapped people, who take part in events such as darts, skittles, quoits, throwing cricket ball, medicine ball activities.

No one is ever left out and in fact this latter group is the most rewarding: in 1978 all won medals for 1st, 2nd and 3rd positions and everyone competing was awarded a certificate. It is for people like this that the club's sports are geared, since the advanced members can compete at the West Midland Sports.

Swimming awards

The club leader, as an STA and ASA examiner, puts the swimming members through various **tests,** but such is the variation between tests that it is difficult to advance from one stage to another without many problems. The only tests tackled easily are those for disabled people. The club leader, realising that there are few tests for the learner, has suggested the following scheme for them.

Learner Scheme Awards. *Learner pool.* Gateway Awards for beginners to help give encouragement as well as water confidence (based on a learner pool).

Stage 1: award 1
1.   Walk around the pool holding the side, not aided (shallow end of big pool, from one side to the other).
2.   Wash face in the water.
3.   Get in and out unaided — using steps.
4.   Holding someone's hands, kick legs from behind.
5.   Support from behind, kick legs in front.

Stage 2: award 2
1.   Walk around not holding sides.
2.   Put head in water.
3.   Get in and out not using steps (unaided).
4.   Use float on front and back, then go ½ width (help can be given).

Stage 3: award 3
1.   Blow bubbles
2.   Kick legs for 15 seconds holding bar
3.   Using floats, swim ½ width.
4.   Swim with helper using one hand and 2 legs (as little assistance as possible).

The next stage would be STA and Swimming Teachers Association Endeavour Award. Anyone testing should have some swimming qualification, e.g. life saving or one of the proficiency awards, etc., to ensure that a good standard is reached.

Badges and certificates should be awarded.

Teaching Keep fit — Newtownards Gateway Club, County Down, Northern Ireland

Points to remember when preparing a lesson for mentally handicapped people:
1.   they may have difficulty in balance;
2.   they may have difficulty in movement;
3.   they may have difficulty in rhythm;
4.   they may have difficulty in hearing;
5.   they may have difficulty in speech;
6.   they have different mental levels;
7.   they like to be treated individually;
8.   try to remember all their names;
9.   try to remember what each individual is capable of;
10.   they will be your friends so make sure that you are their friend.

When starting to teach keep fit, remember to begin with simple movements. These movements are difficult for the class, so don't expect too much from them.

Poise

Since mentally handicapped people have poor poise — this is one aspect of teaching which needs patience.

Co-ordination

Co-ordination of movements eg swinging right arm and then the left, can be very difficult. If they just move their arms, accept that this is the best they can do.

Moving

Moving across the floor, eg skipping and running, is difficult, so accept what they attempt but go on trying to improve the standard.

Floor exercises

Exercises sitting or lying on the floor may not be successful as some members will find it difficult to get up and down. Some may need individual help from class helpers

Balance

Balance exercises are the most difficult, so make sure that your weaker members have a helper nearby to assist them.

Rhythm

Start with very simple movements and don't insist on perfect rhythm or movement at first. Some of the Newtownards class who refused even to move have gradually joined in with the more active members. Remember that 'all' should be encouraged.

Progress

Improvement will be slow, but the class will be keen and willing to try everything they are asked to do. Members who needed support and help at first are now attempting to work by themselves. As the class members gain confidence in themselves, and in the teacher, improvement will be seen, and the teacher's work will be rewarded.

Music

Since music plays a very important part in keep fit, try to engage a good pianist but, if this is impossible, records or tapes may be used. Keep the music very simple, with a definite beat and the class should go 'with a swing'.

Exercises

The following are some simple exercises which can be taught. If possible, take some exercises from each section to give all round movement.

Arm movement   Music: Any waltz tune

1.   Swing right arm forward and back (slowly)
       Swing left arm forward and back (slowly)
       Keep repeating these two movements.

2.   Swing right arm forward and back (slowly)
       Swing right arm forward and circle twice (slowly)
       Repeat these two movements with left arm.
       Repeat all as required.

These exercises are very simple and useful for loosening up. If wrong arms are used, do not worry, the movement is more important.

Poise   Music: Any waltz or polka

Walk tall with shoulders back, head up (not chin out) stretching foot out in front with the toes leading. Repeat with the other foot. Walk slowly at first, and, as class gains confidence quicken the music. This movement may seem exaggerated but will help deportment.

Leg movement and balance   Music: Scotland The Brave

1. Point right toe forward tapping floor.
    Point right toe out to side tapping floor.
    Point right toe behind tapping floor.
    Bring feet together.
    Repeat with left foot.
    Repeat all as required (keep top half of body erect).

2. Swing right leg forward.
    Swing right leg back.
    Swing right leg forward and bring feet together.
    Repeat with left leg.
    Repeat all as required.

This exercise may require help from a partner as balance is necessary.

Floor movement   Music: Waltz

1. Sitting on floor legs stretched out in front.
    Roll on seat from side to side. Repeat.
    Move a little further each time.

2. Using arms for support.
    Bend right leg and bring it up close to seat.
    Bend left leg and bring it up close to seat.
    Repeat as required.

Running and skipping   Music: Polka time

1. 8 runs forward.
    8 skips on the spot.
    Count the runs and tell the class when to skip as some will not be able to count.
    Repeat as required.
    Later encourage class members to count as well.

2. 4 skips forward.
    4 claps standing on the spot.
    Repeat as required.

As the class improves more demanding exercises can be introduced. Here are some suggestions:

Music: Waltz

1. Swing right arm across body and out to right.
    Repeat.
    Circle right arm across body and back out to right.
    Try to get circles larger and bend knees on swings.
    Repeat with left arm.
    Repeat all as required.

2. Feet apart and both arms out to right at shoulder level.
    Swing arms across to left (good swing and bend knees).
    Swing arms across to right.
    Circle both arms out to left and back to left.
    Can be repeated starting out to right side.

3. Facing partner both hands joined at shoulder level (arms slightly bent).
    Swing right arm forward and left back.
    Repeat action left arm forward and right arm back.
    Repeat both movements as required.

4. Facing partner hands joined.
    Swing arms (to bottom of hall) up and stretch overhead and down again.
    Swing arms (to top of hall) up and stretch overhead and down again.
    Swing both arms up and overhead and stretch.
    Repeat as required.

Music: Morningtown ride

5. Facing partner hands joined.
    Swing both arms to top of hall.
    Swing both to bottom of hall.
    Swing both arms to top of hall and turn underneath (Pancake turn).
    (This is a complicated movement but the Newtownards class can now do it very well).
    Repeat all.

Music: John Brown's body

6. 8 walks forward.
    4 knee lifts on the spot (lift right knee as high as possible and back to floor). Repeat.
    Repeat movements are required.

Music: Macnamara's Band

7. In circle facing counter-clockwise.
    Inside hands joined with partner.
    7 runs forward and turn.
    7 runs forward and face partner.
    Clap right hands, clap left hands, clap both hands and own knees.
    Repeat claps. Join hands.
    8 skips round in own small circle.
    Repeat all.

Music: Waltz

8. Sitting on knees on floor.
    Stretch right arm out to right and back.
    Stretch left arm out to left and back.
    Stretch both arms up in front.
    Curl into small ball on floor bringing arms slowly down.
    Repeat as required.

Music: Morningtown ride

9. Kneeling on floor on hands and knees.
    Lift right leg and stretch backwards.
    Lift left leg and stretch backwards.
    Repeat as required.

Music: She'll be coming round the mountain

10. All in large circle facing in, numbered 1 and 2.
    All walk into centre of circle and out again.
    One's into centre and out again (two's clap).
    Two's into centre and out again (one's clap).
    Swing partner.
    Repeat.

FURTHER READING

Further information about Gateway Clubs, their management and administration, leadership and training can be found in Francis Stuart's *Recreation for the retarded. A handbook for leaders,* published by NSMHCA. Available from the NSMHCA Bookshop, 117-123 Golden Lane, London EC1Y 0RT.

CHAPTER FIFTEEN

Facilities, Equipment and Toy Libraries

FACILITIES

Apart from the facilities available at the hospital or ATC, it may be possible to use other community and private facilities if the right approach is made to those in charge of them.

Before making the initial approach, find out to whom the first enquiry should be made, either through the local authority recreation or leisure department or the national or regional sports councils, or through your own personal contacts.

SOME SUGGESTIONS

1. The British Scottish and Welsh Sports Associations for the Disabled. National and regional secretaries will supply local addresses where available.
2. Park facilities — contact the local parks department which is usually based at the town hall (the number will be in the local telephone directory).
3. Sports/leisure centres — contact the director/manager.
4. Swimming baths — contact the baths manager.
5. School halls for use during holidays, evenings, weekends — contact the education office at the local town or county hall.
6. Church halls — contact the vicar or minister in charge.
7. Colleges of further education — contact the principal.
8. Polytechnics — contact the principal.
9. Universities — contact the registrar.
10. Public schools — contact the headmaster/headmistress.
11. Hospitals, e.g. use of swimming pool — outdoor facilities — contact the hospital administrator.
12. Club premises — contact the leader.
13. Industrial sports grounds and indoor facilities for large events — contact the personnel officer.
14. Sports club grounds for large events — contact the secretary.
15. Hotels for use of swimming pool or other facilities — contact the manager.
16. Riding schools — contact the owner/secretary.
17. Halls belonging to other organisations — village halls, dance halls, scout and guide halls and camp sites — contact the secretary.
18. Private facilities — swimming pools, tennis courts, paddocks etc. — contact the owner.

EQUIPMENT

Mentally handicapped people need the same sports equipment as anyone else. It is important that they have sportwear suitable for physical activity in general, shorts, slacks, skirts, T-shirts and track suits are the most common. When a specialised game or sport is practised and a trainee or resident joins a club, sportswear for that sport is essential — he/she must 'look the part'.

Equipment of all kinds is expensive; sports manufacturers produce a great variety of goods. When considering the purchase of equipment it is important to:

(i)   select what is good value for money;
(ii) select equipment which can be used by the maximum number of people.

CHOICE

Before purchasing, investigate what is offered (cheap may not be durable). Seek advice from:
(i)   advisers of physical education or physical education teachers;
(ii) the Sports Council or local governing body of sport;
(iii) catalogues of well-known sports manufacturers of repute.
(iv) local sports shops.

CARE OF EQUIPMENT

When buying equipment, ask for guidance on its care and maintenance and stick to the directions. Durability and safety depend on constant overhaul and repair.

Store equipment carefully when not in use — careful storage can lengthen its life, e.g. balls should hang in nets. A well organised, **tidy** equipment store with clearly labelled shelves saves time and is an excellent way to help trainees and residents to be tidy. It is wise to have a rota of equipment helpers from class members.

OTHER SOURCES OF EQUIPMENT

Used badminton or tennis racquets, golf clubs, fishing tackle, tournament balls, shuttlecocks, may be available either by direct approach to the secretary of the appropriate sports club or through advertisement in the local press. When introducing a new sport it is well worth trying it out with secondhand or loaned equipment before laying out money on equipment which may or may not have any future use. Equipment may also be available on loan from local sports centres, through social services or recreation/leisure departments of the local authority.

If the staff of ATCs, hospitals and clubs in an area want a demonstration of a sport or game and its equipment, some sports manufacturers will send a representative and/or demonstrator either to a joint conference or to make individual visits in an area, e.g. Unihoc.

Coaches and instructors from county or local sports organisations will help to introduce their game or sport by demonstration and group coaching (trainees or residents can have a go!).

168

IMPROVISED EQUIPMENT

Improvised equipment can be used in simple team games and races — and in the early stages of learning skills, e.g. bricks, tins, old tyres can be found, and skittles, bats, stumps, targets, bean bags and soft balls can be made in a workshop. Usually it is possible to find a friend or someone in a hospital (or ATC) who has the 'knack' of making or adapting simple games and play equipment, often from unusual materials and unusual sources.

HAND APPARATUS

Some hand apparatus is used in movement training — balls, hoops, clubs and scarves can be bought or in some cases made.

EQUIPMENT FOR ADVENTURE PLAYGROUNDS

This equipment — fixed, moveable or improvised — should be bought or made to suit the needs of those who will use the adventure playground. Advice is readily available (see p. 182).

PERSONAL SPORTSWEAR

Where possible each individual should have his or her own personal sports gear, particularly sports shoes. It should be regularly laundered and kept in good repair. Shoes should be cleaned. A umber of ATCs and hospitals make some of the personal sportswear, often with the co-operation of parents, and funds seem to be raised for more expensive items such as track suits. If there is space for lockers for sportswear, these should be kept tidy.

Where the teachers, coaches and instructors are themselves immaculately 'turned out', this example sets a standard, usually followed by the class members.

TOY LIBRARIES

WHAT IS A TOY LIBRARY?

A toy library is a centre for lending the best — and sometimes specially adapted — toys to handicapped and socially deprived children. The majority of the 450 Toy libraries in the United Kingdom are organised by voluntary groups with professional advisers; others are in subnormality hospitals, clinics, special schools and assessment centres, with voluntary helpers.

It is widely recognised that the early years of life are vital to the future development of the child; how much more this is true of the handicapped child whose potential has been limited by disability. The handicapped child can have a short span of concentration, the mentally handicapped have an extended childhood — sometimes for life — and the handicapped generally lack the stimulus that normal children receive through exploring their surroundings. They live in a limited world. But the right play material can do a lot to make up for this. These children and adults therefore need more toys and carefully chosen toys to develop their fullest potential by encouraging their imagination, teaching them skills and helping them to become involved socially with other people. Toy libraries fill this need, but their aim is to provide friendship as well as toys. They constitute what is often the only really local meeting place for parents and children.

Toy libraries open their doors to children with any kind of handicap, no matter how young they are. Their sessions are happy occasions with all the toys on display for their parents and children to choose from. Returned toys are cleaned before being returned to stock and most toy libraries will have a helper with a special knowledge of handicap — an occupational therapist, physiotherapist, speech therapist or nurse — who will advise the parents on request on the choice of toys for their children. Tea making facilities are well used and many friendships are formed.

THE TOY LIBRARIES ASSOCIATION

The Toy Libraries Association, based in London, was established as a charitable organisation to assist towns in setting up their own independent toy libraries. The Association's aims include the provision of assistance to aid the development of all handicapped children, beginning in infancy and including every type and degree of disability.

Merchandise

The Association's merchandise includes: badges, balloons, iron-on transfers, toy library posters and Noah's Ark publications (obtainable only from the Association). man inexpensive pamphlets are available, including: *Play for mentally handicapped adults, Do it yourself – Design and make magnetic board toys.*

For particulars and order form write to: The Toy Library Association, Seabrook House, Wyllyotts Manor, Darkes Lane, Potters Bar, Herts EN6 2HL.

Chapter Sixteen

Insurance

Those responsible for sports or recreation projects for mentally handicapped people should consider carefully which insurance they need to cover any liability which might arise as a result of the activities and also the property used.

LIABILITY INSURANCE

Employers

Public liability insurance provides the protection an organisation needs against legal liability claims for injury to people other than employees and for damage to their property. Such a claim could, for instance, arise from an accident caused by the negligence of an employee or voluntary worker and, in view of the greater than normal duty of care which would be owed to mentally handicapped people taking part in sport or physical recreation, the correct arrangement of adequate Public Liability insurance will be essential. Since this cover is important, it is essential that the insurance company is made fully aware of the particular circumstances of the activities to be undertaken. There is always a limit to the amount payable for any one incident and any organisation would be unwise to think of insuring for less than £250,000, in view of the current level of court awards.

Employers' liability insurance protects an organisation against legal liability claims of any amount for injury or disease brought by its employees and is made compulsory by the Employers' Liability (Compulsory Insurance) Act, 1969. It is important to remember that this insurance covers only any legal liability of the employer — it is not Personal Accident and Sickness Insurance described in the next paragraph.

Personal accident and sickness. If any organisation wishes its members or employees to receive a benefit in the event of accident or illness, irrespective of the question of legal liability, it can provide for this by means of a Personal Accident or Personal Accident and Sickness policy on either an individual or a group basis. Accident cover can be for a lump sum payable on death or loss of limbs or sight and a weekly benefit, usually payable for up to two years, while sickness insurance is for a weekly benefit normally payable for up to one year.

Motor insurance. If any motor vehicles are owned by the organisation, they must, by law, be insured against third party personal injury risks. A choice can be made between Third Party, Third Part Fire and Theft and Comprehensive cover. The main distinction between these three versions of motor insurance is that Third Party provides cover against legal liability claims for injury to other people or damage to their property. Fire, Theft and Comprehensive cover are dealt with under property risks below.

Perhaps it is more likely that employees or voluntary workers will use their own vehicle on the organisation's behalf. If so, it would be wise to consider a Contingency Liability policy, which would protect the organisation against claims resulting from an employee's or a voluntary worker's negligence in those circumstances, should there be no other insurance in force. Such a policy would give no protection to the employee or voluntary worker, who must have his own policy — it is really a case of 'belt and braces' by the organisation, just in case.

Should any motor vehicle be taken abroad the insurance company should be told as soon as possible, so that your normal level of cover may be maintained for the trip.

Employees and voluntary workers

Those employed by, or providing voluntary services to a body organising sports or recreation projects for the mentally handicapped should check with that body to see that insurance cover has been arranged to protect them and their charges, so that they know what insurance arrangements they themselves need to make.

An employee's or a voluntary worker's liability for injury to someone or damage to property should be provided for by the organisation's Employer's Liability or Public Liability insurance, as described above, but a voluntary worker may also have cover under a Personal Liability insurance, usually included in a Home Contents policy.

If the organisation does not provide personal accident or sickness cover, an employee or voluntary worker may wish to avoid any hardship, which may arise from being out of action, by taking out his own insurance. He could also consider a Permanent Health insurance which, once granted, stays in force until a previously chosen age — provided the premiums are kept up. To anyone suffering a serious illness, the weekly benefit would be payable continually — until that chosen age if necessary.

An employee or voluntary worker using his own car on the organisation's behalf should tell his motor insurance company exactly what the car is used for and by whom, so that his cover may be extended, if necessary.

PROPERTY RISKS

Of the various property risks, against which different types of insurance may be necessary, are the following:

Fire

Fire insurance is a very important and, at the same time, inexpensive form of cover for both the buildings and their contents. If the building is owned by the organisation using it, that organisation will want its own insurance; if it is leased or simply hired, check the lease or hiring agreement to see whether it requires the hirer or lessee to insure — it might not mention insurance, but simply make them responsible for damage to the building — so do read it carefully. Similar considerations apply to the insurance of the contents of the buildings, for example sports equipment.

Special perils

Special perils insurance is normally added to a Fire policy and can cover both the building and its contents against Explosion, Riot, Earthquake and Impact by Vehicles, Animals and Aircraft and, with the insured being responsible for the first £15 of any damage, Storm, Flood, Burst Pipes and Malicious Damage also.

Theft

Theft insurance is designed to cover loss of, or damage to, contents of the building following a break-in — resultant damage to the building itself will also usually be covered.

'All risks'

'All risks' insurance effectively includes all of the above — and more — by providing accidental loss or damage cover. The wide cover provided makes this type of insurance more expensive and it is usually bought to cover office machines and similar expensive equipment vulnerable to accidental damage.

It is essential to choose very carefully the amount for which buildings and their contents are insured. For a building, it needs to be adequate at the time of taking the cover to provide for full reinstatement or rebuilding, including clearing the site and architects' and surveyors' fees. A reduction would need to be made from this figure for 'betterment', if the building were in poor condition, as it could well be impossible to repair it without improving its condition and insurance law requires that an insured person should not profit from a claim. However, the resulting figure needs to be increased to provide for the expected rise in building costs during the year of insurance and any subsequent period when reliability might be taking place. Contents cover should be for an amount adequate to replace the damaged goods with new. less an amount for wear and tear and, again rising prices must be borne in mind.

Motor insurance

Compulsory Third Party insurance is dealt with under liability insurance above. In addition, Third Party, Fire and Theft and Comprehensive cover are available. Third Party, Fire and Theft cover includes claims for loss of or damage to your car by fire or theft; comprehensive cover brings in claims for accidental damage to your own car.

Personal possession taken to work

There is unlikely to be much, if any, cover for these unless you have your Home Contents insurance extended to provide 'All Risks' cover for them. This should not be very expensive and, of course, the insurance will protect you all the time, not just at work.

CONCLUSION

Anyone discussing insurance with an insurance company or broker must ensure that he tells all there is to tell — if in doubt, tell: otherwise, the insurance could be rendered invalid and have been nothing more than a waste of money. Anyone in doubt about their insurance, whether at the time of taking it out or when claiming, should seek the guidance of the insurance company or broker.

CHAPTER SEVENTEEN

Parents' Views

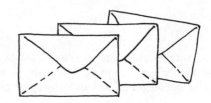

'If only parents would let their sons and daughters have a go, then we could make many more activities available for them — activities which they could enjoy'. How often is this said.

When talking to parents who have encouraged their children to take part in physical recreation, sports and outdoor pursuits it became evident that they should 'speak for themselves' and so share their experiences with others. Comments from parents on particular projects appear throughout the text — the following accounts and letters are more general in character.

SPORT FOR ALL — TRY IT

A father relates how his 17-year-old son has been encouraged throughout his life to take part in various sporting activities with the rest of the family.

'Peter, who is now 17, has from his earliest days taken part in all family activities in which he was able to participate. From children's party games, hide-and-seek and putting, he has graduated via trampolining, swimming, table tennis and family football and hockey, to carpet bowls and badminton. Like all of us, he takes part because of the pleasure and sense of achievement which he gets and which are not necessarily — and certainly not always! — related to excellence in performance or winning. Like all of us too, as a bonus, he gets healthy exercise, improved co-ordination and companionship.

'Nothing unusual about the story so far — and there shouldn't be! But Peter is mentally handicapped having Down's Syndrome and, unfortunately, many like him have been denied the opportunity to take part in any physical activity. For them, mental handicap has come, for some inexplicable reason, to be equated with complete physical disability. Parents, I regret to say, have often acquiesced in this view. To them I would say **"give your child the chance to enjoy physical recreation and add a new dimension to his or her life"**.

'How then was Peter encouraged to participate and develop his ability in specific sports, such as swimming and badminton? Truth to tell, there is no ingenious secret or deliberate plan. It has simply been a case of taking advantage of what opportunities and facilities exist.

'Thus, so far as swimming is concerned, we were fortunate to be able to make use in the early days of the facilities obtained by the swimming club organised by our local branch of the Scottish Society for the Mentally Handicapped. There Peter (and I might add two of his sisters!) learnt to swim in the usual way — playing in the water, swimming with supports and, eventually, (at about age 7) swimming unaided. Family outings to the local swimming pools are just part of our normal activities and, whilst none of us are dedicated swimming enthusiasts, all, including Peter, thoroughly enjoy them.

'Badminton is the latest sport in which Peter has been given the opportunity to take part. It is one of the activities provided at an evening class for the mentally handicapped run by the local Further Education College. He is still at the initial stage of hitting (or attempting to hit!) the shuttle back over the net,

but he is enthusiastic and improving all the time. Provided his enthusiasm for his new love continues, there is no reason why he should not be able to go to the local Church Badminton Club and enjoy both the sport and the company there'.

RISK TAKING

A mother recounts the advantages of allowing her son to take calculated risks like other young people.

'I am the mother of an educationally sub-normal son of twenty-nine, called Christopher. My husband and I both have a genetic abnormality which has affected eight out of eleven pregnancies, three sons aged twenty to thirty-five are normal, two babies died two months after birth and the others were spontaneously aborted at three to four months.

'At two year Chris was blind, brain damaged, weighed ten pounds, had cirrhosis of the liver and kidney stones. He spent most of his first three years in the Hospital for Sick Children, Great Ormond Street, where he received wonderful treatment. Next came daily speech and physiotherapy, travelling daily from home to the hospital. After many eye operations he was registered eventually as partially sighted and learned to use a white cane.

'He started at the local Educationally Sub-Normal (M) School at six years and made good progress. He learned to read and cope with numbers and money, but his writing is still poor. He was promoted from the school but to public transport at 14 — this was one of the early risks!

Living dangerously

'When Chris was eight-years-old I joined the local group of the national Society for Mentally Handicapped Children. I met a widow at the first meeting who said: 'Do your best to feel it is better that Chris might die young living dangerously, rather than wrap him in cotton wool until he's eighty'. This made a great impression on me and, while it is still difficult to let him take risks, I have tried very hard to put it into practice. I know that as a result Chris has gained in self-confidence and independence and developed as a person of whom the whole family are proud.

'He joined the handicapped swimming club at 14, travelling alone and very slowly learned to swim. Eventually he progressed to helping other learners, besides helping others to dress and pushing wheelchairs. He had the normal need to be needed and was invaluable on outings, while the physically handicapped members gave him immense support and stimulation. The risk in this case was often in finding him safely at 2 a.m. after a long day trip, perhaps to Liverpool as a member of the swimming team. Chris started a Saturday job at the age of 15, filling shelves at a local store. This time we risked him being rejected by the other staff. He was, but he survived for 18 months.

'On leaving school at 16, he attended a three-month residential course for school leavers. He then worked his way through the three graded workshop/training establishments in Croydon, ending up in six years on a special assembly line for mentally handicapped at a local factory. He has an hour's journey on two buses, and this work at present seems the limit of his capabilities because he can't cope with pressure or crises. He has done a typing course and tried clerical work, but not very successfully. Incidentally, his sight in one good eye gets him by.

Leaving home

'Three years ago he left home, after much heart searching, to live in a mixed hostel for 29 young people. Our local parents' group had helped to raise the money for the hostel, and I preached 'to all and sundry' as their Chairman how necessary it was for the residents to leave home while still young enough to be flexible. When the day came, and for weeks after, I was very tearful and felt I had thrown Chris out of the family. Chris came home to supper every night for about three weeks, unable to talk but obviously unhappy. It was very hard to send him off to the hostel every night when his old bedroom was still upstairs, but by the end of the month he had settled down and began to drop in only sporadically. Looking back and talking to Chris we know that this experience has matured him and he has enjoyed his independence as his brothers do. He acts as an elder brother to the other less able residents, helps with their money, teaches bus travel, how to order a meal in a restaurant, etc.

'He has also enjoyed being a volunteer at the old people's home on Sundays. He comes home weekly, but does not ever want to live at home again. We are now looking forward, once again with mixed feelings, to Chris leaving the hostel with four friends to live in a house independantly, but we hope with some support from the hostel staff. I accept intellectually that this is the next logical step towards a flat of his own eventually, but I still worry emotionally about how they will cope in an emergency. Unless we give them the opportunity to cope with crises, they will never learn.

'I think back to al the emergencies and risks that have arisen — going to Cub and Scout camps and mixing his own synthetic milk; being lost on Victoria Station three times before he learned to travel safely to London and back; the day he took six hours and seven buses to reach Guildford just as the MCC stopped play for the day and the excitement on his return last year from a caving and riding adventure holiday on Dartmoor. We used to worry, ten years ago, about marriage and children and wanted to have him sterilised. He's now decided he doesn't want to marry, but to enjoy his brothers children.

Important things learned

'The most important things I have learned in these 30 years are firstly, that I shall never accept the fact that I gave birth to Chris, but I have learned to live with all that mental handicap means and hopefully am a better person for that knowledge. Secondly, other people are much better at risk-taking with Chris than I can ever be, because they are not emotionally involved. I can quite happily encourage risk-taking with other people's children or adults in my work as the Co-ordinator of Voluntary Services in a very large sub-normality hospital. I find too that my reactions as a parent can be both helpful and constructive when talking to other professionals in this field'.

CARRICKFERGUS (NORTHERN IRELAND) ATC's PROJECT

The Centre's manager, describes a scheme to increase parent involvement in the provision of leisure time pursuits.

'As Manager of Carrickfergus Adult Centre I invited the parents/guardians of the trainees to a meeting at the Centre to discuss the setting up of a Parents' Group and a Tuesday evening Social Club.

'After a lengthy discussion parents were very keen on the idea. A committee of six was elected with the responsibility for:

> raising funds,
> organising transport to and from the Centre
> organising and supervising trainees.

Senior staff from the Centre are always in attendance to guide and assist.

'Every Tuesday evening (7-9.30 p.m.) approximately 30 trainees and 12 parents (on rota) are involved with other groups invited from the community (adult centre, Schools, police cadets, etc.).

'Our Club closes for summer recess in June and re-opens in September.

Encourage parents' participation

'It is most important that parents should be encouraged to participate and are given responsibilities so that they become part of everything thus giving them self-satisfaction and a feeling of achievement.

'Many managers do not encourage parents to attend clubs or social evenings because some parents tend to be over-protective in the presence of their son or daughter, and managers feel that more adventurous activities can be attempted if parents are not present. I believe that, despite this valid point, parents have much to offer in the formation of a family atmosphere. **First,** parents provide the much needed transport, not only to bring their son or daughter to the club, but also friends who live near them. **Second,** many adult mentally handicapped people learn by example — it is hoped that the mature behaviour of the parents will be copied.

'The growing number of parents and friends at meetings illustrates how parents are interested in helping in a practical way, not only with their own children but with other families as well.

'Parents know much about the background of their children and it is wise to listen to constructive suggestions and criticism.

'Trainees enjoy every Tuesday evening in the Centre, but not all wish to take part in vigorous activities. Provision should be made for this group to sit in a quiet room playing card games or discussing topics with parents.

'Parents perform a much needed service in helping with the provision and preparation of refreshments at club meetings.

'The many activities include: disco, table tennis, billiards, darts, bowls, drama, yoga, choir, music, discussion etc.

'It is essential that trainees embark on activities that are adult in outlook, purposeful, and as far as possible on terms similar to normal people.

'Our club is a tremendous success — it helps to make parents more aware of the activities of the Centre, creates better relations with the staff, thus ensuring that many benefits are gained by the people who matter, *our trainees'*.

TEN PIN BOWLING

An appreciation by a mother of a community bowling scheme.

'In opening the doors of the ABC Ten-Pin Bowling Alley (free of charge) to the trainees of the mentally handicapped Senior Occupation Centres in Aberdeen, the managers, Mr.

and Mrs. Ron Parry, have opened the doors to a wider and more fulfilling life for our handicapped people.

'This weekly, lively activity is stimulating our retarded sons and daughters to realise an undreamed of potential and quality of life. It encourages effort, team spirit, and healthy friendly rivalry with ordinary people, *on equal terms.*

'The bowling T-shirts, donated by BP Oil, are proudly worn and matches are played against teams from Grampian ITV, the local newspaper *The Press and Journal* and the local BBC.

'In May this year, Lord Provost Fraser and his wife presented a beautiful trophy to the winners of the final match, the Grampian ITV team, but they also honoured our mentally handicapped teams by presenting each member with an inscribed 'Runners Up' plaque and an LP record autographed by the artiste.

'Working in the centes, bowling, swimming and dancing at their club discos, etc. means a better deal for mentally handicapped people with the co-operation of and integration within the community. In the field of sport, the horizon for our trainees has no limits.

'What Mr. and Mrs. Parry have done *is just the beginning'.*

CONCLUSION

As a Gateway Club helper and mother of a severely hyperactive boy says: 'In the early days of learning to cope with the everyday problems of a mentally handicapped child one feels so very much alone, even within one's own family circle. It is as though yours was the only family with a handicapped child. But there are many of us, one in every hundred so statistics tell us. Most are very willing to pass on the benefit of their experience to new parents and that is generally done through membership of a Society formed to help the mentally handicapped and their families'.

CHAPTER EIGHTEEN

Co-operation within the Community

In the past mentally handicapped people were treated as a group unto themselves; they were seldom seen and their abilities were sadly under-estimated. This section contains examples of the ways in which hospitals (Brockhall and Offerton house Hospitals), adult training centres (Woodford, Oakbank, Brighouse and Marlborough ATCs) and clubs (the Keep Fit Association in Sheffield) have co-operated and integrated with the local community to the benefit of all concerned.

BROCKHALL HOSPITAL, OLD LANGHO, BLACKBURN

In 1959, Dr. Bland, the present Headmaster of the school at Brockhall Hospital, started an Evening Centre as a club for residents. In spite of initial difficulties the club has grown over the past 20 years. It maintains a close liaison with the Lancashire Education Authority which provides further education services under the terms of the 1959 Mental Health Act.

Music and movement

Music and movement classes attract a large number of moderately and profoundly mentally handicapped adults. Traditional or modern dance and music making with self-made instruments are included in the class activities. Two teachers practise team teaching with this group — one, the school secretary, is an accomplished pianist, the other a former member of the school teaching staff who now teaches in the community.

PE classes

The physical education classes are taken by specialist teachers on the day school staff. Senior students from local secondary schools play a game against the students after school and local works send their teams after work hours. The hospital authority provides hospitality. The students appreciate this contact with the community, and there is little doubt that the visitors derive tremendous satisfaction too. They are more than willing to visit annually or several times a year. Swimming session take place at a public bath with the public present. Activities such as yoga, physical fitness and gymnastics are attended by both males and females.

Dancing

Regular dancing classes are taught by a male teacher, an ex-plumber in the hospital who is qualified in ballroom dancing and has taught within the evening school for many years. He is assisted by a young American undergraduate working locally as a social services volunteer; she is a professional folk singer and guitarist. Modern ballroom dancing, olde tyme and sequence dancing are included in preparation for the entertainments for all the evening school population and the talents of the folk singer guitarist are used fully.

Each session of the evening school ends with free and informal dancing for all, when teachers are expected to dance with the students. The activities of the various music and dancing classes greatly contribute to its success.

Co-operation with local education authority

The local education authority finds and pays all teachers. In addition, the authority assists in the further training of tutors and the centre is fully integrated into the educational work of the local authority. Certain classes for non-ambulant people are held on wards at the request of the nursing staff.

Helpers

Voluntary helpers are always welcome although, at the present time, most of their efforts are being utilised in the wards.

The hospital authority provides the premises, the materials with which the students work, the refreshments and any hospitality which is afforded to outside visitors. No fees are charged to the students.

PHYSICAL ACTIVITIES AT OFFERTON HOUSE HOSPITAL, STOCKPORT

This, is a much smaller hospital than Brockhall, managers to maintain a well-balanced programme of recreational activities and sports in spite of the fact that they too have lost their more able residents. Through the energetic efforts of the recreation officer, supported by other staff members, the hospital is well known in the community; this ensures a healthy supply of helpers to the hospital and opportunites for the residents to be absorbed into the community.

Over the years various physical activites have taken place. Residents have competed in 'Inter-Hospital' sports Days and the cricket and football teams have been second to none.

However, in line with government policy, all the more able residents now live in the community and most of those left behind are severely mentally handicapped — but for all that, many physical activities are still practised and enjoyed.

In the first year a cup was won for 'the best effort' which was quite an achievement at the team came last in everything except the skittles, in which it was first. In the second year, the young men and women did not have the competitive spirit needed to take part in such a well organised day. Now, after discussion, it has been decided not to participate in this sports day again, until a 'special-care' section is included; at the present time the residents are just not capable of reaching that standard.

Mini Sports

A 'Mini' Sports Day is held at the hospital each year. In 1978 it was held in co-operation with local Gateway Clubs, The usual track events, e.g. sack race — relay race, were included together with javelin throwing (with brush stakes), 'Welly throwing' (all the Wellington Boots painted or decorated with coloured paper), 'Tossing the broom' (the ladies version of throwing the hammer). A rope is tied round the brush head and it is twisted above the head and then released — plenty of room is needed for this event as the broom head goes off in all directions (that is, if the competitor lets go of the rope).

Everyone enjoyed the day which ended with a disco — even the wheelchair residents participated by either wriggling feet or waving arms in the air. They had a great time bursting the 200 balloons in 5 minutes which had taken the staff hours to blow up!

WRVS dance

A team of WRVS ladies organises dances usually to recorded music, but on special occasions like Valentine's

Day a band plays. These ladies have taught the residents many dances including the Barn Dance, The Russian Ballet, Veleta Waltz, Foxtrot, the Slosh and Boomps-a-Daisy. Pop dancing just seems to come naturally.

Music and movement

Music and movement is another popular pastime — it encourages movement of all the joints and muscles. Jimmy Shand's records are used and wheelchair residents join in and move as much of themselves as they can.

Sand and water play is popular, but it is usually taken out-of-doors because of the mess. The boys tend to fill their pockets with sand leaving long trails everywhere, much to the consternation of the domestic staff!

Games and gymnastics

Football is very popular. The staff and residents play a football match once each week.

There are only one or two cricketers left but sometimes the boys from a local school play for an hour or so with interested residents after school.

A qualified physical education teacher comes in for one session each week to teach gymnastics — a few selected residents don PE kit and track suits and spend an hour doing simple exercises, then jog around the field. They take part in the British Amateur Gymnastic Association awards scheme.

Camping

Camping was started by selecting six residents to 'camp out' under canvas in the hospital field. The boys enjoyed this so much that residents from all over the hospital kept appearing with a pillow under their arm asking if they could sleep in a tent!

For the past three or four years ten boys and girls have spent four days under canvas at a scout camp site with a member of staff and some students from the local College of Technology. They help erect tents, sleep under canvas and take part in many 'adventure' activities. Since a minibus is available, residents with slight physical handicaps can be involved in camping.

Table games

A technical instructor made some giant-sized Ludo and snakes and Ladders boards — about 1m square. Forked sticks are used to push the counters around the floor. This is fun, and the spastic residents find it easier to manage the larger dice and counters.

A voluntary worker comes along twice a week to play 'putting' or 'bowls' and 'dominoes' when it rains.

All the play equipment is maintained by residents under the supervision of their technical instructor.

Walking

Walking is popular, and every week end groups are taken to the local park.

Horse-riding

This was tried some time ago, but as most of the residents do **not** like taking their feet off the ground, this did not prove successful.

The aim of this hospital programme is to stimulate the residents and fill their days with interesting pastimes and joyful activities — the rewards are many and a marked decrease in incontinence has been noticed.

WOODFORD (SHEFFIELD) ATCs WEEKLY PROGRAMME OF PHYSICAL ACTIVITIES

This centre has provided an example of an overall programme of physical activities and sport as planned for the trainees. It illustrates what is possible using the expertise of the centre staff to the full together with the community resources of personnel and facilities.

Day	Activity	Venue	Comment
Monday	Movement training	Concord Sports Centre	Taken by a teacher of Physical Education and one other member of staff.
Tuesday	Swimming	Local swimming baths	Staff ratio including qualified swimming teachers 1 : 6.
Wednesday (alternate weeks)	Outdoor pursuits	This centre links up with the Sheffield ATC Outdoor Pursuits scheme under the direction of Roy Briggs. (See Outdoor Pursuits p. 146).	
Thursday	Badminton	Concord Sports Centre	Sports clothes, made by the women in the Centre's sewing department.
Friday	Weight training	Concord Sports Centre	Taken by two members of staff, one is a qualified teacher of weight lifting.

The manager says:
'The activities, movement training, badminton, swimming, weight lifting and outdoor pursuits are all structured to allow as many trainees as possible to experience activities of their choice. In addition, there is a recreational period each day which includes if the weather is good, cricket and rounders, if the weather is bad, table tennis, snooker, darts, football game and table games such as draughts, dominoes and ludo. There is also a disco session. A fishing club is organised by one of the centre staff. The members spend at least 4 full days (centre time) fishing under licence. An inter-centre fishing match is arranged and trophies presented to the winners'.

OAKBANK TRAINING CENTRE, CHADDERTON, OLDHAM: LUNCH-BREAK RECREATIONAL ACTIVITIES

Informal leisure activities play a major part in the free time after lunch, when facilities are provided for those who wish to join in voluntarily. Sometimes gentle persuasion is used, but it is a period of free time and as adults the choice is theirs.

The actual choice of activities depends on time and playing space. Equipment must be easy to 'set up' and dismantle and the equipment used should be cost effective.

Space

Use is made of the dining room, a workshop and a blanked-off corridor in inclement weather. Outside, a bowling green, a putting green and the car park are used when conditions allow. Both greens were laid by the staff and trainees and are maintained by the gardening section as part of the work programme.

Activities: bowls, carpet bowls, putting, gold skittles, badminton, music, dancing.

BRIGHOUSE ADULT TRAINING CENTRE, WEST YORKSHIRE: 5–7 CLUB *

Brighouse ATC run a 5–7 club in co-operation with the Eastfield Secondary School. Between 5–7 p.m. trainees meet at the club based in the school. The overall responsibility is shared by members of the staff and students of both establishments.

The 5–7 Club was estabished in 1970 and the structure of the Club and its activities has expanded through a wide range of hobbies and pastimes. What makes the Club of special interest is the relationship between the Training Centre and Eastfield Secondary School. At first the Club was formed to provide an experience for the trainees at the Centre and the pupils in the fourth and fifth years at Eastfield, in which both groups could share their experiences and individual skills.

Relationships

The relationships developed between the pupils and the Club and the trainees and pupils is evident in the continued attendance of some of the previous pupils who have moved to the sixth form, college courses and open employment. Whilst the attendance of the trainees is more captive, several who were transferred to a neighbouring authority still attend the Club with transport provided by that authority. The involvement within the school has spread to second and third year pupils, and recently includes some first years. The number of trainees has grown from the original 25 to 30, to 50 or more. This is matched in the school by 20 to 30 pupils on a regular basis. The staff situation is excellent, approximately eleven teachers, six centre staff and a couple of social workers take part along with the more recent involvement of the Hostel staff.

Activities

The activities are graded to meet the needs of individuals, and groups are formed so that the participants get the maximum benefit from them. Specialist activities covered are canoeing, climbing, boat-building, fell-walking, camping, judo, archery, cookery, doll-making (period costume), drama and dance, art and woodwork.

---

*Reprinted from NSMHCA Year Book.

Affiliation

The affiliation and registration with the Youth and Community Education Service has proved of immense value. Facilities have been provided for specialist courses, with qualified instructors. A group of trainees joined the authority's Unit 4 + 1 activity weekend recently at Lakeside (the National YMCA centre). This integrated and involved the group with the different uniformed and open youth organisations around Calderdale.

One problem arises from the inclusion of ESN(M) clients into the Centre. It is now necessary to provide activities to this level of sophistication and while this leaves the truly mentally handicapped adult with a wider scope in the experiences offered, the individual needs of the more mature club members are not being catered for, because the stimulus offered is not of their choice or within their physical capabilities. Consideration should be given to what provision and physical resources are required to enable the mature (chronologically) to gain as much satisfaction from the Club as those under thirty who are more active.

With this in mind, it is necessary to be more outward looking and for this provision in particular more community orientated.

MARLBOROUGH ADULT TRAINING CENTRE: SIXTH FORM INVOLVEMENT IN PHYSICAL ACTIVITIES

Marlborough Adult Training Centre works in the reverse way from the Brighouse ATC (see above) — sixth formers from St. John's Comprehensive School help with physical activities on one afternoon each week under the supervision of their physical education teacher.

First contact

The manager of the Centre contacted the physical education adviser in 1975 to ask for the use of a school swimming pool. The possibility of sixth formers from the adjacent St. John's Comprehensive School giving some help with the swimming was explored at the same time. This proved impractical due to the travelling time involved. Swimming for the trainees went ahead nevertheless, and other ways in which the sixth formers could help at the Centre were found, including some extension of the physical activities programme on Wednesday afternoons, a plan readily agreed to by the headmistress.

Co-operation

A lecturer in physical education and dance at King Alfred's College, Winchester, started movement training which proved helpful to a group of shy young women trainees. A teacher at the Adult Training Centre has continued this movement work and netball is now played as well as the traditional football, with rounders, cricket and athletics in the summer. Sixth form girls work with the trainees in movement training, netball and rounders.

Matches

Inter-centre matches have provided an undoubted stimulus in widening the range of physical and social activities. The manager is concerned that the value of physical work and its contribution to the personal and social development shall be made available to as many people as possible. There has been an improvement in the way the young women move and hold themselves, and opportunities to increase language vocabulary and understanding have been created.

Daily activity

A daily activity session is now taken by a member of the ATC staff to develop body and spatial awareness and co-ordination.

Organisation

No sixth form boys are involved in this particular project although they help with other projects in the county. Careful liaison between all the people concerned is essential because of the many interruptions in sixth form life — interviews, exams — and the need for continuity of help in the Centre. The sixth formers themselves agree that they have learned a lot about getting to know and understand people who at first talk and appear to communicate very little.

Future development

This project and others involving people from the community coming into the Centre is seen as a first step in helping men and women to go out from the Centre into the community in ways which are suitable for them.

CO-OPERATION BETWEEN THE CITY OF SHEFFIELD EDUCATION DEPARTMENT, THE FAMILY AND COMMUNITY SERVICES AND THE KEEP FIT ASSOCIATION

The national movement and dance organisations are becoming more aware of the need for their activities for mentally handicapped adults. Some Keep Fit, League of Health and Beauty, Medau, Sesame and dance teachers are working in hospitals, adult training centres and clubs. One such scheme under the guidance of an adviser of physical education is described.

A percentage of mentally handicapped people are physically handicapped and/or elderly. The following account draws attention to the need to train keep fit teachers and other specialists to appreciate the special needs of physically and mentally handicapped people and the elderly.

A number of keep fit teachers and experienced class members in Sheffield have been interested for some time in helping special groups. These include physically handicapped and mentally handicapped people in day and residential care.

This work began in a small way with just a few keep fit teachers who had a natural instinct for the quality and type of work needed when they entered any special field, who learnt quickly, and readily sought advice and help from those with expertise in the care of handicapped people. It is a matter for concern that these teachers are in the minority and that some form of training should be provided for those wishing to be involved in this kind or work.

The Education Authority, the Family and Community Services and the Keep Fit Association have held meetings and introductory days for teachers to make them aware of the need for some form of training before working with handicapped people.

The 'extras' which these teachers need to know include some basic knowledge of physical and mental handicaps and of the ageing process; a simple knowledge of physiology and anatomy related to handicapped people; an understanding of the support services available, some simple knowledge of nursing, First Aid and general care; practical sessions on suitable work to be undertaken with specific groups, opportunities for discussion, supervised teaching practice and opportunities to work with experienced teachers.

Teachers and experienced class members have responded well to courses and meetings. The result has been that an even greater demand for teachers has been received from other establishments. Most of the work is done on a voluntary basis, although some efforts to obtain funds through adult education have been successful but estimates do not always allow for this. Though talks have been held with various agencies, this aspect of finance is still unsatisfactory and the leaders are relied upon to give their help without financial reward.

Two leaders visited Conisbrough Adult Training Centre and the special care unit, to work with the mentally handicapped trainees and patients. The staff have been most appreciative.

Appendices

Information in the following appendices generally relates to England only. For relevant information in Northern Ireland, Scotland and Wales apply to the appropriate Sports Council.

Information correct at the time of going to press (January 1981).

Titles of books on specific topics appear at the end of each chapter. a separate list of films and videotapes appears in Appendix 5.

For further reading on the general aspects of mental handicap information can be obtained from the National Association of Mentally Handicapped Children and Adults and MIND (see Appendix 4). For general information about all aspects of physical activities and sport, contact the appropriate Governing Body of Sport, the Sports Councils, and the Sports Associations for the Disabled (see Appendix 3), and the Physical Education Association (see Appendix 2). Lists of publications are available from most Governing Bodies of Sport.

Useful periodicals concerned with mental handicap or physical recreation and sports are published by many of the organisations listed in the appendices.

Appendix One

STEERING GROUP AND ORGANISATION OF THE PROJECT

STEERING GROUP September 1976 – February 1980

LADY HAMILTON CBE MA (Chairman)	Chairman, Disabled Living Foundation
W. D. ABERNETHY OBE	Consultant for Handicapped Children and Play, National Playing Fields Association
C. ATKINSON MCSP	Technical Officer, British Sports Association for the Disabled
G. BUCKLEY Dip TMH MISW	Manager, Brixton Adult Training Centre
MISS B. L. BUSHELL TMAOT	Retired Principal, Botleys Park School of Occupational Therapy, Chertsey, Surrey
MISS E. DENDY DipPE	Senior Executive Officer, The Sports Council
MISS K. EVANS MBE MCSP DipPE	Project Officer, Disabled Living Foundation
DR. RACHEL FIDLER MRCS LRCP DPH	Assistant Controller Health, Non-Hospital Services, London Borough of Harrow
T. FRENCH JP SRN RNMS RNT	Nursing Officer (Mental Health) Department of Health and Social Security
C. T. HEDDITCH SEN	Physical Recreation Officer, St. Lawrence's Hospital, Caterham, Surrey
DR H. HUNTER MD DPM	Medical Superintendent, Balderton Hospital, Newark
R. PRICE MA B.ED DipPE	Physical Education Association of Great Britain & Northern Ireland until January 1979
MISS B. NORRICE DipPE	Senior Lecturer in Physical Education, Keswick Hall College of Education, Norwich Physical Education Association of Great Britain & Northern Ireland from January 1979
K. R. PUGSLEY SRN	Divisional Nursing Officer, Hertfordshire Area Health Authority, South West District
MRS. JOAN RUSH SRN DipSoc	Project Officer, The King's Fund Centre
W. LLOYD DMA OHA	Project Training Officer, Trent Regional Health Authority (Regional Training Section)
DR VIVIENNE SIMMONS MRCS LRCP DCH	Medical Officer, Department of Health and Social Security
F. A. STUART MA	National Officer, National Federation of Gateway Clubs
R. STUART BA DipPE	Development officer, Scottish Sports Association for the Disabled
P. THODAY MSc NDH MI Biol	Lecturer in Amenity Horticulture, University of Bath, School of Biological Sciences
DR THERESE VANIER MB B.Chir MRCP	Trustee, Disabled Living Foundation Regional Co-ordinator, L'Arche Ltd.
J. WYATT JP DPA	General Secretary, Disabled Living Foundation

Observers

MRS. E. CAVE	Department of Education and Science until June 1979
J. R. FISH BSc	Department of Education and Science from June 1979
MRS. K. LATTO DipPE MCSP	Project Officer, Sport and Physical Recreation for Mentally Handicapped People, Disabled Living Foundation
MRS. J. DUVAL MRS. H. WILSKER	Secretaries to Project
MRS. ELAINE BATT	Illustrator

180

ORGANISATION OF THE PROJECT

The Steering Group, representing organisations concerned with the daily living of mentally handicapped people and those who have contributed to the development of sport and physical activities for them, was formed in autumn 1976.

The Terms of Reference

To prepare a manuscript for publication to serve as guide for parents, families and friends, for staff and helpers, teachers, leaders and coaches responsible for organising fitness training, games and sports, and outdoor activities in hospitals, adult training centres, Gateway Clubs and hostels in the community generally.

Questionnaire

A simple questionnaire was sent to all hospitals for mentally handicapped people and to all directors of social services for distribution to adult training centres and hostels in England, Northern Ireland, Scotland and Wales.

The purpose of the questionnaire was to discover what physical activities and sports were provided for mentally handicapped people, what facilities were available and what personnel were employed to teach these activities. As a result of the information received the author selected various establishments to visit. In making her choice, she took the following factors into consideration:

(i)   the nature and variety of activities being practised, the interesting and constructive comments made on the value, planning and content of the individual programme;
(ii)   the need to give as wide a coverage as possible to the four countries within the limits of time and financial resources;
(iii)   the need to see as many mentally handicapped people as possible taking part in a wide variety of physical activities, sports and outdoor pursuits;
(iv)   the information gathered as a result of the Press Release and information obtained from the Disabled Living Foundation Information Service and from other sources.

Organisation of Visits

Arrangements to visit hospitals and adult training centres were made through the hospital administrators and directors of social services and through the latter to managers of the training centres.

All arrangements for visits in Scotland were made by the Development Officer of the Scottish Sports Association for the Disabled, for the visit in Ireland by the Sports Council of Northern Ireland in association with the area health boards and for the visit to Wales by the Sports Council for Wales.

Visits were made to adult training centres, hostels and Gateway Clubs and several events, sports days, swimming sports, inter-hospital matches and sports days, displays and finals days were attended. Many meetings were held with representatives of the medical and ancillary professions, hospital administrators, nursing staff and recreative officers together with managers, staff and helpers of adult training centres. Where possible contact was made with the physical education departments of the training establishments running the 1-year diploma course for instructors of adult training centres.

During the visits small groups of specialists were brought together for discussion and consultations were held with many individuals.

APPENDIX 2

ORGANISATIONS CONCERNED WITH SPORT AND PHYSICAL RECREATION

1. **Organisations which promote sports and physical recreation (activities) for people with any form of handicap**

   British Sports Association for the Disabled, Sir Ludwig Guttmann Sports Centre, Harvey Road, Aylesbury, Bucks HP21 8PP. (Swimming Division, BSAD HQ.) *Water Sports for the Disabled Division,* Co-ordinator Len Warren, 29 Ironlatch Avenue, St. Leonard's, East Sussex TN38 9JE.

   Disabled Living Foundation (Project, Sport and Physical Recreation), Project Officer, Disabled Living Foundation, 346 Kensington High Street, London W14 8NS.

   Scottish Sports Association for the Disabled, Secretary Mr. R. C. Brickley, Fife Institute of Physical and Recreational Education, Viewfield Road, Glenrothes, Fife KY6 2RA.

   Special Olympics UK., Director Miss Nancy Wise, Michael House, 47 Baker Street, London W1.

   United Kingdom Sports Association for people with Mental Handicap, c/o The Sports Council, 70 Brompton Road, London SW3 1EX.

   Welsh Sports Association for the Disabled, Mrs. Pamela Williams, c/o Sports Council for Wales, National Sports Centre for Wales, Sophia Gardens, Cardiff CF1 9SW.

2. **Sports Councils concerned with the development of sport and physical recreation for all including disabled people**

   The Central Council of Physical Recreation, Francis House, Francis Street, London SW1 P1DG.

   The Sports Council, 70 Brompton Road, London SW3 1EX.

   The Sports Council for Northern Ireland, 49 Malone Road, Belfast BT9 6RZ.

   The Scottish Sports Council, 1 St. Colme Street, Edinburgh EH3 6AA.

   Sports Council for Wales, National Sports Centre for Wales, Sophia Gardens, Cardiff CF1 9SW.

3. **Professional organisations concerned with the development of physical education and recreation in schools and adult education**

   British Association of Advisers and Lecturers in Physical Education, The Secretary, 19 Broughton Avenue, Bournemouth, Dorset BH10 6HS.

   The Physical Education Association of Great Britain and Northern Ireland, Ling House, 10 Nottingham Place, London W1M 4AX.

4. **Organisations concerned with the provision and landscaping of play areas and the training of play leaders**

   Handicapped Adventure Playground Association, Fulham Palace, Bishops Avenue, London SW6.

   National Playing Fields Association, 25 Ovington Square, London SW3 1LQ.

5. **Professional organisations which include sport and physical activities as a means of rehabilitation**

   British Association of Occupational Therapists, 20 Rede Place, London W2.

   The Chartered Society of Physiotherapy, 14 Bedford Row, London WC1R 4ED.

   Health Education Council, 78 New Oxford Street, London WC1A 1AH.

   Society of Remedial Gymnasts, c/o Northampton Town F.C., County Ground, Northampton.

APPENDIX 3

GOVERNING BODIES OF SPORT, OUTDOOR PURSUITS, MOVEMENT AND DANCE

ANGLING

National Anglers' Council
Secretary: P. H. Tombleson FZS
          National Anglers' Council
          5 Cowgate
          Peterborough
          Cambridgeshire PE1 1LR
          Tel. (0733) 54084

Committee for Disabled Anglers
          Address as above

National Federation of Anglers
Secretary: J. W. Warner
          National Federation of Anglers
          Haig House
          87 Green Lane
          Derby
          Tel. (0332) 362000

National Federation of Sea Anglers
Secretary: R. W. Page
          National Federation of Sea Anglers
          26 Downsview Crescent
          Uckfield
          East Sussex TN22 1UB
          Tel. (0825) 3589

Salmon and Trout Association
Secretary: J. Rose CMG MBE DFC
          Salmon and Trout Association
          Fishmongers' Hall
          London Bridge
          London EC4R 9EL
          Tel. (01) 626 3531

ARCHERY

Grand National Archery Society
Secretary: J. J. Bray
          Grand National Archery Society
          The National Agricultural Centre
          Stoneleigh
          Kenilworth
          Warwickshire CV8 2LG
          Tel. (0203) 23907

Disabled   John Burgess
Archery   7 New Street, Shefford
Co-   Bedfordshire
ordinator: SG17 5BW

ATHLETICS

Amateur Athletic Association
Secretary: B. E. Willis
          Frances House
          Frances Street
          London SW1P 1DL
          Tel. (01) 828 3163/4

Women's Amateur Athletic Association
Secretary: Miss M. Hartmann MBE
          Francis House
          Francis Street
          London SW1P 1DL
          Tel. (01) 828 3163/4

BADMINTON

Badminton Association of England
Secretary: J. B. H. Bisseker
          Badminton Association of England
          44/45 Palace Road
          Bromley
          Kent BR1 3JU
          Tel. (01) 464 0031/2/3

BASKETBALL

English Basket Ball Association
Secretary: K. K. Mitchell
          Department of Physical Education
          The University
          Leeds LS2 9JT
          Tel. (0532) 31751 ext. 282

English Mini Basket Ball Association
Secretary: K. G. Charles
          English Mini Basket Ball Association
          The Greneway School
          Garden Walk
          Royston
          Hertfordshire SG8 7JF
          Tel. (0763) 43650

BILLIARDS AND SNOOKER

Billiards and Snooker Foundation
Secretary: Mrs. S. B. Cuming
          Billiards and Snooker Foundation
          145 Oxford Street
          London W1R 1TB
          Tel. (01) 437 7281

BOWLS

British Crown Green Bowling Association
Secretary: E. M. Elson
          British Crown Green Bowling Association
          21 Beechwood Road
          Bedworth
          Nuneaton
          Warwickshire CV12 9AG
          Tel. (0203) 314447

English Bowling Association
Secretary: J. F. Elms
          English Bowling Association
          2a Iddesleigh Road
          Bournemouth
          Dorset BH3 7JR
          Tel. (0202) 22233

English Bowls Council

Secretary: E. J. Crosbie MBE JP
English Bowls Council
150 Wellington Road
Enfield
Middlesex
Tel. (01) 360 7669

English Women's Bowling Federation

Secretary: Mrs. D. Ellis
English Women's Bowling Federation
22 Bloomfield Park
Bath
Avon
Tel. (0225) 312560

English Indoor Bowling Association

Secretary: B. Telfer
English Indoor Bowling Association
730 Romford Road
London E12
Tel. (01) 553 5539

English Women's Indoor Bowling Association

Secretary: Mrs. P. M. White
English Women's Indoor Bowling Association
'Whitehaven'
1 Bayley's Caravan Site
Lent Rise
Burnham
Buckinghamshire SL1 7HS
Tel. (062 86) 63687

CAMPING

The Camping Club of Great Britain and Ireland

Secretary: G. A. Cubitt MBE
Camping Club of Great Britain and Ireland
11 Lower Grosvenor Place
London SW1W 0EY
Tel. (01) 828 1012

The Youth Camping Association of Great Britain and Ireland

Secretary: Mrs. C. A. Clark
Youth Camping Association of Great Britain and Ireland
91 Hurst Drive
Waltham Cross
Hertfordshire

CANOEING

The British Canoe Union

Secretary: J. G. Richards MBE
British Canoe Union
Flexel House
45-47 High Street
Addlestone
Weybridge, Surrey KT15 1JV
Tel. (97) 41341

The Canoe Camping Club

Secretary: G. Halfacree
Canoe Camping Club
9 Glebe Road
Sandy
Bedfordshire SG19 1LS
Tel. (0767) 80712

CAVING

National Caving Association

Secretary: D. Judson
National Caving Association
Bethel Green
Calderbrook Road
Littleborough
Lancs
Tel. (0706) 78581

CRICKET

The Cricket Council

Secretary: D. B. Carr
The Cricket Council
Lord's Cricket Ground
London NW8 8QN
Tel. (01) 289 1611

Women's Cricket Association

Admin   Mrs. M. Archer
Officer: Women's Cricket Association
70 Brompton Road
London NW3 1HA
Tel. (01) 584 7213

CROQUET

The Croquet Association

Secretary: R. F. Rothwell
The Croquet Association
Hurlingham Club
Ranelagh Gardens
London SW6 3PR
Tel: (01) 736 3148

CYCLING

The British Cycling Federation

Secretary: L. A. Unwin
British Cycling Federation
70 Brompton Road
London SW3 1EN
Tel. (01) 584 6706/7

Cyclists' Touring Club

Secretary: L. Warner
Cyclists' Touring Club
Cotterell House
69 Meadrow
Godalming
Surrey GU7 7HS
Tel. (048 68) 7217/8

DANCE AND MOVEMENT

The Dalcroze Society

Secretary: Mrs. A. Heron
The Dalcroze Society
89 Highfield Avenue
London NW11 9TU
Tel. (01) 455 1263

English Folk Dance and Song Society

Contact: Mrs. Jean Howard
English Folk Dance and Song Society
Cecil Sharp House
2 Regent's Park Road
London NW1 7AY
Tel. (01) 485 2206

Imperial Society of Teachers of Dancing
Secretary: P. J. Pearson FCA
              Imperial Society of Teachers of Dancing
              Euston Hall
              Birkenhead Street
              London WC1H 8BE
              Tel. (01) 837 9967

Keep Fit Association
Secretary: Miss Janet Hilderley
              Keep Fit Association
              70 Brompton Road
              London SW3 1HE
              Tel. (01) 584 3271

Laban Art of Movement Guild
Secretary: Mrs. M. Kershaw
              Laban Art of Movement Guild
              'Mullions'
              Eastcombe
              Stroud
              Gloucestershire GL6 7EA
              Tel. (045 277) 416

Margaret Morris Movement
              Suite 3/4
              39 Hope Street
              Glasgow G2 6AG

Medau Society of Great Britain and Northern Ireland
Secretary: Mrs. H. Hewitt
              Medau Society of Great Britain and Northern
              Ireland
              8b Robson House
              East Street
              Epsom
              Surrey KT17 1HH
              Tel. (78) 29056

Sesame (Movement and Drama)
Hon.   Hon. Director
              Christchurch
              27 Blackfriars Road
              London SE1 8NY
              Tel. (01) 633 9690

Women's League of Health and Beauty
Secretary: H. N. Mussen
              Women's League of Health and Beauty
              c/o Neville Russell and Co
              30 Artillery Lane
              London E1 7LT

              EXTEND (Exercise Training for Elderly and
              Disabled)
              Secretary: Mrs. P. Copple SRN
              Conway House
              5 Conway Road
              Sheringham
              Norfolk NR26 8DD
              Tel. (0263) 822479

DARTS

British Darts Organisation
Secretary: O. A. Croft
              British Darts Organisation
              47 Creighton Avenue
              Muswell Hill
              London N10 1NR
              Tel. (01) 883 5055

FENCING

Amateur Fencing Association
Secretary: Commander F. A. Booth RN
              Amateur Fencing Association
              83 Perham Road
              West Kensington
              London W14 9SP
              Tel. (01) 385 7442

Ladies Amateur Fencing Union
Secretary: Mrs. P. Casey
              42 Grove Crescent
              Kingston-on-Thames
              Surrey
              Tel. (01) 546 9200

FIELD STUDIES

The Field Studies Council
              9 Devereux Court
              London WC2R 3JR
              Tel. (01) 583 7471

FOOTBALL

The Football Association
Secretary: E. A. Croker
              The Football Association
              16 Lancaster Gate
              London W2 3LW
              Tel. (01) 262 4542

FRISBEE

United Kingdom Frisbee Association
Secretary: J. B. Way
              United Kingdom Frisbee Association
              28 Gilray House
              Gloucester Terrace
              Lancaster Gate
              London W2
              Tel. (01) 262 4945

GAMES

New Games UK
Secretary: C. Lloyd
              60 Park Road
              Dartford
              Kent

GOLF

Golf Development Council
Secretary: D. Hughes
              Golf Development Council
              3 The Quadrant
              Richmond
              Surrey TW9 1BY
              Tel. (01) 940 0038

The Golf Foundation
Director: Miss Lesley Attwood
              The Golf Foundation
              Allington House
              136-142 Victoria Street
              London SW1E 5LD
              Tel. (01) 834 4688

English Ladies' Golf Association
Secretary: Miss L. H. Peters
English Ladies' Golf Association
Flat 3
28 Shepherd's Hill
Highgate
London N6 5AH
Tel. (01) 340 5984

GYMNASTICS

British Amateur Gymnastics Association
Secretary: Lt Cmdr B. W. C. Middleton RN RTD
British Amateur Gymnastics Association
95 High Street
Slough
Berkshire SL1 1DH
Tel. (75) 32763

HANDBALL

British Handball Association
Secretary: J. D. Timmins
British Handball Association
90 Penryn Avenue
Fishermead
Milton Keynes
Buckinghamshire MK6 2BG
Tel. (0908) 678339

HOCKEY

The Hockey Association
Secretary: Colonel D. M. R. Eagan
The Hockey Association
70 Brompton Road
London SW3 1HB
Tel. (01) 584 2584

All England Women's Hockey Association
Secretary: Miss T. Morris
All England Women's Hockey Association
160 Great Portland Street
London W1N 5TB
Tel. (01) 636 0264

JOGGING

National Jogging Association
Secretary: T. McNab
35 Bruton Street
London W1X 7DD
Tel. (01) 491 3276

JUDO

British Judo Association
Secretary: A. C. G. Johnson
British Judo Association
70 Brompton Road
London SW3 1DR
Tel. (01584) 3273

KARTING
Contact: Motor Sports Division
Royal Automobile Club
31 Belgrave Square
London SW1X 8QH
Tel. (01) 235 8601

KITE FLYING

British Kite Flyers' Association
Secretary: R. Moulton
c/o Model and Allied Publications
P.O. Box 35
13-15 Bridge Street
Hemel Hempstead
Hertfordshire HP1 1EE
Tel. (0442) 41221

KORFBALL

British Korfball Association
Secretary: Mrs. J. Sage
British Korfball Association
46 Ashtree Avenue
Mitcham
Surrey
Tel. (01) 640 3068

LAWN TENNIS

The Lawn Tennis Association
Secretary: J. U. C. James
Lawn Tennis Association
Barons Court, West Kensington
London W14 9EG
Tel. (01) 385 2366

The Lawn Tennis Foundation of Great Britain
Manager: J. Moore
Lawn Tennis Foundation of Great Britain
The Queen's Club
West Kensington
London W14
Tel. (01) 385 4233/4

LIFE SAVING

Royal Life Saving Society
Director & O. S. M. Bayley
Secretary: Royal Life Saving Society
Desborough House
14 Devonshire Street
London W1N 2AT
Tel. (01580) 5678/9

MOUNTAINEERING

British Mountaineering Council
Secretary: D. Gray
British Mountaineering Council
Crawford House
Precinct Centre
Booth Street East
Manchester M13 9RZ
Tel. (061 275) 5835/5839

NETBALL

All England Netball Association
Director: Miss E. Nicholl
Francis House
Francis Street
London SW1 1DE
Tel. (01) 828 2176

ORIENTEERING

British Orienteering Federation
Prof. B. Porteous
Officer: British Orienteering Federation
Lea Green
Nr. Matlock
Derbyshire DE4 5GJ
Tel. (062 984) 628

OUTDOOR EDUCATION

National Association for Outdoor Education
Bewerley Park Centre (Outdoor Pursuits)
Pateley Bridge
Nr. Harrogate
North Yorkshire
Tel. Harrogate 611287

PETANQUE

British Petanque Association
Secretary: L. R. Brooks
British Petanque Association
'Farthings'
Church Street
Seal
Sevenoaks, Kent
Tel. (07320) 61612

National Headquarters
160 New Bond Street
London W1Y 0SE
Tel. (01) 493 7252

PLATFORM TENNIS

British Platform Tennis Association
Secretary: D. E. Cuin
British Platform Tennis Association
P.O. Box 3
Radcliffe-on-Trent
Nottingham NG12 1BJ

RACQUETBALL

British Racquetball Association
Secretary: Mrs. J. Francis
British Racquetball Association
Mapledrakes Farm
Ewhurst
Surrey GU6 7QP

RIDING

British Horse Society
Secretary: J. E. Blackmore
British Horse Society
National Equestrian Centre
Stoneleigh
Kenilworth
Warwickshire CV8 2LR
Tel. (0203) 27192/5

English Riding Holiday and Trekking Association
Secretary: L. Moore
English Riding Holiday and Trekking Assoc.
The British Horse Society
National Equestrian Centre
Stoneleigh
Kenilworth
Warwickshire CV8 2LR
Tel. (0203) 27192/5

The Pony Club
Secretary: Miss C. Moir
The Pony Club
National Equestrian Centre
Stoneleigh
Kenilworth
Warwickshire CV8 2LR
Tel. (0203) 27192

Riding for the Disabled Association
Director: Miss C. Haynes
Riding for the Disabled Association
Avenue 'R'
National Agricultural Centre
Stoneleigh
Kenilworth
Warwickshire CV8 2LR
Tel. (0203) 56107

RAMBLING

Ramblers' Association
Secretary: A. Mattingly
Ramblers' Association
1-4 Crawford Mews
York Street
London W1H 1PT
Tel. (01) 262 1477

ROUNDERS

National Rounders Association
Secretary: Miss S. McNab
National Rounders Association
3 Felbridge Court
311 High Street
Harlington
Middlesex
Tel. (01) 897 1194

ROWING

Amateur Rowing Association
Secretary: D. Lunn-Rockliffe
Amateur Rowing Association
6 Lower Mall
Hammersmith
London W6 9DJ
Tel. (01) 748 3632

Women's Rowing Committee
Secretary: Mrs. P. Sly
Women's Rowing Committee
Old Place
Remenham Lane
Henley-on-Thames
Oxon
Tel. (04912) 77925

RUGBY

British Amateur Rugby League Association
Secretary: T. Keaveney
British Amateur Rugby League Association
Britannic Building
3 Upperhead Row
Huddersfield
West Yorkshire HD1 2JL
Tel. (0484) 44131

Rugby Football Union
Secretary: Air Commodore R. H. G. Weighill CBE DFC
Rugby Football Union
Whitton Road
Twickenham
Middlesex TW2 7RQ

SAILING

Royal Yachting Association
Secretary: J. Durie
Royal Yachting Association
Victoria Way
Woking
Surrey GU21 1EQ
Tel. (048 62) 5022

SKATING

National Skating Association of Great Britain (including Roller Skating)
Secretary: J. B. Duncan
National Skating Association of Great Britain
117 Charterhouse Street
London EC1M 6AT
Tel. (01) 253 3824/5

SKI-ING

British Ski Club for the Disabled
H. Sturges
Corton House
Corton
Warminster
Wiltshire
Tel. (098 55) 321

National Ski Federation of Great Britain
Secretary: P. B. C. Watson
National Ski Federation of Great Britain
118 Eaton Square
London SW1W 9AF
Tel. (01) 235 8227/8

SQUASH

Squash Rackets Association
Secretary: E. P. Woods
Squash Rackets Association
70 Brompton Road
London SW3 1DX
Tel. (01) 584 2506

Women's Squash Rackets Association
Secretary: Miss C. S. Myers
Women's Squash Rackets Association
345 Upper Richmond Road West
Sheen
London SW14 8QN
Tel. (01) 876 6219

SURFING

British Surfing Association
Administrator: G. E. Dimmer
British Surfing Association
16-18 Bournemouth Road
Parkstone
Poole
Dorset BH14 0ES
Tel. (0202) 746154

SWIMMING

Amateur Swimming Association
Secretary: N. Sarsfield MC
Amateur Swimming Association
Harold Fern House
Derby Square
Loughborough
Leics LE11 0AL
Tel. (0509) 30431

Development officer for the Disabled: Miss S. Green (address as above)

Association of Swimming Therapy
Secretary: J. T. Wrighton
Association of Swimming Therapy
10 West Way
Wheelback
Sandbach
Cheshire
Tel. (093 67) 2724

British Swimming Coaches' Association
Secretary: H. Bland
British Swimming Coaches' Association
Dormer House
13 Dormer Place
Leamington Spa
Warwickshire CV32 5AA
Tel. (0926) 35428

National Association of Swimming Clubs for the Handicapped
Secretary: D. E. V. Braham
National Association of Swimming Clubs for the Handicapped
4 Hillside Gardens
Northwood
Middlesex
Tel. (65) 27784

National Co-ordinating Committee on Swimming for the Disabled
Secretary: Mrs. S. Barrie
Swimming Teachers Association
Birmingham Road
West Bromwich
West Midlands BT1 4JQ
Tel. (021 553) 5828/9

Swimming Teachers' Association
Secretary: D. L. Brailsford MSTA
             Swimming Teachers' Association
             1 Birmingham Road
             West Bromwich
             West Midlands
             Tel. (021 553) 5828/9

TABLE TENNIS

English Table Tennis Association
Secretary: A Shipley
             English Table Tennis Association
             21 Claremont
             Hastings
             East Sussex TN34 1HA
             Tel. (0424) 433121

TENNIS AND RACKETS

Tennis and Rackets Association
Secretary: R. N. Bruce CBE TD
             Tennis and Rackets Association
             'Fairwater'
             7 Orchard Gate
             Esher
             Surrey KT10 8HY
             Tel. (01) 398 3135

TEN PIN BOWLING

British Ten Pin Bowling Association
Secretary: M. Glazer MBE
             British Ten Pin Bowling Association
             19 Canterbury Avenue
             Ilford
             Essex IG1 3NA
             Tel. (01) 554 9173

TRAMPOLINING

British Trampoline Federation Ltd
Secretary: R. C. Walker
             British Trampoline Federation Ltd
             152a College Road
             Harrow
             Middlesex
             Tel. (01) 863 7278

TUG OF WAR

Tug of War Association
Secretary: P. J. O. Edlin
             Tug-of-War Association
             Spire Gate
             Steep Hollow
             Dinton
             Salisbury
             Wiltshire
             Tel. (072 287) 549

VOLLEYBALL

English Volleyball Association
General   Miss E. Pratt
Admini-   English Volleyball Association
strator: 128 Melton Road
             West Bridgford
             Nottingham NG2 6EP
             Tel. (0602) 816324

WATER SKI-ING

British Water Ski Federation
Secretary: Miss J. Hill
             British Water Ski Federation
             70 Brompton Road
             London SW3 1EG
             Tel. (01) 584 8262

WEIGHT LIFTING

British Amateur Weight Lifters' Association
Secretary: W. Holland
             British Amateur Weight Lifters' Association
             3 Iffley Turn
             Oxford
             Tel. (0865) 778319

YOGA

British Wheel of Yoga
Secretary: Patchitandanda
             British Wheel of Yoga
             445 High Road
             Ilford
             Essex

FRISBEE *(See also p. 185)*

United Kingdom Frisbee Disc Association
Director: Maureen A. Faulkner
             9b Marlborough Road
             Richmond-upon-Thames
             Surrey TW10 6JT

APPENDIX 4

ORGANISATIONS WITH AN INTEREST IN SPORT AND PHYSICAL ACTIVITIES

Association for Professions for the Mentally Handicapped	c/o The King's Fund Centre 126 Albert Street London NW1 7NF
Association of Recreation Managers	Berry House 41 High Street Over Cambs
British Red Cross Society	9 Grosvenor Crescent London SW1X 7EJ
Duke of Edinburgh's Award Scheme	5 Prince of Wales Terrace London W8 5PG
Girl Guides Association	17 Buckingham Palace Road London SW1 W0PT
Inland Waterways Association	114 Regents Park Road London NW1 8UQ
Institute of Baths Management	Giffard House Sherrard Street Melton Mowbray Leicestershire LE13 1XJ
Institute of Mental Subnormality	Wolverton Road Kidderminster DY10 3PP
Institute of Park and Recreation Administration	Lower Basildon Reading Berks RG8 9NE
Institute of Recreation Management	200 Shorncliffe Road Folkestone Kent CT20 3PH
King's Fund Centre	126 Albert Street London NW1 7NF
Methodist Association of Youth Clubs	2 Chester House Pages Lane Muswell Hill London N10 1PR
MENCAP National Society for Mentally Handicapped Children and Adults	117-123 Golden Lane London EC1 Y0RT
MIND National Association for Mental Health	22 Harley Street London W1N 2ED
Mobility International	2 Colombo Street Leicester
National Association of Teachers of the Mentally Handicapped	Secretary: Mr. David Myatt The Court House Stapledon Lane Ashburton, Devon
National Council for Special Education	Beacon Wood Boidon Hill Stratford-upon-Avon Warwickshire CV37 9RX
National Federation of Gateway Clubs	117-123 Golden Lane London EC1 Y0RT
National Youth Bureau	17 Albion Street Leicester LE1 6GD
Outward Bound Trust	Avon House 360 Oxford Street London W1
RADAR Royal Association for Disability and Rehabilitation	25 Mortimer Street London W1N 8AB

Royal Society for the Prevention of Accidents	Cannon House Priory Queensway Birmingham B4 6QS
Scouts Association	Baden Powell House Queen's Gate London SW7 5JS
Spastics Society	12 Park Crescent London W1N 4EQ
Women's Royal Voluntary Service	17 Old Park Lane London W1Y
Youth Hostels Association	Trevelyan House 8 St. Stephen's Hill St. Albans Herts AL1 3DY

APPENDIX 5

FILMS AND VIDEOTAPES

Films and Videotapes on specific sports can be recommended by the governing bodies of sport (see Appendix 3).

1. **Films and videotapes showing mentally handicapped people taking part in physical activities**

   NORRICE, BARBARA
   Physical activities for severely mentally handicapped adults in hospitals and Adult Training Centres
   Two 1-hour videotapes divided into sections which can be shown separately.

   Tape 1
   Part 1 Introductory Session showing a good relationship between the leader and the group through (a) floorwork activities; (b) group tasks; (c) use of games equipment — 35 mins.
   Part 2 Session 1. Awareness of knees, showing nursing staff and residents working together — 20 mins.

   Tape 2 Session 2. Awareness of the centre of the body and back — 35 mins.
   Part 3 The observation of six residents using the soft play area for the first time — 15 mins.
   Note: These tapes are primarily teaching aids.

   Tape 3
   Gymnastic skills for ATC students — 30 mins with sound.
   Twelve students doing an initial teacher training course are working with twelve ATC students. The college students are studying the educational needs of severely mentally retarded people. They are **not** specialising in physical education. This film is an edited record of the 3rd session. It demonstrates the range of activities attempted and the progressions from floor work to the development of skills using apparatus.
   Age range 19 – 35 years.

   Folk dancing for ATC students — 30 mins with sound.
   Twelve students doing an intial teacher training course are working with students from two ATCs. It is an edited record of a single one hour session showing how folk dance music can be used to stimulate physical activity and increase concentration. The learning of specific dances is of secondary important. This film shows that given the stability of working with those who are not handicapped ATC students can derive much educational value combined with enjoyment.
   Age range 19 – 32 years.

   The above films are recorded on both ½" Sony High Density Open Reel tape and VHF cassettes.

   Enquiries concerning the purchase of any of the above tapes on either ½" Sony high Density Open Reel tape or VHF cassettes should be made to: Miss B. Norrice, 1 Irving Road, Norwich, Norfolk NR4 6RA.

   SHERBORNE, VERONICA
   A Sense of Movement 16mm colour 40 mins.
   Explorations 16mm black & white 29 mins.
   In Touch 16mm black & white 30 mins.
   These films are based on Movement Training. Available from Concorde Film Council Ltd., Nacton, Ipswich, Suffolk IP10 0JZ.

2. **Films showing disabled people taking part in sport and physical recreation**

   Not just a spectator
   Recreative physical activities for disabled people from climbing to wheelchair dancing — 16mm colour 35 mins.

   Riding for the disabled
   How to start a group for teaching riding to disabled children — 16mm colour 30 mins.

   Riding towards freedom
   (The range of facilities provided by the Riding for the Disabled Association in rural and urban areas) — 16mm colour 33 mins.

   The right to choose
   A visual commentary as discussed between members of the medical and para-medical profession and distinguished teachers of riding, on the risks and rights of temporary and permanently disabled people to enjoy horse riding as a recreation — 16mm colour 35 mins.

   Swimming
   Three audio sound programmes to illustrate important techniques for handicapped people of all types and ages in water.
   (i)   position and balance in water;
   (ii)   movement in water;
   (iii) group activities and formations in water.
   Each programme is approximately 35 slides with tape in cassette.

192

Water free
A detailed explanation of methods and techniques by which disabled people of different ages are able to enjoy the support and freedom of movement that only water can give. — 16mm colour 35 mins.

The above are available from: Town and Country Productions Ltd., 21 Cheyne Row, London, SW3 5HP.

An adventure playground for the handicapped — 16mm colour 25 mins.
Available from: The Central Film Library, Government Building, Bromyard Avenue, Acton, London, W3 7JB.

It's ability that counts
Sport for the physically handicapped, available from: British Sports Association for the Disabled, Sir Ludwig Guttmann Sports Stadium, Harvey Road, Aylesbury, Bucks HP21 8PP.

Note: Although these films are concerned primarily with physically handicapped individuals, there are ideas and material relevant to mentally handicapped people.

3. **Safety**

Water safety — 16mm colour   28 mins.
A visual appreciation of the factors affecting the safety of those people who enjoy recreation both in and out of the water available from: The Royal Society for the Prevention of Accidents, Cannon House, The Priory, Queensway, Birmingham B4 6BS.

4. **Some films showing shots of physical activities for handicapped people**
Available from: The British Red Cross Society; The Duke of Edinburgh Award Scheme; National Society of Mentally Handicapped Children and Adults; Scouts Association; The Spastics Society; Town & Country Productions Ltd.

5. **Special and Mini-olympics**
(a) *Special Olympics* — 16mm   21 mins.
Shows the achievements of the British competitors in the Special Olympics in New York in 1979 (they won 60 medals).
Video cassette can be *hired* from Concord Film Council Ltd., Nacton, Ipswich, Suffolk IP10 0JZ.
Video copies can be *bought* from Special Olympics U.K., Michael House, 47 Baker Street, London W1.

(b) *Mini-Olympics picture show and commentary 1979* — 20 mins.
Slides can be hired from J. O'Brien, Havering Training Centre, Spilsby Road, Harold Hill, Romford, Essex. Please give alternative dates when writing for slides. Details of equipment required and method of showing slides will be provided.

Index

Notes